Innovations and New Developments in Craniomaxillofacial Reconstruction

Julio Acero

Editor

Innovations and New Developments in Craniomaxillofacial Reconstruction

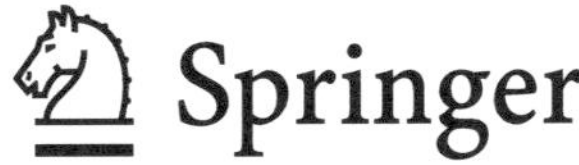 Springer

Editor
Julio Acero
Department of Oral and Maxillofacial Surgery
University Hospital Ramón y Cajal
University of Alcala
Madrid, Spain

ISBN 978-3-030-74324-6   ISBN 978-3-030-74322-2   (eBook)
https://doi.org/10.1007/978-3-030-74322-2

This Springer imprint is published by the registered company Springer Nature Switzerland AG
The registered company address is: Gewerbestrasse 11, 6330 Cham, Switzerland

Preface

"It is important to realize that if certain areas of science appear to be quite mature, others are in the process of development, and yet others remain to be born."— **Santiago Ramón y Cajal,** *Advice for a Young Investigator*. *Reglas y Consejos sobre Investigación Biológica* (1916).

The importance of the facial image for each person is obvious. The perception by a person of the normality of their face, the most visible region of the body and also involved in the social relationship, is of great importance for the personal balance of the individual. Not only aesthetics but also important functions such as vision, speech, swallowing, or chewing depend on the integrity of the craniomaxillofacial region. The loss of harmony as well as the alteration of the aforementioned functions will cause an impact on the person that can have devastating consequences both on a psychic and social level. Due to the complexity of the anatomy and function of this region, reconstruction of the craniomaxillofacial region has been a challenging task for the surgeons throughout history. Attempts to repair lost tissues and restore facial normality have been a constant among surgeons from ancient times to the present day. The exciting journey through the history of facial reconstruction begins in ancient India where the technique of flaps for nasal reconstruction is described in the Vedas, the sacred texts of Hinduism. In the Renaissance another important milestone is the realization of an arm flap for the reconstruction of the nose by Gasparo Tagliacozzi (1546–1549) in Bologna. In the nineteenth century, authors such as Dieffenbach or Lisfranc developed the use of local skin flaps for facial reconstruction. A breakthrough in head and neck reconstruction occurred in 1979, when Stephan Ariyan described the pectoralis major myocutaneous pedicled flap. Despite the progress made by the introduction of myocutaneous and osteomyocutaneous pedicled flaps, their relative lack of versatility and the lack of predictability in the results of bone reconstruction in the craniomaxillofacial region were a major disadvantage. A significant step in the progress of head and neck reconstructive surgery was the introduction in the last decades of the twentieth century of microvascular flaps, based on the transfer of free tissue with microvascular anastomosis with the antecedent of the first transplant of an inguinal flap to the oral cavity by Kaplan and Buncke in 1971. Microsurgical flaps are today considered state of the art in oro-craniomaxillofacial reconstruction due to their versatility, ability to provide different types of tissue (skin, fascia, muscle, or bone), and the high success rate. The historical review of facial reconstruction cannot finalize without mentioning the first facial transplant in history. This impressive advance in the history of science was performed in 2005 by Bernard Devauchelle, author of one of the chapters of this book.

Advances in surgery have frequently occurred in the context of the history and today we live in the Digital Age. The future is becoming the present almost instantaneously, and the reconstructive surgeon needs to be aware of what this technological revolution means for humanity. The digital age can be defined as the period of the history characterized by the existence of the digital technologies, which are associated with a fast knowledge turnover and increased technological functionalities offering amazing tools with a high impact in the progress of Sciences including Surgery. The world is immersed in the Digital Revolution, a shift from mechanical and analogic technology to digital electronics. The technological innovations in this period have transformed our world, opening new ways for global communication and information sharing. Digital information can be stored, managed, and shared in an interactive way in a global scenario. The new technologies together with the progress in regenerative medicine and biomaterials can impact very especially in the field of craniomaxillofacial surgery due to the complex anatomy of this region. Computer-assisted surgery including preoperative virtual planning of tumor excision and reconstruction, design and manufacturing of three-dimensional (3D) models of the patient or patient-specific implants, surgical navigation and digital intraoperative imaging, robotic surgery, augmented reality, and virtual reality are technologies which open a new world. These innovative techniques help the surgeon to enhance treatment's safety as well as to obtain potentially better aesthetic and functional results in the different fields of oral and craniomaxillofacial surgery such as the management of congenital or acquired malformations, facial trauma, temporomandibular joint surgery as well as head and neck tumors resection and reconstruction. Today the final responsibility of the application of the technological advances belongs to the surgeon, working in a multidisciplinary team with other specialists like biomedical engineers, radiologists, etc. Health professionals need to understand that the technological evolution is a fast evolving process. Progress in Computer Science seems to be leading to a new world since the development of digital computers started in 1940. Large amounts of clinical and biological data can be collected and managed at an unprecedented scale. Big data technologies and artificial intelligence defined as the capability of a machine to mimic intelligent human behavior including decision-making will offer new applications in the field of Biomedical Sciences including Surgery but also will open a number of concerns.

This book aims to offer a comprehensive review of the most updated innovations and new technological developments that have affected the complex field of craniomaxillofacial reconstruction. An impressive group of outstanding authors, all of them pioneers representing the most experienced and innovative surgeons working in this field, discuss the basis and the impact of the new technologies in their areas of expertise. We hope that this book can provide the reader the most up-to-date reference in this field and contribute to spread the knowledge shared by the authors, thus determining an influence on the advancement of clinical practice.

My sincere gratitude to our contributors for their commitment to this project. All of them are highly prestigious and busy specialists and their enthusiastic support is deeply recognized. Our thanks also are extended to the editorial team at Springer, in particular to Ms Smitha Diveshan, project coordinator, for her patience and technical assistance. Finally, a very special thanks to our beloved families. Without their great support, our dedication to our patients and our scientific projects would not have been possible.

Madrid, Spain   Julio Acero

Contents

Contributors

Julio Acero, MD, DMD, PhD, FDSRCS, FEBOMS Department of Oral and Maxillofacial Surgery, University Hospital Ramón y Cajal, University of Alcala, Madrid, Spain

Fernando Almeida, MD, DMD, PHD Department of Maxillofacial Surgery, Ramon y Cajal University Hospital, Madrid, Spain

R. Bryan Bell, MD, DDS Head and Neck Cancer Program, Providence Cancer Institute, Portland, OR, USA

E. Belli, PhD Maxillo-Facial Unit, MESMOS Department, Ospedale S. Andrea "Università La Sapienza", Rome, Italy

Federico Biglioli, MD Maxillofacial Surgery Unit, San Paolo Hospital, University of Milan, Milan, Italy

J. Collin Department of Oral and Maxillofacial Surgery, Bristol Royal Infirmary, Bristol, UK

Marcus Couey, MD, DDS Head and Neck Cancer Program, Providence Cancer Institute, Portland, OR, USA

Sophie Cremades, MD Department of Psychiatry, University Hospital Amiens Picardie, Amiens Cedex 1, France

Research Unit UR7516 Chimere, Facing Faces Institute, Amiens, France

Stéphanie Dakpe, MD, PhD Department of Maxillofacial Surgery, University Hospital Amiens Picardie, Amiens Cedex 1, France

Research Unit UR7516 Chimere, Facing Faces Institute, Amiens, France

Patricia de Leyva, MD, PhD Department of Oral and Maxillofacial Surgery, University Hospital Ramón y Cajal, University of Alcala, Madrid, Spain

Bernard Devauchelle, MD, PhD Department of Maxillofacial Surgery, University Hospital Amiens Picardie, Amiens Cedex 1, France

Research Unit UR7516 Chimere, Facing Faces Institute, Amiens, France

R. Fernandes Division of Head and Neck Surgery, Department of Oral and Maxillofacial Surgery, University of Florida, Jacksonville, FL, USA

Joël Ferri, MD, PhD, HDR Department of Oral and Maxillo Facial Surgery, Lille University Nord de France, Lille, France

Departement of Stomatology and Oral and Maxillofacial, Roger Salengro Hospital, INSERM U 1008, CHRU, Lille Cedex, France

Andreas M. Fichter, PhD, DMD, MD, FEBOMFS Department of Oral and Maxillofacial Surgery, Klinikum rechts der Isar, Technical University Munich, Munich, Germany

Ana Isabel Romance, MD Maxillofacial Surgery Department, 12 de Octubre University Hospital, Madrid, Spain

Michael P. Grant, MD, PhD Department of Plastic and Reconstructive Surgery, Johns Hopkins Hospital, Baltimore, MD, USA

Division of Plastic, Maxillofacial, and Reconstructive Surgery, R Adam Cowley Shock Trauma Center, Baltimore, MD, USA

Barbara Hersant, MD, PhD Department of Plastic and Maxillofacial Surgery, Hôpital Universitaire Henri-Mondor, Créteil, France

Jean Christophe Hornez, PhD Laboratoire des Matériaux Céramiques et Procédés Associés (LMCPA), Université Polytechnique Hauts-de-France (UPHF), Maubeuge, France

Vincent Hornez CryoBeryl Software, ETH, France

A. Kapitonov, MD Maxillo-Facial Unit, MESMOS Department, Ospedale S. Andrea "Università La Sapienza", Rome, Italy

Ludovic Lauwers, DDS, MSc Department of Stomatology, Oral and Maxillo-facial Surgery, Roger Salengro-CHRU, Lille Cedex, France

Luis Ley, MD Department of Neurosurgery, Ramon y Cajal University Hospital, Madrid, Spain

Joseph Lopez, MD, MBA Department of Plastic and Reconstructive Surgery, Johns Hopkins Hospital, Baltimore, MD, USA

Division of Plastic, Maxillofacial, and Reconstructive Surgery, R Adam Cowley Shock Trauma Center, Baltimore, MD, USA

Jean-Paul Meningaud, MD, PhD Department of Plastic and Maxillofacial Surgery, Hôpital Universitaire Henri-Mondor, Créteil, France

Shannath L. Merbs, MD, PhD Department of Ophthalmology and Visual Sciences, University of Maryland Medical Center, Baltimore, MD, USA

Emmanuel Morelon, MD, PhD Department of Immunology and Transplantation, University Hospital of Lyon, Lyon, France

Jorge Núñez, MD Department of Maxillofacial Surgery, Ramon y Cajal University Hospital, Madrid, Spain

Ashish Patel, MD, DDS Head and Neck Cancer Program, Providence Cancer Institute, Portland, OR, USA

Manuel Picón, MD Department of Maxillofacial Surgery, Ramon y Cajal University Hospital, Madrid, Spain

Martin Rachwalski, MD, DDS Department of Plastic and Maxillofacial Surgery, Hôpital Universitaire Henri-Mondor, Créteil, France

Majeed Rana, MD, DDS Department of Craniomaxillofacial Surgery, University Hospital Düsseldorf, Heinrich Heine University (HHU), Düsseldorf, Germany

Gwénael Raoul, MD, PhD Departement of Stomatology and Oral and Maxillofacial, Roger Salengro Hospital, INSERM U 1008, CHRU, Lille Cedex, France

Marta Redondo, MD Maxillofacial Surgery Department, 12 de Octubre University Hospital, Madrid, Spain

Ana Isabel Romance, MD Maxillofacial Surgery Department, 12 de Octubre University Hospital, Madrid, Spain

Gregorio Sánchez-Aniceto, MD, PhD Maxillofacial Surgery Department, 12 de Octubre University Hospital, Madrid, Spain

Eduardo Sánchez-Jáuregui, Medical Degree Department of Oral and Maxillofacial Surgery, Ramón y Cajal University Hospital, Madrid, Spain

Alexander Schramm Department of Oral, Maxillofacial and Plastic Surgery, German Armed Forces Hospital of Ulm, Ulm, Germany

Department of Oral and Maxillofacial Surgery, University Hospital, Ulm University, Ulm, Germany

Sylvie Testelin, MD, PhD Department of Maxillofacial Surgery, University Hospital Amiens Picardie, Amiens Cedex 1, France

Research Unit UR7516 Chimere, Facing Faces Institute, Amiens, France

Luis Vega, DDS Department of Oral and Maxillofacial Surgery, Vanderbilt University Medical Center, Nashville, TN, USA

Frank Wilde Department of Oral, Maxillofacial and Plastic Surgery, German Armed Forces Hospital of Ulm, Ulm, Germany

Department of Oral and Maxillofacial Surgery, University Hospital, Ulm University, Ulm, Germany

Max Wilkat, MD, DDS Department of Craniomaxillofacial Surgery, University Hospital Düsseldorf, Heinrich Heine University (HHU), Düsseldorf, Germany

Thomas Wojcik, MD ENT Cancerology Department, Lille, France

Klaus-Dietrich Wolff Department of Oral and Maxillofacial Surgery, Klinikum rechts der Isar, Technical University Munich, Munich, Germany

M. Zappalà, MD Maxillo-Facial Unit, MESMOS Department, Ospedale S. Andrea "Università La Sapienza", Rome, Italy

Fundamental Concepts in Regenerative Medicine: Structural Fat Grafting (SFG) and Platelet-Rich Plasma (PRP)

Barbara Hersant, Martin Rachwalski, and Jean-Paul Meningaud

1.1 Introduction

Since the introduction of liposuction by Illouz [1] in 1980 and the standardization of the technique by Coleman [2], the injection of autologous fat (lipofilling) has largely developed in maxillofacial and plastic surgery and currently represents a real revolution in our activity. Indeed, the fatty tissue was initially used by plastic surgeons as autologous filling or even volumizer but quickly it has demonstrated healing trophic properties that are very useful in reconstructive surgery. The discovery of fat mesenchymal stem cells in 2001 by Zuck et al. [3] helped to explain and validate the hypothesis that fat had trophic properties. Lipofilling is currently considered as an advanced biotherapy and the techniques have largely developed and become more complex: macro-lipofilling, micro-lipofilling, and nanofat. Indeed, adipose tissue (AT) is a source of mesenchymal stem cells, preadipocytes, and mature adipocytes. The autologous and extemporaneous nature of this adipose tissue preparation raises no legal or ethical problem, unlike embryonic stem cells.

At the same time, autologous and extemporaneous cell therapies are booming in the field of plastic surgery: platelet-rich plasma (PRP), vascular stromal fraction (VSF), injection of mesenchymal stem cells from fatty tissue or bone marrow. PRP is a simple and economical way to obtain several autologous growth factors at the same time. For example, PRP is one of the innovative methods used in regenerative medicine to biologically improve tissue healing and regeneration. Therapeutic combinations are currently under evaluation and appear promising in the area of tissue regeneration [4]. The growing interest for these autologous methods in the field of surgery is reflected in recent years by the large number of publications (1585 articles over the last 5 years) and the increasing number of congresses dealing exclusively with regenerative medicine.

1.2 Platelet-Rich Plasma (PRP)

Platelet-rich plasma (PRP) is defined as an autologous biological product derived from the patient's blood, and in which, following a centrifugation process (Fig. 1.1), a plasma fraction is obtained with a higher platelet concentration than circulating blood [5]. This therapeutic technology process is gaining interest in regenerative medicine because of its potential to stimulate and accelerate tissue healing [6].

B. Hersant (✉) · M. Rachwalski · J.-P. Meningaud
Department of Plastic and Maxillofacial Surgery,
Hôpital Universitaire Henri-Mondor, Créteil, France
e-mail: barbara.hersant@aphp.fr;
jean-paul.meningaud@aphp.fr

© Springer Nature Switzerland AG 2021
J. Acero (ed.), *Innovations and New Developments in Craniomaxillofacial Reconstruction*,
https://doi.org/10.1007/978-3-030-74322-2_1

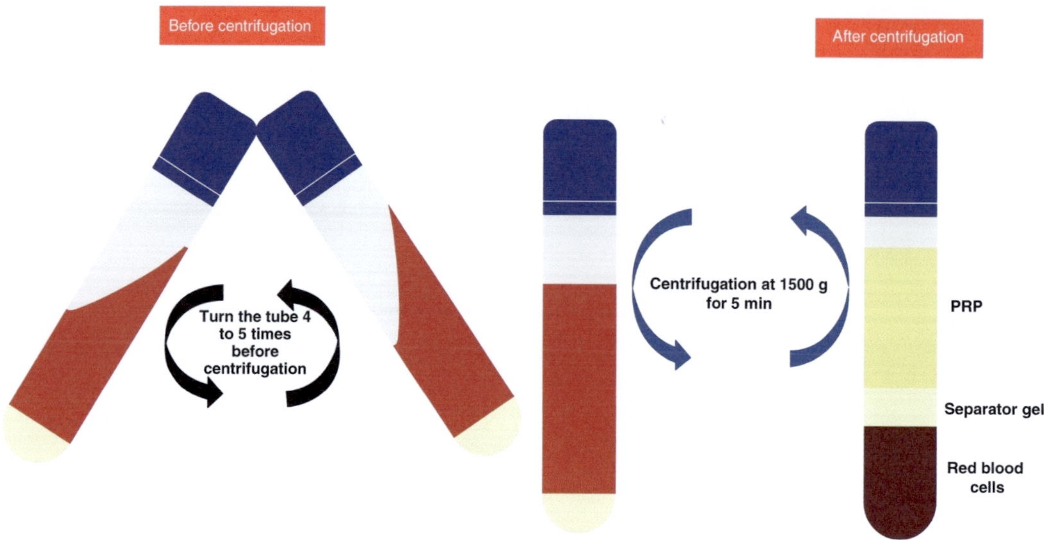

Fig. 1.1 Preparation of PRP from a blood sample (8Ml) with the RegenKI-BCT® device. The preparation of PRP requires a blood sample. Before centrifugation, 8 mL of blood are taken from a tube containing an anticoagulant (sodium citrate). After centrifugation at 1500 × g for 5 min, the PRP is separated from the red blood cells which settles at the bottom of the tube as sediment. The tube is inverted several times to resuspend the platelets contained in the plasma

1.2.1 Physiology and Platelet Function

A blood sample on average contains 93% red blood cells, 6% platelets, and 1% white blood cells [7]. Platelets are small disc-shaped cells with a lifespan of about 7–10 days. After an injury that causes bleeding, the platelets are activated and aggregate to release their granules containing growth factors that stimulate the inflammatory cascade and the healing process (Fig. 1.2). Platelets are responsible for hemostasis, the construction of new connective tissue and revascularization, and most research in the last century has focused on this primary function [11].

The use of growth factors to promote skin healing has existed since the 1940s and can be applied in different ways, either topically or intralesionally, using specific scaffolds or even as gene therapy [12]. The ideology of PRP treatment is the reversal of the platelet/red blood cell ratio by decreasing red blood cells to 5% (which are less useful in the healing process) and especially by concentrating platelets containing a potent mixture of growth factors to 94%. A nor-mal platelet count in a healthy individual is between 150,000 and 450,000 cells per microliter of blood. Platelet concentrations in the PRP below 1000×10^6/mL were unreliable to improve healing [5] and most studies suggest tissue repair efficacy with PRP having a minimal increase of five times the normal platelets (approximately one million platelets/μL) [13] while much higher concentrations showed no improvement in healing. The ideal concentration remains to be defined. The wide variability of the devices used to isolate PRP [14] in different studies may alter the characteristics of platelet degranulation that could affect clinical outcomes [15, 16]. The key growth factors of PRP (Fig. 1.3) include transforming growth factor (TGF)-β, platelet derived growth factors (PDGF-αβ and PDGF-ββ), growth factor insulin (insulin growth factor; IGF), vascular endothelial growth factor (VEGF), epidermal growth factor (EGF), and fibroblast growth factor (FGF-2) [18–20]. PRP also contains a variety of plasma proteins, which are known to be essential components in the connective tissue healing mechanism [21]. In contrast to serum, plasma contains fibrinogen and other coagulation factors, which can be activated

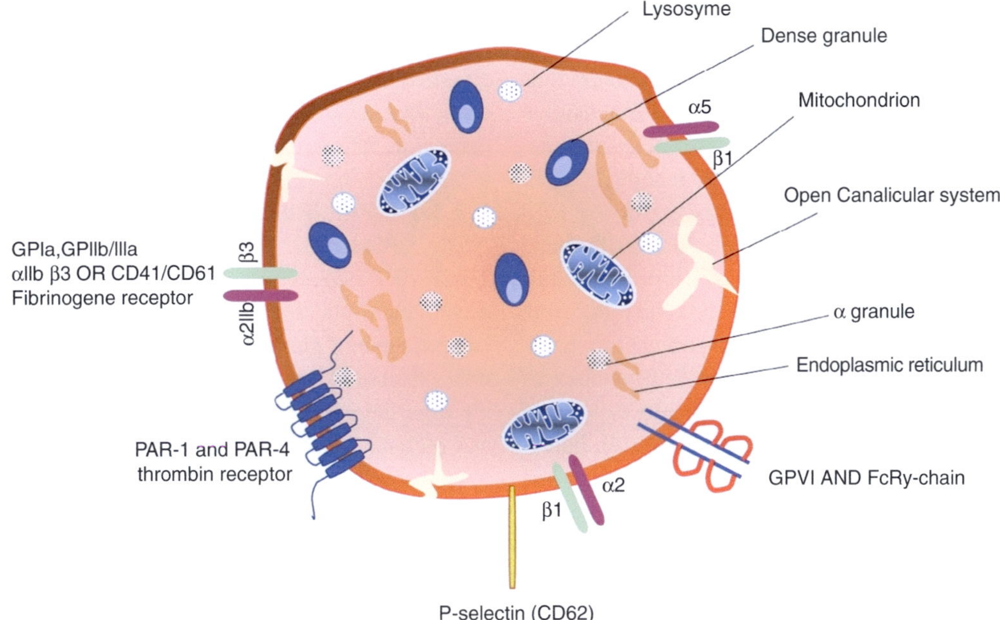

Fig. 1.2 Diagram of a platelet with organelles, showing key surface receptors, aggregation factors and an overview of known α-granule release factors. A-granules of adhesive proteins, coagulation factors and their inhibitors, fibrinolytic factors and their inhibitors, proteases and antiproteases, growth factors and mitogenic factors, chemokines, cytokines, membrane glycoproteins and antimicrobial proteins. In addition, platelet lysate can be used as a biomaterial in many applications of regenerative medicine [8]. Only in the last two decades have we learned that platelet activation releases growth factors [9]. There are many growth factors with various functions, among which is the acceleration of the healing of tissues and wounds [10]

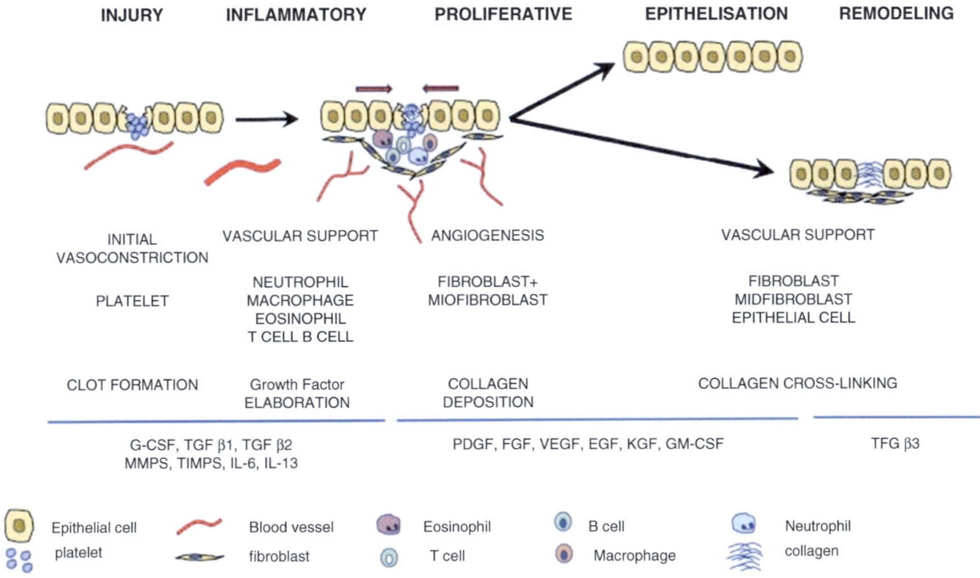

Fig. 1.3 Growth factors and cytokines involved in the signaling process of wound healing (*G-CSF* granulocyte colony stimulating factor, *TGF* transforming growth factor, *MMPS* matrix metalloproteinases, *TIMPS* tissue inhibitor of MMP, *IL* interleukin, *PDGF* platelet derived growth factor, *FGF* fibroblast growth factor, *VEGF* vascular endothelial growth factor, *EGF* epidermal growth factor, *KGF* keratinocyte growth factor, *GM-CSF* granulocyte macrophage colony stimulating factor [17]). https://www.mdpi.com/2079-4983/9/1/10#cite. This figure is licensed under the Creative Commons Attribution 4.0 International: https://creativecommons.org/licenses/by/4.0/legalcode

to form a temporary fibrin scaffold allowing cells to adhere, migrate, and proliferate [22]. Since platelets aggregate along fibrin fibers during coagulation, the resulting three-dimensional scaffold can also act as a reservoir of growth factors that exert favorable effects on cells [22, 23]. In addition, the clinical advantages of the PRP fibrin matrix are well known in maxillofacial surgery and tissue healing of chronic wounds [10, 24]. Each growth factor can have different effects on the healing process and acts by binding to specific receptors on the cell membranes of the target cells [25]. These effects include chemotaxis (cell attraction in the wound), inducing migration and proliferation of cells, and stimulating cells to upregulate protein production [26]. These growth factors regulate not only cell migration and proliferation, but also remodeling of the extracellular matrix and promote angiogenesis, creating an ideal environment that promotes the skin healing process [27].

1.2.2 Methods of PRP Preparation

The American Association of Blood Banks Technical Manual [28] states that "platelet-rich plasma is separated from whole blood by centrifugation." The centrifugation process separates the blood components because of their different densities, that is to say that the red blood cells are heavier (are trapped thanks to the separator gel), followed by platelets contained in the plasma and which are the lightest. Centrifugation is carried out at $1500 \times g$ for 5 min. The platelet yield depends mainly on certain parameters such as the size and shape of the container used, the speed and the centrifugation time, and the anticoagulant used. There is a significant lack of comparative studies to standardize the procedural parameters of PRP.

1.2.3 Classification of Platelet Concentrates

The development of a wide range of preparation protocols, devices, and centrifuges for various indications has led to a number of different platelet concentrates. Ehrenfest et al. [29] proposed a classification of platelet concentrates into four categories according to their leucocyte and fibrin content as follows:

1.2.3.1 P-PRP (Pure Platelet-Rich Plasma)

The P-PRP concentrate consists of an undetermined leuco-platelet layer fraction, containing a large number of platelets, but most leucocytes are not collected. After the first centrifugation, only the superficial leucocyto-platelet layer is pipetted and prepared for the next centrifugation in order to concentrate the platelets a second time.

1.2.3.2 L-PRP (Leukocyte and Platelet-Rich Plasma)

L-PRP consists of most platelets, as well as leukocytes and some residual red blood cells, suspended in fibrin-rich plasma. It differs from P-PRP only on the buffy coat collection means in which PRP with the entire buffy coat and the buffy coat outer layer of 1–2 mm are pipetted.

1.2.3.3 P-PRF (Pure Fibrin Rich in Platelets)

The term PRF is used as a synonym for platelet-rich fibrin matrix (PRFM). When P-PRP is mixed with the activator (calcium or athrombin) and allowed to incubate for a certain period of time, a stable PRFM clot can be collected, which has useful applications as described below.

1.2.3.4 L-PRF (Platelets Rich in Fibrin and Leucocytes)

In this category, the blood is collected without anticoagulant and immediately centrifuged. A natural coagulation process occurs and three layers are formed: the buffy coat basecoat, the acellular plasma top layer, and the L-PRF clot in the middle, which harvests the platelet and leukocyte growth factors in the cell. fibrin matrix (Fig. 1.4). There is no biochemical modification of the blood, i.e., no anticoagulant, thrombin or $CaCl_2$ (sodium chloride) is required. When the gel is pressed between two gauzes, it becomes a membrane that also has

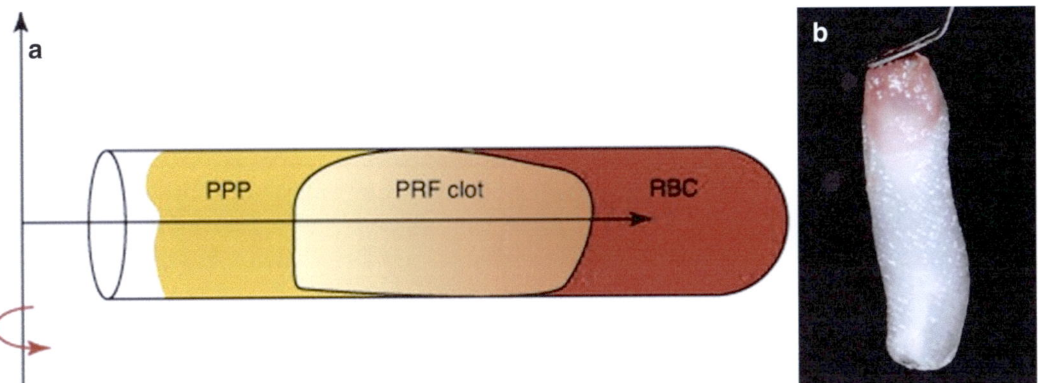

Fig. 1.4 Choukroun platelet-rich fibrin (PRF) method. (**a**) The blood is gently centrifuged without anticoagulants, and coagulation begins rapidly. The blood is separated into three components with the formation of a fibrin clot in the middle of the tube. This clot acts as a plug that traps most light blood components, such as platelets and leukocytes, as well as circulating molecules, such as growth factors and fibronectin. This method leads to the natural production of a leukocyte-rich PRF clot (L-PRF). (**b**) After compression of the L-PRF clot, it can be easily used as a membrane (actual length indicated: 3–4 cm) [29]. (*TRENDS in Biotechnology*)

potential applications described in oral [30] or maxillofacial [31–34] surgery, and plastic surgery [13].

1.3 Adipose Tissue and Different Approaches

Adipose tissue (AT) develops during the last trimester of intrauterine life and is derived from the mesodermal layer. Adipose tissue is among the most important tissues of the human body since it can reach 15–25% of the total weight, and up to 50% in cases of morbid obesity. AT plays a key role in the storage and release of lipids, managing the body's energy reserves according to needs and supplies. It also functions as an endocrine organ that synthesizes and secretes adipokines, which can act at the local or systemic level and influence the glucose and lipid regulation system [35]. The characteristic cells of adipose tissue are adipocytes. In mammals, there are three types of adipose tissue: marrow adipose tissue, brown adipose tissue, and white adipose tissue (Fig. 1.5).

In vitro, white adipose tissue cells can be separated after enzymatic digestion into two populations: mature adipocytes and vascular stromal fraction (VSF) or stromal vascular fraction (SVF) containing inter alia stem cells of mesenchymal origin.

1.3.1 Lipofilling or AT Graft: An Advanced Therapy

Interest in lipofilling was long regarded to be due to volumizing but the discovery of its trophic character made lipofilling the most used regenerative medicine treatment.

Recent studies have shown that the stroma-vascular fraction of adipose tissue represents a reservoir of precursor cells whose pro-angiogenic potential was comparable to that of stem cells derived from bone marrow [36, 37]. In addition, it has been shown that mesenchymal stem cells are also present in adipose tissue. The latter therefore represents a new potential reservoir of pluripotent cells that could be used in regenerative medicine.

Autologous adipose tissue transfer is a procedure already applied to achieve increased soft tissue volume loss. The adipose tissue grafts are taken by liposuction and reinjected subcutaneously to restore the volumes of the defect areas. In this type of approach, the main obstacle lies in the partial resorption of the transplanted tissue, which is due to necrosis of the adipose tissue after implantation. This necrosis is the consequence of the damage caused to the tissue during its removal on the one hand, and the lack of availability of nutrients in the center of the adipose tissue particles on the other hand. In order to

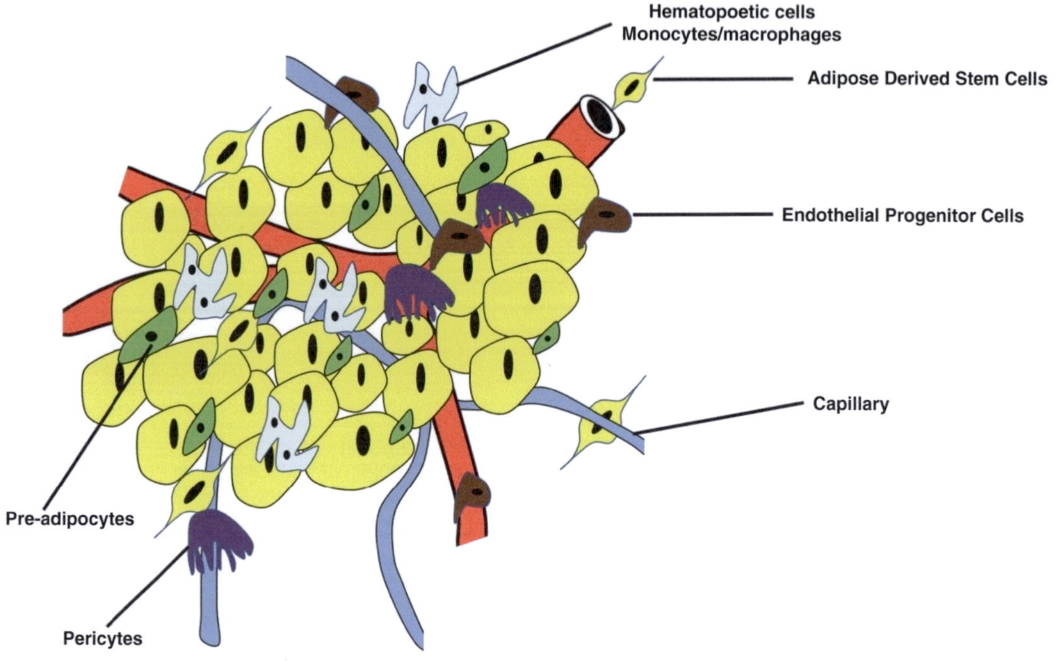

Fig. 1.5 Schematic representation of white adipose tissue [35]

guarantee the survival of the adipocytes, it is necessary to create an optimal microenvironment which allows a correct architectural distribution of the adipocytes also facilitating the interaction between cells, their growth and their differentiation, and which offers an early protection of the surrounding inflammatory phenomena, as well as a capillary network capable of delivering adequate levels of nutrients.

Several techniques have been proposed for the removal of adipose tissue. Coleman et al. [2] have described a technique minimizing the trauma of adipocytes. With a 2-hole, 3 mm, rounded-edge cannula attached to a 10 mL syringe, the grease is manually aspirated by removing the plunger. The cannula is pushed through the sampling site, the surgeon pulls on the plunger of the syringe and creates a slight negative pressure that allows shreds of fat to pass through the cannula and the Luer-Lok opening into the barrel of the syringe. Once filled, the syringe is disconnected from the cannula, which is replaced by a plug that seals the Luer-Lok end of the syringe. The fat sucked into the syringes is centrifuged at 3000 RPM (rotations per minute)

for 3 min to isolate the fat. However, the decrease in centrifugation time to 1 min recently showed an increase in cell viability [38].

1.3.1.1 Macrofat

Macrofat is characterized by fat lobules with a diameter of 2.4 mm. Macrofat is more structural in nature and is easily injected through an 18 or 19 G (gauge) cannula. Macrofat is used for structural enhancement in the temporal regions and deep fatty compartments of the cheek (medial and prezygomatic, pyriform region, mandible, lateral region of the eyebrows, nasal bridge and columella as well as chin and the lips). This type of graft is at risk of resorption, cystosteatonecrosis, oily cysts, and infection [39–41].

1.3.1.2 Microfat

Microfat is characterized by fat lobules with a diameter of 1 mm and is obtained by removing the fat with cannulas of 2 mm diameter whose multiple holes are each less than 1 mm. The sample microcannula has orifices designed specifically to provide a fat sample consisting of adipocyte lobules calibrated in volume. The microcannula deposition has a diameter calibrated on the size of the cell units obtained with the sampling cannula. Microfat is used for trophicity but also for filling.

1.3.1.3 Nanofat

Nano-fat (nanofat) is characterized by fat lobules of 400–600 μm. The nano-fat is obtained by taking the emulsified microfat and passing it between two 10 mL syringes connected together by a female-female Luer-Lok connector (Fig. 1.6). After 3 min of continuous transfer (20–30 passages), the fat becomes an emulsified liquid with a whitish appearance rich in FCS. The emulsified fat is subsequently filtered through a superfine filter to obtain the nanofat [42]. Nanofat can be easily injected using a 27, 30, 32 G needle. This cell seeding is used to improve the trophicity.

Nano-fats can be centrifuged in order to remove free fatty acids and create a gel that can be applied in combination with a cream that promotes dermal penetration and can be applied by mesotherapy techniques after laser resurfacing or facelift. A combination of the three types of fat grafts is used in facial cosmetic surgery or facial fat grafting [43–45].

Tonnard et al. sought to determine the cellular content of nanofat grafts [46]. In their study, they showed that nanofat grafts were devoid of mature adipocytes and that the native architecture was disrupted. However, nanografts retained a rich supply of adipose stem cells, which were similar to macro and micro samples in terms of stem cell

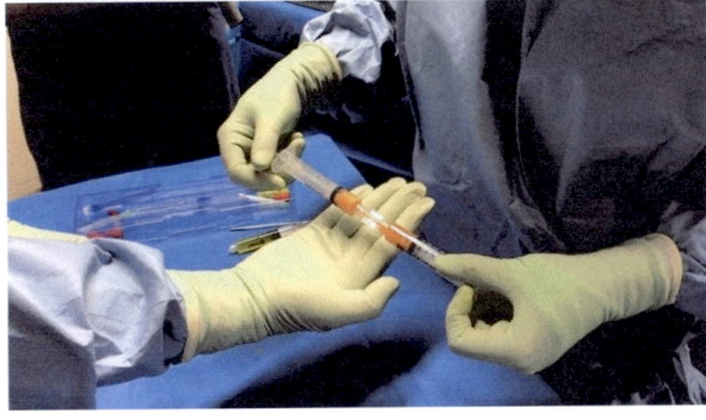

Fig. 1.6 Microfat emulsified mechanically to obtain the nanofat

proliferation and differentiation. Several clinical cases using nanofat grafts showed an improvement in skin quality 6 months after the procedure. Therefore, the authors suggest that even though nanografts do not contain viable adipocytes, their high stem cell content is clinically useful in indications of skin rejuvenation. Emulsified fat thus appears to be a simple alternative to cell therapy processes and the preparation of VSF (Vascular Stroma Fraction) [47, 48]. The injection of fragmented adipocytes present in the emulsified fat and released cytokines could therefore have a stimulating effect on differentiation and tissue regeneration [49]. In addition, an increase in elastin synthesis and dermal remodeling could be induced by the secretory activity of mechanically stimulated stem cells by the emulsion method [50, 51].

Mesguich Batel et al. [48] reported in one study an improvement in fine lines after treatment with the nanofat method (Fig. 1.7). Furthermore, the authors characterized the stem cell composition of this method and showed the presence in 1 cm^3 of emulsified fat of 23,712 ± 7832 cells/cm^3 compared to non-emulsified adipose tissue with a cell viability of 85.1 ± 6.84% and a proportion of 18.77 ± 6.2% of regenerative cells.

In addition, the intradermal injection of emulsified fat was found to be safe. No erythema, skin discoloration or inflammatory reaction was found in all patients [48].

1.3.1.4 Vascular Stroma Fraction (VSF)

The most widely used technique for isolating VSF from lipoaspirate is the digestion of the lipid portion of lipoaspirate by collagenase, separating the content into two distinct phases: the floating fraction of mature adipocytes and the cellular components of interest in the lower fraction [52, 53]. This separation can be improved by centrifugation; however, separation can be achieved also by phase separation and gravity filtration [54]. Although centrifugation is more efficient, it will also sediment all cells present, while filtration can be designed to capture only the important cell types based on their size, thus enriching the

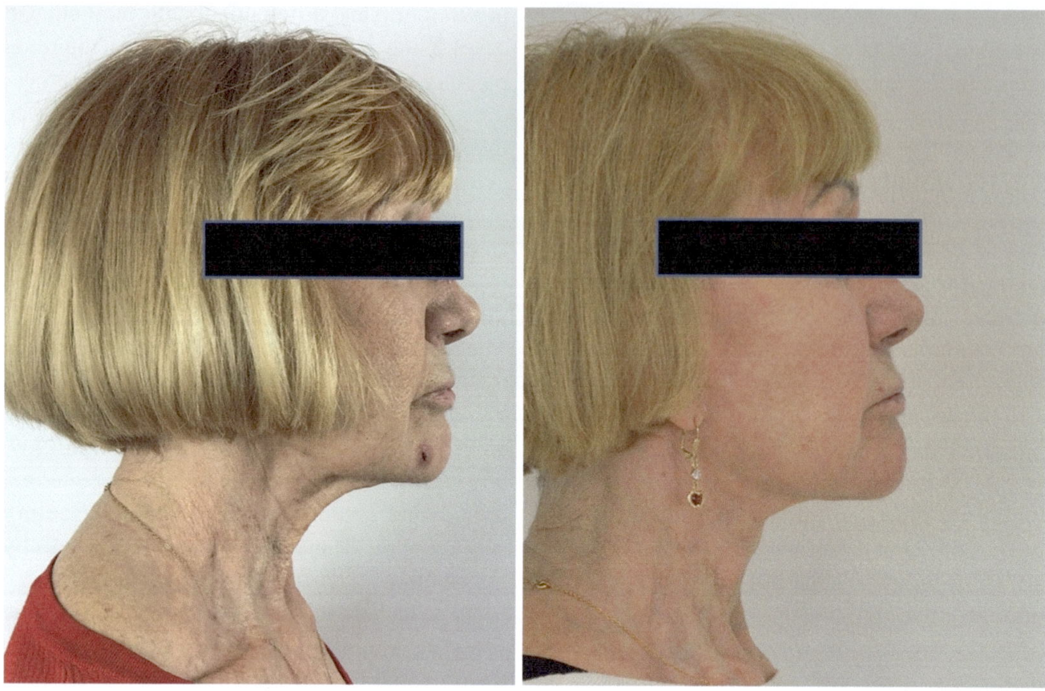

Fig. 1.7 Nanofat injections as an adjunct therapy for facelifts for 80-year-old lady: notice the improvement of skin trophicity

specific cell mix. Centrifugation of the aqueous fraction gives a reddish pellet which contains VSF cells. Erythrocytes, a major contaminant present in the VSF pellet, can be lysed to isolate a more pure population of VSF cells if they are intended for in vitro expansion [55]. VSF contains a variety of cells: mesenchymal stem cells, pericytes, vascular cells, fibroblasts, preadipocytes, monocytes, macrophages, red blood cells, fibrous tissues, and extracellular matrix (ECM) [56] (Fig. 1.8).

The number of stem cells contained in the fat VSF can fluctuate considerably. In adipose tissue, the number of nucleated cells may range from 500,000 to 2,000,000 cells per gram (g) of adipose tissue, and from 1 to 10% ADSCs (Adipose-Derived Stem Cells) [56]. The number of ADSCs in 1 g of adipose tissue can vary from 5000 to 200,000 stem cells [57]. Theoretically, in 100 g of adipose tissue, 0.5–20 million ADSCs can be extracted as VSF. One of the reasons for this variation can be attributed to individual differences. Patients have different texture and density of adipose tissue [58].

1.3.1.5 Stem Cells of Adipose Tissue

Adipose-Derived Stem Cells (ADSCs) were first characterized in 2001 and since then have been extensively studied and used as a major source of cells with regenerative potential, with similar characteristics to those of mesenchymal stem cells (MSCs) [59–62]. Stem cells are cells capable of self-renewal generating identical daughter cells to maintain the stem cell pool and to differentiate into multiple cell lines (progenitors with smaller potential). We then speak of asymmetric differentiation since after each cell division, one cell is renewed while the other enters into differentiation and acquires the characteristics of the tissue concerned. The discovery of mesenchymal stem cells was initiated by the work of Friedenstein et al. in 1968 [63], which showed that rat bone marrow cells contained a small population of plastic-adherent stromal cells capable of forming fibroblast-like colonies. These cells were first named Colony-Forming Unit Fibroblast (CFU-F). Subsequently, in the 1980s, several teams demonstrated their ability to differentiate into cells belonging to mesenchyme lineages (an

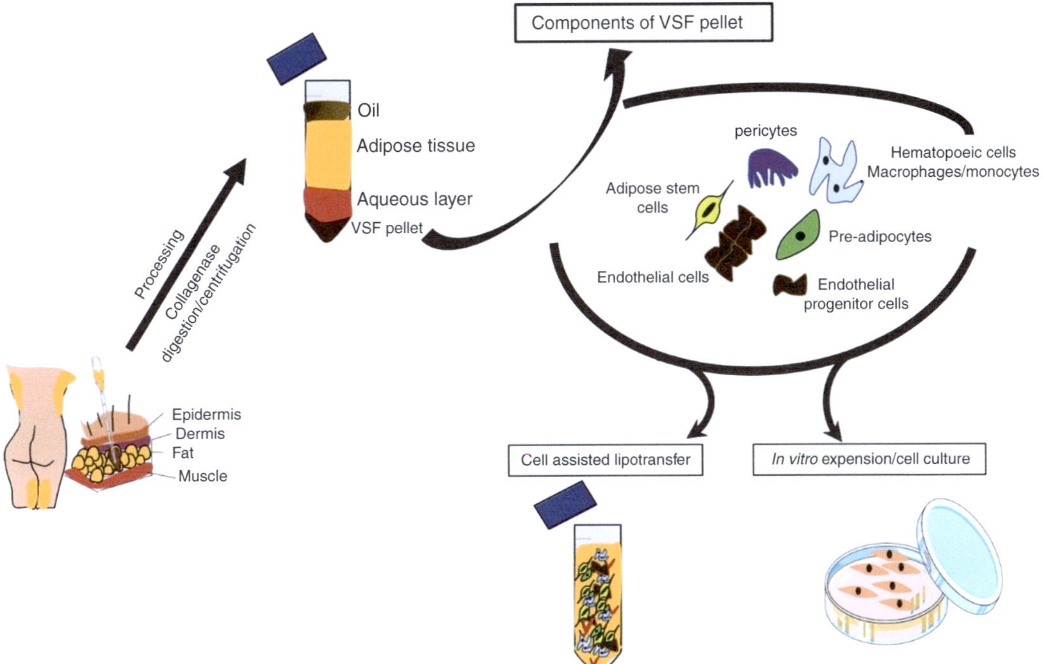

Fig. 1.8 Composition of the VSF. Diagrammatic diagram illustrating the lipoaspiration procedure of the subcutaneous fat is performed, followed by the separation of the different layers by centrifugation. The adipose tissue and the infranatant are recovered and then digested with collagenase. VSF can be used for tissue culture or added to a lipoaspirate [37]

embryonic support tissue derived from the mesoderm and the origin of certain tissues in adults such as vessels, cartilage, or bone), such as chondrocytes, adipocytes, and osteoblasts. The term "mesenchymal stem cell" was then introduced by Caplan in 1991 [64].

For the sake of harmonization, the International Society for Cellular Therapy (ISCT) decided in 2006 to refer to these cells as multipotent mesenchymal stromal cells and to determine minimum criteria to define them [35]: adhesion to plastic under standard culture conditions with the presence of antigen specific to their surface at greater than 90%: CD73 (5′ ectonucleotidase), CD90 (thy-1), CD105 (endoglin); at least 98% of them do not express the following hematopoietic markers: CD45, CD34, CD14, CD19, CD11a, and HLA-DR (Human Leukocyte Antigen-DR) and show the in vitro ability to give rise to cell lines derived from the mesenchyme such as adipocytes, osteoblasts, and chondrocytes.

Bone Marrow MSCs (BM-MSC for Bone Marrow-Mesenchymal Stem Cells) were a reference since they were the first described and used in the field of regenerative medicine. However, the recovery of these stem cells presents constraints because cell sampling is invasive and causes pain, sometimes requiring general anesthesia. In addition, the bone marrow contains few stem cells. Other sources of multipotent stem cells beside bone marrow and adipose tissue are skin, liver, intestine, muscles, synovial tissue, lung tissue, umbilical cord blood, or the cornea [65, 66]. Today, ADSCs are recovered directly from fat "surgical waste" after careful dermolipectomy or lipoaspiration 10–100 million stem cells can be obtained from 300 mL of lipoaspirate of which more than 90% would be viable [67]. A large number of stem cells can be obtained in a few passes. Thus, the risk of chromosomal abnormalities related to senescence and induced by culture is low [35]. In addition, it is possible to preserve the frozen cells and to constitute important stocks. Finally, their use poses fewer ethical problems, unlike embryonic stem cells for example. Summarizing, since their discovery, numerous articles have been published using different terminology, such as adipose-derived stem cells (ADSCs), term defined by the International Federation for Adipose Therapeutics and Science (IFATS), adipose-derived adult stem cells (ADAS), adipose-derived mesenchymal stem cells (AD-MSCs), adipose MSCs (AMSCs), and stromal adipose/stem cells (ASC) [68].

References

1. Illouz YG. The fat cell "graft": a new technique to fill depressions. Plast Reconstr Surg. 1986;78(1):122–3.
2. Coleman SR. Structural fat grafts: the ideal filler? Clin Plast Surg. 2001;28(1):111–9.
3. Zuk PA, et al. Multilineage cells from human adipose tissue: implications for cell-based therapies. Tissue Eng. 2001;7(2):211–28.
4. Gurtner GC, Chapman MA. Regenerative medicine: charting a new course in wound healing. Adv Wound Care (New Rochelle). 2016;5(7):314–28.
5. Marx RE. Platelet-rich plasma (PRP): what is PRP and what is not PRP? Implant Dent. 2001;10:225–8.
6. Anitua E, Alkhraisat MH, Orive G. Perspectives and challenges in regenerative medicine using plasma rich in growth factors. J Control Release. 2012;157:29–38.
7. Marx RE, Garg AK. Dental and craniofacial applications of platelet-rich plasma. Carol Stream: Quintessence Publishing Co., Inc.; 2005.
8. Scully D, Naseem KM, Matsakas A. Platelet biology in regenerative medicine of skeletal muscle. Acta Physiol (Oxf). 2018;223(3):e13071.
9. Werner S, Grose R. Regulation of wound healing by growth factors and cytokines. Physiol Rev. 2003;83:835–70.
10. Anitua E, Sánchez M, Nurden AT, Nurden P, Orive G, Andía I. New insights into and novel applications for platelet-rich fibrin therapies. Trends Biotechnol. 2006;24:227–34.
11. Sampson S, Gerhardt M, Mandelbaum B. Platelet rich plasma injection grafts for musculoskeletal injuries: a review. Curr Rev Musculoskelet Med. 2008;1:165–74.
12. Zielins ER, Atashroo DA, Maan ZN, Duscher D, Walmsley GG, Hu M, Senarath-Yapa K, McArdle A, Tevlin R, Wearda T, et al. Wound healing: an update. Regen Med. 2014;9:817–30.
13. Marx RE. Platelet-rich plasma: evidence to support its use. J Oral Maxillofac Surg. 2004;62:489–96.
14. Dohan Ehrenfest DM, Rasmusson L, Albrektsson T. Classification of platelet concentrates: from pure platelet-rich plasma (P-PRP) to leucocyte-and platelet-rich fibrin (L-PRF). Trends Biotechnol. 2009;27:158–67.
15. Weibrich G, Kleis WK, Hafner G, Hitzler WE, Wagner W. Comparison of platelet, leukocyte, and growth factor levels in point-of-care platelet-enriched plasma, prepared using a modified Curasan kit, with preparations received from a local blood bank. Clin Oral Implants Res. 2003;14:357–162.
16. Gonshor A. Technique for producing platelet-rich plasma and platelet concentrate: background and process. Int J Periodontics Restorative Dent. 2002;22:547–57.
17. Chicharro-Alcántara D, Rubio-Zaragoza M, Damiá-Giménez E, Carrillo-Poveda J, Cuervo-Serrato B, Peláez-Gorrea P, et al. Platelet rich plasma: new insights for cutaneous wound healing management. J Funct Biomater. 2018;9(1):10. https://doi.org/10.3390/jfb9010010.
18. Yu W, Wang J, Yin J. Platelet-rich plasma: a promising product for treatment of peripheral nerve regeneration after nerve injury. Int J Neurosci. 2011;121(4):176–80.
19. Borrione P, Gianfrancesco AD, Pereira MT, Pigozzi F. Platelet-rich plasma in muscle healing. Am J Phys Med Rehabil. 2010;89:854–61.
20. Christgau M, Moder D, Hiller KA, Dada A, Schmitz G, Schmalz G. Growth factors and cytokines in autologous platelet concentrate and their correlation to periodontal regeneration outcomes. J Clin Periodontol. 2006;33:837–45.
21. Mann KG. Biochemistry and physiology of blood coagulation. Thromb Haemost. 1999;16:165–74.
22. Xie X, Wang Y, Zhao C, Guo S, Liu S, Jia W, Tuan RS, Zhang C. Comparative evaluation of MSCs from bone marrow and adipose tissue seeded in PRP-derived scaffold for cartilage regeneration. Biomaterials. 2012;16:7008–18.
23. Kang YH, Jeon SH, Park JY, Chung JH, Choung YH, Choung HW, Kim ES, Choung PH. Platelet-rich fibrin is a bioscaffold and reservoir of growth factors for tissue regeneration. Tissue Eng Part A. 2011;16:349–59.
24. O'Connell SM, Impeduglia T, Hessler K, Wang XJ, Carroll RJ, Dardik H. Autologous platelet-rich fibrin matrix as cell therapy in the healing of chronic lower-extremity ulcers. Wound Repair Regen. 2008;16:749–56.
25. Roubelakis MG, Trohatou O, Roubelakis A, Mili E, Kalaitzopoulos I, Papazoglou G, Pappa KI, Anagnou NP. Platelet-rich plasma (PRP) promotes fetal mesenchymal stem/stromal cell migration and wound healing process. Stem Cell Rev. 2014;10:417–28.
26. Cross KJ, Mustoe TA. Growth factors in wound healing. Surg Clin N Am. 2003;83:531–45.
27. Demidova-Rice TN, Hamblin MR, Herman IM. Acute and impaired wound healing: Pathophysiology and current methods for drug delivery, part 2: role of growth factors in normal and pathological wound healing: therapeutic potential and methods of delivery. Adv Skin Wound Care. 2012;25:349–70.
28. American Association of Blood Banks Technical Manual Committee. Method 6.11: preparation of

platelets from whole blood. In: Vengelen-Tyler V, editor. AABB technical manual. 13th ed. Bethesda, MD: American Association of Blood Banks; 1999. p. 725.

29. Ehrenfest DM, Rasmusson L, Albrektsson T. Classification of platelet concentrates: from pure platelet-rich plasma (P-PRP) to leucocyte- and platelet-rich fibrin (L-PRF). Trends Biotechnol. 2009;27:158–67.

30. Choukroun J, Diss A, Simonpieri A, Girard MO, Schoeffler C, Dohan SL, Dohan AJ, Mouhyi J, Dohan DM. Platelet-rich fibrin (PRF): a second-generation platelet concentrate. Part IV: clinical effects on tissue healing. Oral Surg Oral Med Oral Pathol Oral Radiol Endod. 2006;101:56–60.

31. Diss A, Dohan DM, Mouhyi J, Mahler P. Osteotome sinus floor elevation using Choukroun's platelet-rich fibrin as grafting material: a one-year prospective pilot study with microthreaded implants. Oral Surg Oral Med Oral Pathol Oral Radiol Endod. 2008;105:572–9.

32. Choukroun JI, et al. Influence of platelet rich fibrin (PRF) on proliferation of human preadipocytes and tympanic keratinocytes: a new opportunity in facial lipostructure (Coleman's technique) and tympanoplasty? Rev Laryngol Otol Rhinol. 2007;128:27–32.

33. Braccini F, Dohan DM. The relevance of Choukroun's platelet rich fibrin (PRF) during facial aesthetic lipostructure (Coleman's technique): preliminary results. Rev Laryngol Otol Rhinol (Bord). 2007;128:255–60. Implantodontie. 2001;42:55–62.

34. Eppley BL, Pietrzak WS, Blanton M. Platelet-rich plasma: a review of biology and applications in plastic surgery. Plast Reconstr Surg. 2006;118:147e.

35. Cousin L, Planat-Benard V, Laharrague P, Casteilla B. Adipose-derived stromal cells: their identity and uses in clinical trials, an update. World J Stem Cells. 2011;3(4):25–33.

36. Wronska A, Kmiec Z. Structural and biochemical characteristics of various white adipose tissue depots. Acta Physiol (Oxf). 2012;205(2):194–208.

37. Zimmerlin L, Donnenberg VS, Pfeifer ME, Meyer EM, et al. Stromal vascular progenitors in adult human adipose tissue. Cytometry A. 2010;77:22–30.

38. Hoareau L, Bencharif K, Girard AC, Gence L, Delarue P, Hulard O, Festy F, Roche R. Effect of centrifugation and washing on adipose graft viability: a new method to improve graft efficiency. J Plast Reconstr Aesthet Surg. 2013;66(5):712–9.

39. Eto H, Kato H, Suga H, Aoi N, Doi K, Kuno S, Yoshimura K. The fate of adipocytes after nonvascularized fat grafting: evidence of early death and replacement of adipocytes. Plast Reconstr Surg. 2012;129:1081.

40. Alexander D, Bucky LP. Breast augmentation using preexpansion and autologous fat transplantation—a clinical radiological study. Plast Reconstr Surg. 2011;127:2451–2.

41. Spear SL, Pittman T. A prospective study on lipoaugmentation of the breast. Aesthet Surg J. 2014;34(3):400–8.

42. Wei H, Gu SX, Liang YD, Liang ZJ, Chen H, Zhu MG, Xu FT, He N, Wei XJ, Li HM. Nanofat-derived stem cells with platelet-rich fibrin improve facial contour remodeling and skin rejuvenation after autologous structural fat transplantation. Oncotarget. 2017;8(40):68542–56.

43. Cohen SR, Hewett S, Ross L, Delaunay F, Goodacre A, Ramos C, Leong T, Saad A. Regenerative cells for facial surgery: biofilling and biocontouring. Aesthet Surg J. 2017;37(Suppl_3):S16–32.

44. Dasiou-Plakida D. Grosses injections pour le rajeunissement du visage: 17 ans d'expérience chez 1720 patients. J Cosmet Dermatol. 2003;2:119–25.

45. Mazzola RF. Injection de graisse: du remplissage à la régénération. St. Louis, MO: Quality Edition Médicale; 2009. p. 373–422.

46. Tonnard P, Verpaele A, Peeters G, Hamdi M, Cornelissen M, Declercq H. Nanofat grafting: basic research and clinical applications. Plast Reconstr Surg. 2013;132:1017–26.

47. Bertheuil N, Chaput B. A novel and effective strategy for the isolation of adipose-derived stem cells: minimally manipulated adipose-derived stem cells for more rapid and safe stem cell therapy. Plast Reconstr Surg. 2015;135(2):454–5.

48. Mesguich Batel F, Bertrand B, Magalon J, François P, Velier M, Veran J, Mallet S, Jouve E, Sabatier F, Casanova D. [Treatment of wrinkles of the upper lip by emulsified fat or "nanofat": biological and clinical study about 4 cases]. Ann Chir Plast Esthet. 2018;63(1):31–40.

49. Mahdavian Delavary B, van der Veer WM, van Egmond M, Niessen FB, Beelen RHJ. Macrophages in skin injury and repair. Immunobiology. 2011;216(7):753–62.

50. Banyard DA, Sarantopoulos CN, Borovikova AA, Qiu X, Wirth GA, Paydar KZ, et al. Phenotypic analysis of stromal vascular fraction after mechanical shear reveals stress-induced progenitor populations. Plast Reconstr Surg. 2016;138(2):237e–247.

51. Osinga R, Menzi NR, Tchang LAH, Caviezel D, Kalbermatten DF, Martin I, et al. Effects of intersyringe processing on adipose tissue and its cellular components: implications in autologous fat grafting. Plast Reconstr Surg. 2015;135(6):1618–28.

52. Matsumoto D, Sato K, Gonda K, et al. Cell-assisted lipotransfer: supportive use of human adipose-derived cells for soft tissue augmentation with lipoinjection. Tissue Eng. 2006;12:3375–82.

53. Zuk PA, Zhu M, Mizuno H, et al. Multilineage cells from human adipose tissue: implications for cell-based therapies. Tissue Eng. 2001;7:211–28.

54. SundarRaj S, Deshmukh A, Priya N, et al. Development of a system and method for automated isolation of stromal vascular fraction from adipose tissue lipoaspirate. Stem Cells Int. 2015;2015:1–11.

55. Riis S, Zachar V, Boucher S, et al. Critical steps in the isolation and expansion of adipose-derived stem cells for translational therapy. Expert Rev Mol Med. 2015;17:11.

56. Shukla L, Morrison WA, Shayan R. Adipose-derived stem cells in radiotherapy injury: a new frontier. Front Surg. 2015;2:1.
57. Baer PC, Geiger H. Adipose-derived mesenchymal stromal/stem cells: tissue localization, characterization, and heterogeneity. Stem Cells Int. 2012;2012:812693.
58. Martin AD, Daniel MZ, Drinkwater DT, Clarys JP. Adipose tissue density, estimated adipose lipid fraction and whole body adiposity in male cadavers. Int J Obes Relat Metab Disord. 1994;18(2):79–83.
59. Bourin P, Bunnell BA, Casteilla L, Dominici M, Katz AJ, March KL, Redl H, Rubin JP, Yoshimura K, Gimble JM. Stromal cells from the adipose tissue-derived stromal vascular fraction and culture expanded adipose tissue-derived stromal/stem cells: a joint statement of the International Federation for Adipose Therapeutics and Science (IFATS) and the International Society for Cellular Therapy (ISCT). Cytotherapy. 2013;15:641–8.
60. Gimble JM, Bunnell BA, Frazier T, Rowan B, Shah F, Thomas-Porch C, Wu X. Adipose-derived stromal/stem cells: a primer. Organogenesis. 2013;9(1):3–10.
61. Nguyen A, Guo J, Banyard DA, Fadavi D, Toranto JD, Wirth GA, Paydar KZ, Evans GR, Widgerow AD. Stromal vascular fraction: a regenerative reality? Part 1: current concepts and review of the literature. J Plast Reconstr Aesthetic Surg. 2016;69:170–9.
62. Bunnell BA, Flaat M, Gagliardi C, Patel B, Ripoll C. Adipose-derived stem cells: isolation, expansion and differentiation. Methods. 2008;45(2):115–20.
63. Friedenstein AJ, Petrakova KV, Kurolesova AI, Frolova GP. Heterotopic of bone marrow. Analysis of precursor cells for osteogenic and hematopoietic tissues. Transplantation. 1968;6:230–47.
64. Caplan AI. Mesenchymal stem cells. J Orthop Res. 1991;9:641–50.
65. Calloni R, Cordero EA, Henriques JA, Bonatto D. Reviewing and updating the major molecular markers for stem cells. Stem Cells Dev. 2013;22(9):1455–76.
66. Smadjaa D, Silvestre JS, Lévy BI. Genic and cellular therapy for peripheral arterial diseases. Transfus Clin Biol. 2013;20(2):211–20.
67. Locke M, Windsor J, Dunbar PR. Human adipose-derived stem cells: isolation, characterization and applications in surgery. ANZ J Surg. 2009;79:235–44.
68. Dominici M, Le Blanc K, Mueller I, Slaper-Cortenbach I, Marini F, Krause D, et al. Minimal criteria for defining multipotent mesenchymal stromal cells. Int Soc Cell Ther. 2006;8:315–7.

New Developments and Biomaterials in Reconstruction of Defects of the Alveolar Ridge in Implant Surgery: Part 1—Biomaterials

Thomas Wojcik, Vincent Hornez, Jean Christophe Hornez, and Joël Ferri

2.1 Introduction: Bone Biology and Healing Process

Bone is a tissue that has the ability of self-regeneration leading this healing process in most of the cases to a fully morphologic and functional regeneration.

The knowledge of bone biology is essential to understand the required conditions for a successful reconstruction. The more evident function of the bone skeleton is to allow the locomotion and protection of internal organs, but the bone is also the siege of the hematopoiesis and an essential component in the homeostasis of the phosphor-calcic equilibrium of the organism. Thus, the bone is in a perpetual renewal cycle through resorption and regeneration, allowing the ionic release and capture and response to biomechanical demands [1, 2]. Although the main components of the bone remain homogeneous, including an inorganic mineralized matrix of apatites associated to a protein matrix mainly composed of type 1 collagen, the bone can present different architectural and biological properties, showing the cortical bone a compact structure while the trabecular bone has spongy structure.

In order to understand the prerequisites for a successful bone reconstruction, it is also interesting to know the bone healing process. A bone injury is firstly leading to the formation of an hematoma associated to an inflammatory response and the recruitment of signaling molecules (BMPs, ILs, VEGFs, FGFs,…) involved in bone homeostasis. Thereafter, the process continues by the formation of a callus undergoing chondrogenesis and progressive calcification. Finally, the blood vessels growth into the callus carries both chondroclasts, which resorb the calcified cartilage, and osteoprogenitor cells initiating the bone formation process. It is also important to notice that to complete the bone healing process the stability of the callus is essential, otherwise, the cartilaginous callus is not replaced and results in pseudarthrosis. Thus, bone has strong regenerative capacities, nevertheless, in case of large defects or pathological local condition (infection, insufficient vascularization, instability of the

T. Wojcik
ENT Cancerology Department, Lille, France

V. Hornez
CryoBeryl Software, ETH, France
e-mail: contact@cryoberyl.com

J. C. Hornez
Laboratoire des Matériaux Céramiques et Procédés Associés (LMCPA), Université Polytechnique Hauts-de-France (UPHF), Maubeuge, France
e-mail: jean-christophe.hornez@uphf.fr

J. Ferri (✉)
Department of Oral and Maxillo Facial Surgery, Lille University Nord de France, Lille, France

© Springer Nature Switzerland AG 2021
J. Acero (ed.), *Innovations and New Developments in Craniomaxillofacial Reconstruction*,
https://doi.org/10.1007/978-3-030-74322-2_2

callus,…) the healing process can be compromised which can have an impact in graft's success. In these cases, four elements are essential in the bone graft's healing process and shall be taken in account in every bone grafting procedure: presence of osteogenic cells, osteoconductive scaffold, mechanical environment, and growth factors [3]. Furthermore, a fifth element can't be ignored, the vascularization of the graft and its surrounding tissues.

2.2 Bone Grafts

A bone graft can be defined as an implanted material that promotes osteogenesis through osteoconduction, osteoinduction, and osseointegration. The osteogenesis is the property to produce new bone, whereas osteoconduction is the capability of a grafted material to allow bone growth on its surface or down into pores. Osteoinduction is the capability to recruit and stimulate differentiation of immature cells into bone forming cells and osseointegration is the ability to bind the graft to the surrounding bone without interposition of fibrous tissue [4–7]. All bone grafts or substitute materials can be compared through these characteristics.

The bone grafting procedure is a very common procedure with up to 2.2 million performed worldwide each year while the bone is the second most transplanted tissue after blood. The cost of these procedures is estimated around $2.5 billion per year [8, 9] being the craniofacial field one of the most popular indications for bone grafting [10]. The concept of **autologous graft** means that the tissue is collected of and grafted on the same patient. Due to its biological properties, the autologous bone graft remains the gold standard in bone reconstruction for decades.

The grafted bone brings to the reconstructed site cells, matrix and molecules, guiding and improving the bone healing process. Depending on the type of bone, two type of grafts can be considered concerning its structural features, the cancellous and the cortical bone. The cancellous bone shows high porosity having strong osteogenic properties whereas, on the other hand, the cortical bone has higher density and thus better mechanical properties. The cancellous bone is frequently used to fill limited defects with low mechanical strength while the cortical bone is frequently used as an onlay graft in order to increase the alveolar ridge. It is exposed to a lower vascularization and mechanical constraints of the surrounding mucosa. Indeed during the healing process, mucosa induces an increase of the pressure on the underlying grafted bone and so a higher resorption rate. In fact, many factors are involved in the resorption process but it seems clear that the cortical bone graft has a higher resorption rate. The autograft can be harvested from different sites (Fig. 2.1); however, despite its biological and mechanical properties, the autograft presents a major disadvantage which is the morbidity of the donor sites [11–13], with possible impact on patient quality of life. Moreover, the potential amount of bone that can be harvested is limited especially in case of pediatric or geriatric patient. That is why alternatives as allografts and xenografts have been considered.

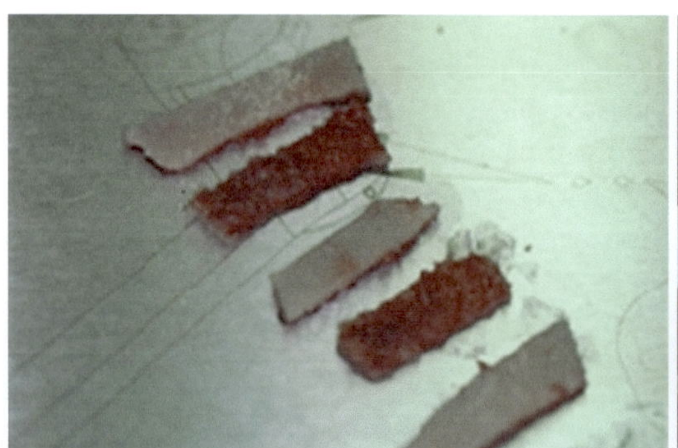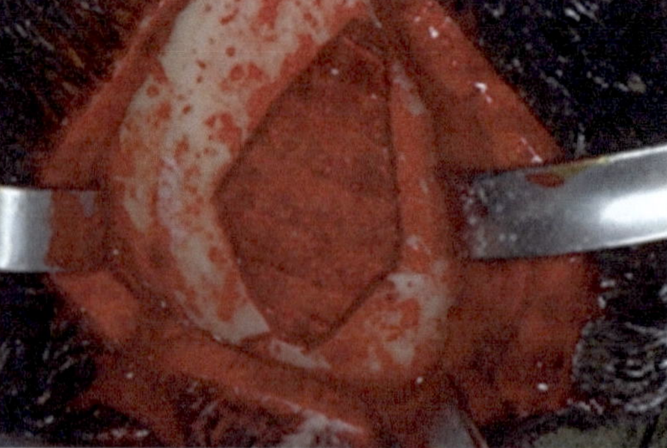

Fig. 2.1 Calvarial bone sample for bone graft

Allografts are tissue harvested from one individual and transplanted to another individual of the same species with a different genotype, whereas **xenografts** are harvested from other species. They both eliminate the donor site morbidity and are available in large quantity having also osteoconductive and osteoinductive properties but in comparison with the autologous grafts, allografts and xenografts present a lower osteogenic potential, increase the rejection risk due to the immune response and present a risk of disease transmission. Furthermore, the procedure required to decrease the risk of disease transmission also negatively impact in their biological and mechanical properties. Today, allografts are rarely used for implant surgery in comparison with the popularity of xenografts in this field due to their easy access for practitioners.

Thus, due to the multiple problems related to the use of bone grafts, research is carried out in order to find an ideal bone substitute which should present the biological properties of the autograft combined with unlimited amount and limited cost. In order to reach that goal, different approaches are possible including tissue engineering [14, 15]. Tissue engineering is based on the use of cells, molecules, and matrix that can be used independently or combined aiming to maintain, reestablish, or improve tissue architecture and function. Considering the specific Bone Tissue Engineering (BTE) field, some key points have to be taken into account: a scaffold shall mimic the bone extracellular matrix with osteoinductive properties facilitating osteogenic cell adhesion, it shall differentiate the cells to the desirable phenotype through osteoinductives properties and allow sufficient vascularization and nutrition of the construct to complete the healing process [14].

2.3   Biomaterials and Scaffolds

Scaffolds are to date the most important issue in bone tissue engineering. Scaffolds are materials designed to support and facilitate the bone healing process by allowing the undifferentiated cells migration and specialization, sequestration of extracellular matrix components, vascularization development, and three-dimensional tissue organization. They also shall provide structural stability to the reconstructed site, withstanding mechanical strength supported by the bone. Biomaterials are materials of natural or synthetic origin suitable to be implanted and interact with living tissue.

Scaffolds can be divided in organic and inorganic, with biological or synthetic origin. The advantages of biological scaffolds are that they have better biocompatibility, bioresorption ability, and regenerative properties (osteoconduction, osteoinduction, osteogenesis, and osseointegration) in comparison with synthetic materials although they also can present immune response. The immune reaction and mechanical failures are the two main causes of failure in bone reconstruction protocols.

2.3.1 Natural-Origin Biomaterials

Collagens are one of the most widely present proteins in the human body and provide stability and strength to many tissues from skin till bones [16]. Type I collagen is the main component of the extracellular matrix of the bone and is one of the most popular organic biological material for bone tissue engineering. Integration of collagen on the surface of scaffolds improves cellular proliferation and osteoblastic differentiation. Collagens can also be used as carriers for other molecules as bone morphogenetics proteins, enhancing the new bone formation [17]. However, collagens present poor mechanical properties as a major limitation for bone tissue engineering which can be improved combining them with other materials with better mechanical features.

Chitosan is another example of organic biological material which can be used for bone tissue engineering. It's a linear polysaccharide with bending ability but poor mechanical properties. Chitosan modifies its structure depending on the acid-base environment. Thus, in a neutral environment, chitosan maintains its structure but solubilizes and degrades in an acidic medium. Chitosan can be used as a carrier in polymeric nanoparticles and is used in combination with other materials for bone tissue engineering [18, 19]. However, the resorption of the polymer can lead to aseptic inflammation which negatively affects the bone healing process.

Summarizing, even if they are used for implant procedures, the major limitations in the use of natural-origin biomaterials are the difficulties in refining them, their potential immunogenicity and the poor mechanical properties in comparison to the bone. Thus they shall be considered as an alternative when bone grafts are not possible.

2.3.2 Synthetic Biomaterials

In order to reduce the problems related to the use of natural-origin biomaterials, a challenging field has been the development of polymeric synthetic biomaterials [20–22] like polyglycolic acid (PGA), polylactic acid (PLA), or polylactic-*co*-glycolic acid (PLGA) that are very promising in bone tissue engineering field but are not today included in practitioners' current practice.

The synthetic bone substitutes share several advantages over allografts, including unlimited supply, easy sterilization and storage but their biocompatibility, biodegradability, and regenerative properties are lower than those of natural scaffolds [15]. Since the initiation of bone tissue engineering procedures more than three decades ago, different options have been considered but calcium phosphate matrix (hydroxyapatite, beta-tricalcium phosphate) and bioactive glasses remain as the most used currently because of their morphological and biological similarities to the inorganic part of bone [23]. In fact, bone is a composite material composed of both mineral (calcium phosphate) and protein matrix. The proteins provide its flexibility to the bone while calcium phosphate gives its compressive strength, although linked to their low plasticity, the calcium phosphate matrix (CaP) can be also fragile.

Biological apatites (BA) are the mineral phase of bone. They have a very flexible composition linked to their ability to chemical substitution. In fact, other components such as Mg, Na, Si, Cl, K, CO_3 and F can be included in their structure, leading to variations in their chemical and mechanical properties [24]. On the other hand, synthetic apatites like synthetic hydroxyapatite (S-HA) have a stable composition and do not include "impurities." Moreover, crystals of S-HA are much bigger than the BA [25]. This induces variations in their biological and mechanical properties in comparison to the BA and even if they are considered to be biocompatible, osteoconductive bioactive and have a great affinity for growth factors and proteins, they have a lower solubility and low osteoinductive potential. Furthermore, a lot of parameters also influence the biological and physical properties of the S-HA scaffolds, like sinterization temperature and pore size (micro- and macroporosity). In order to simplify, we may say that for synthetic phosphocalcic matrix, the microporosity and resorption potential vary inversely with the increase of the sintering temperature and the increase of mechanical resistance [26–28] .

The beta-tricalcium phosphate (β-TCP) is another synthetic calcium phosphate that presents a less stable crystalline phase than S-HA and thus a higher degradation rate and better osteoinductive property. Moreover, its mechanical properties like compression and tensile strength are very similar to that of cancellous bone, which make β-TCP one of the most popular options for bone tissue engineering. The most recent and promising approach to date in phosphocalcic matrix is the development of biphasic calcium phosphates (BCP) to combine the properties of both materials, hydroxyapatite and tricalcium phosphate. Two different approaches are possible to produce that BCP. The most popular and the easier is to mix HA and β-TCP powder and modify their ratio to modulate their mechanical and physiological properties. However, the inhomogeneity of the proportions of these two phases in the material may lead to variation of the mechanical and biological properties inside the matrix. The second approach consist in a molecular mix of HA and β-TCP during the synthesis process which is supposed to guaranty a higher homogeneity of the material and its physicochemical properties [29, 30].

Multiple studies on S-HA, beta-tricalcium phosphate (β-TCP), and bicalcium phosphate (BCP) have shown that a fast resorption is beneficial concerning osteoinduction properties; however, a stability of the surface is necessary for bone formation. By modulating S-HA/β-TCP proportions in the BCP, it is possible to modulate their resorption rate and mechanical properties and thus to mimic the properties of the repaired bone defect [31]. A high proportion of β-TCP has been demonstrated to be better to develop early bone formation [32]. Like other calcium phosphate (CaP) matrix, the porosity and architecture of the BCP matrix also play a major role in their properties [33, 34]. Thus, to reproduce the biological properties of the bone, an adequate architecture is essential. In fact, it has been well documented that the pore size plays a major role in neoangiogenesis, osteoconduction, and new bone formation [35, 36]. Today, apatite materials are frequently used in implants surgery to fill bone defect. They can be used alone or in association with bone graft depending on the procedures.

2.4　The Impact of the New Technologies on CaP Matrix

The computer assisted design (CAD) associated with addictive technologies known as 3D printing is probably a "game changer" in the conception of our matrix. In fact, CAD procedure allows to anticipate the control of both macro and micro architectures of the matrix (Fig. 2.2a, b), virtually reproducing the architectural characteristics of trabecular and cortical bones (Fig. 2.3). In a near future, bone defects could be repaired through the accurate reproduction of the previous architecture in order to simplify and to increase the precision of the reconstruction procedures (Figs. 2.4 and 2.5).

Different printing techniques are possible to create a calcium phosphate matrix. The most promising to date seems to be the stereolithography,

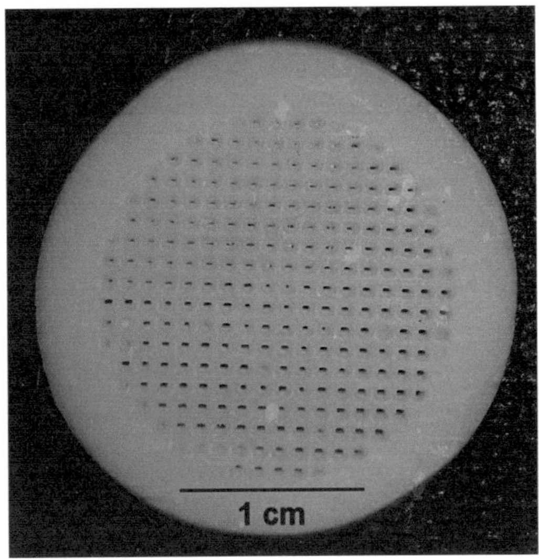

Fig. 2.3 Hydroxyapatite architecture of trabecular (macroporous) and cortical (dense) bones printed by ceramic stereolithography

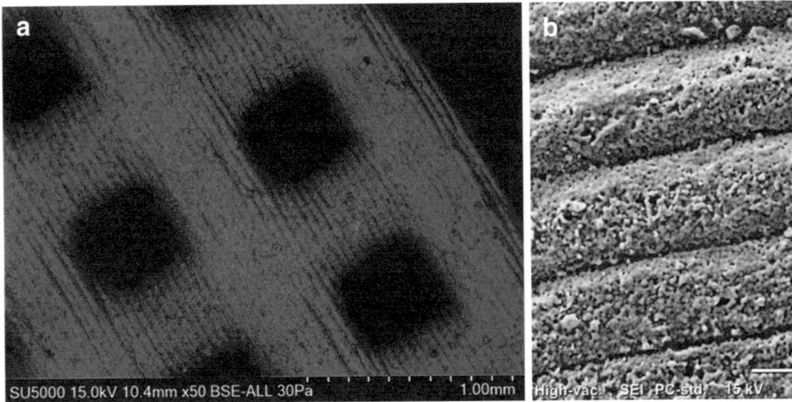

Fig. 2.2 (**a**) SEM morphology of BCP macroporous structure produced by ceramic stereolithography. (**b**) SEM morphology of β-TCP microporous structure produced layer by layer by ceramic stereolithography

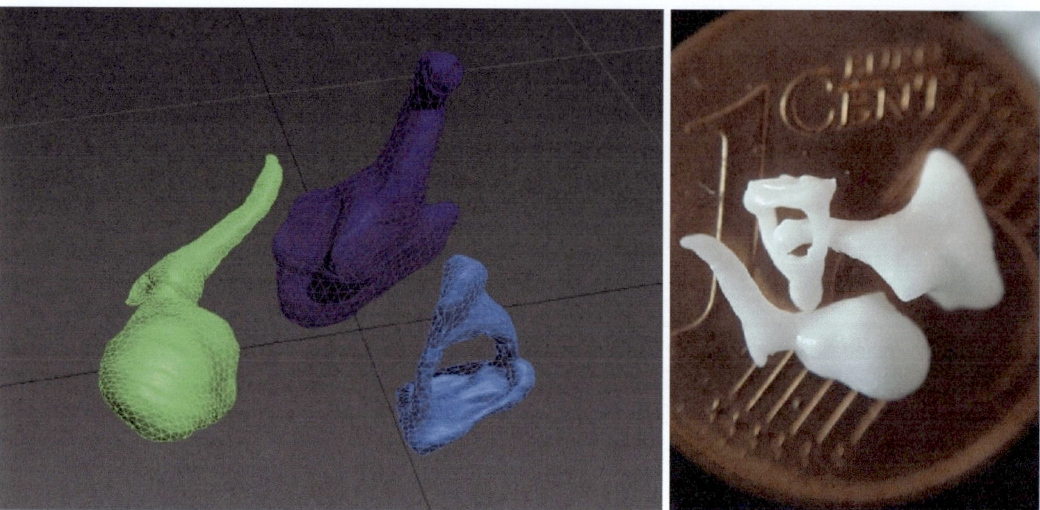

Fig. 2.4 The smallest bones in the human body (of the middle ear) produced by stereolithography with a resolution of less than 50 µm of dense hydroxyapatite

Fig. 2.5 Demonstration of a bone defect reconstructed with printed phosphocalcic matrix

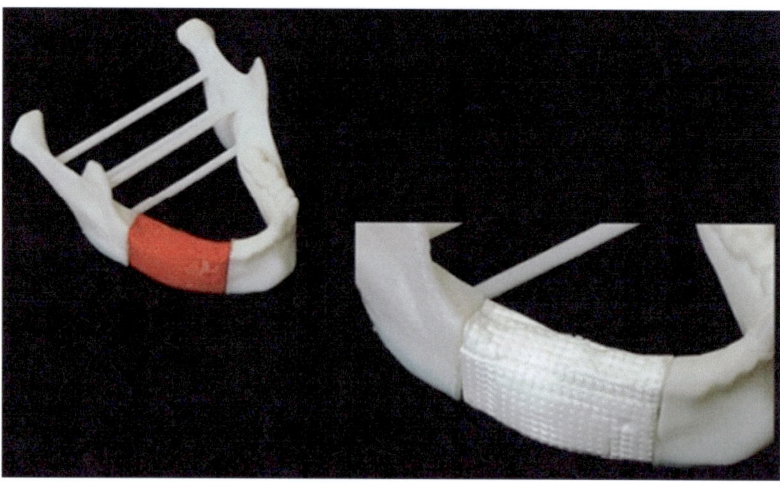

consisting in the polymerization layer by layer of a photo-curable resin mixed with phosphocalcic particles. After the end of the printing process, matrix has to be sintered in order to finish the shaping process (Fig. 2.6). Main advantage of this technique is its high resolution (under 100 µm) but it involves potential contamination of the product from resin. The laser casting technique uses a high resolution laser to produce a selective layer by layer thermal binding of the particles. Like the ste- reolithography, the main advantage of that technique is its resolution but remains expensive to date. Finally, the third and most popular technique is the material extrusion 3D printing. It consists in a continuous material deposit through an extruder. The layer by layer deposit finally results in a 3D structure that need to be sintered to complete the shaping process. The limit of the extrusion technique is its lower resolution compared to stereolithography and laser casting [37, 38].

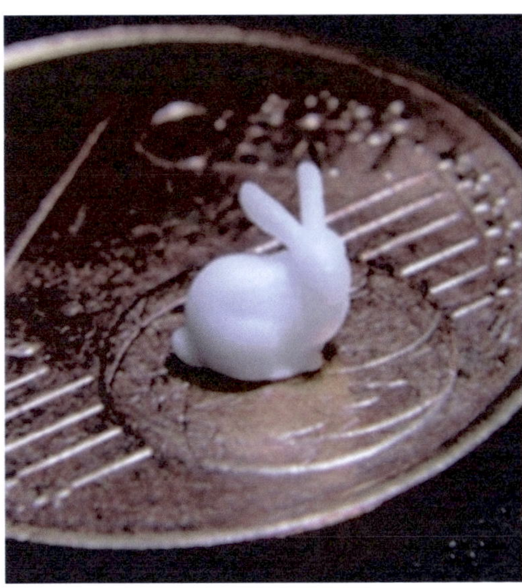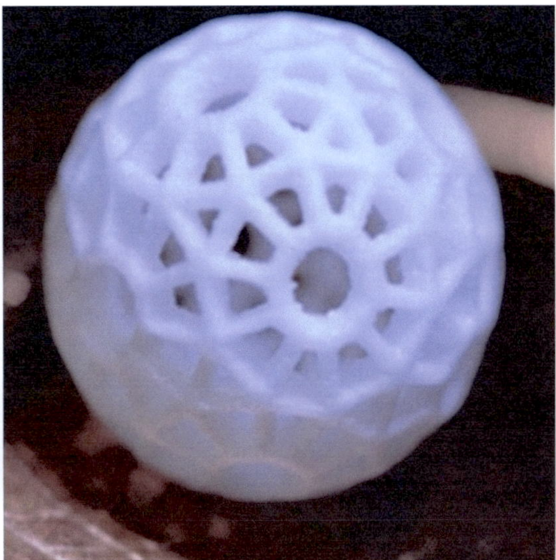

Fig. 2.6 Examples of phosphocalcic matrices printed using stereolithography. Note the high resolution of the produced pieces and the complex design achieved

2.5 Conclusion

To date, the autologous bone graft shall remain the gold standard in the treatment of bone defects in implant surgery. However, the needs in terms of bone regeneration are constantly increasing and the autologous graft can't be the only answer. Allografts and xenografts are useful but not ideal alternatives as they present a risk of disease transmission and rejection, that's why the development of synthetic grafting material has been introduced.

Tissue engineering including CaP matrix associated with 3D printing techniques seem to be promising for the next future. However, these techniques should certainly combine composite materials and introduce a cellular and molecular approach in order to mimic the bone structure and function to become the new gold standard in bone reconstruction.

References

1. Zuo C, Huang Y, Bajis R, Sahih M, Li Y-P, Dai K, et al. Osteoblastogenesis regulation signals in bone remodeling. Osteoporos Int. 2012;23(6):1653–63.
2. Fazzalari NL. Bone fracture and bone fracture repair. Osteoporos Int. 2011;22(6):2003–6.
3. Giannoudis PV, Einhorn TA, Marsh D. Fracture healing: the diamond concept. Injury. 2007;38(Suppl 4):S3–6.
4. Albrektsson T, Johansson C. Osteoinduction, osteoconduction and osseointegration. Eur Spine J. 2001;10(Suppl 2):S96–101.
5. Zarb G, Albrektsson T. Osseointegration: a requiem for the periodontal ligament? An editorial. J Periodont Rest Dent. 1991;11:88–91.
6. Brånemark PI, Hansson BO, Adell R, Breine U, Lindström J, Hallén O, et al. Osseointegrated implants in the treatment of the edentulous jaw. Experience from a 10-year period. Scand J Plast Reconstr Surg Suppl. 1977;16:1–132.
7. Wilson-Hench J. Osteoconduction. In: Williams DF, editor. Definitions in biomaterials, Progress in biomedical engineering. Amsterdam: Elsevier; 1987. p. 29.
8. Baroli B. From natural bone grafts to tissue engineering therapeutics: brainstorming on pharmaceutical formulative requirements and challenges. J Pharm Sci. 2009;98(4):1317–75.
9. Bureau UC. Section 3. Health and nutrition [Internet]. The United States Census Bureau. [cited 2019 Dec 14]. Available from https://www.census.gov/library/publications/2011/compendia/statab/131ed/health-nutrition.html.
10. Elsalanty ME, Genecov DG. Bone grafts in craniofacial surgery. Craniomaxillofacial Trauma Reconstr. 2009;2(3):125–34.
11. Ebraheim NA, Elgafy H, Xu R. Bone-graft harvesting from iliac and fibular donor sites: techniques and complications. J Am Acad Orthop Surg. 2001;9(3):210–8.

12. Touzet S, Ferri J, Wojcik T, Raoul G. Complications of calvarial bone harvesting for maxillofacial reconstructions. J Craniofac Surg. 2011;22(1):178–81.

13. Banwart JC, Asher MA, Hassanein RS. Iliac crest bone graft harvest donor site morbidity. A statistical evaluation. Spine. 1995;20(9):1055–60.

14. Amini AR, Laurencin CT, Nukavarapu SP. Bone tissue engineering: recent advances and challenges. Crit Rev Biomed Eng. 2012;40(5):363–408.

15. Oryan A, Alidadi S, Moshiri A, Maffulli N. Bone regenerative medicine: classic options, novel strategies, and future directions. J Orthop Surg. 2014;9(1):18.

16. Pastorino L, Dellacasa E, Scaglione S, Giulianelli M, Sbrana F, Vassalli M, et al. Oriented collagen nanocoatings for tissue engineering. Colloids Surf B Biointerfaces. 2014;114:372–8.

17. Hamilton PT, Jansen MS, Ganesan S, Benson RE, Hyde-Deruyscher R, Beyer WF, et al. Improved bone morphogenetic protein-2 retention in an injectable collagen matrix using bifunctional peptides. PLoS One. 2013;8(8):e70715.

18. Agnihotri SA, Mallikarjuna NN, Aminabhavi TM. Recent advances on chitosan-based micro- and nanoparticles in drug delivery. J Control Release. 2004;100(1):5–28.

19. Nguyen DT, McCanless JD, Mecwan MM, Noblett AP, Haggard WO, Smith RA, et al. Balancing mechanical strength with bioactivity in chitosan-calcium phosphate 3D microsphere scaffolds for bone tissue engineering: air- vs. freeze-drying processes. J Biomater Sci Polym Ed. 2013;24(9):1071–83.

20. Mistura DV, Messias AD, Duek EAR, Duarte MAT. Development, characterization, and cellular adhesion of poly(L-lactic acid)/poly(caprolactone triol) membranes for potential application in bone tissue regeneration. Artif Organs. 2013;37(11):978–84.

21. Ortega-Oller I, Padial-Molina M, Galindo-Moreno P, O'Valle F, Jódar-Reyes AB, Peula-García JM. Bone regeneration from PLGA micro-nanoparticles. Biomed Res Int. 2015;2015:415289.

22. Yang Y-L, Chang C-H, Huang C-C, Kao WM-W, Liu W-C, Liu H-W. Osteogenic activity of nanonized pearl powder/poly (lactide-co-glycolide) composite scaffolds for bone tissue engineering. Biomed Mater Eng. 2014;24(1):979–85.

23. Damien CJ, Parsons JR. Bone graft and bone graft substitutes: a review of current technology and applications. J Appl Biomater. 1991;2(3):187–208.

24. Boanini E, Gazzano M, Bigi A. Ionic substitutions in calcium phosphates synthesized at low temperature. Acta Biomater. 2010;6(6):1882–94.

25. Rh Owen G, Dard M, Larjava H. Hydoxyapatite/beta-tricalcium phosphate biphasic ceramics as regenerative material for the repair of complex bone defects. J Biomed Mater Res B Appl Biomater. 2018;106(6):2493–512.

26. Will J, Melcher R, Treul C, Travitzky N, Kneser U, Polykandriotis E, et al. Porous ceramic bone scaffolds for vascularized bone tissue regeneration. J Mater Sci Mater Med. 2008;19(8):2781–90.

27. Kasten P, Luginbühl R, van Griensven M, Barkhausen T, Krettek C, Bohner M, et al. Comparison of human bone marrow stromal cells seeded on calcium-deficient hydroxyapatite, beta-tricalcium phosphate and demineralized bone matrix. Biomaterials. 2003;24(15):2593–603.

28. Rodríguez-Lugo V, Karthik TVK, Mendoza-Anaya D, Rubio-Rosas E, Villaseñor Cerón LS, Reyes-Valderrama MI, et al. Wet chemical synthesis of nanocrystalline hydroxyapatite flakes: effect of pH and sintering temperature on structural and morphological properties. R Soc Open Sci. 2018;5(8):180962.

29. Wagoner Johnson AJ, Herschler BA. A review of the mechanical behavior of CaP and CaP/polymer composites for applications in bone replacement and repair. Acta Biomater. 2011;7(1):16–30.

30. Willie BM, Petersen A, Schmidt-Bleek K, Cipitria A, Mehta M, Strube P, et al. Designing biomimetic scaffolds for bone regeneration: why aim for a copy of mature tissue properties if nature uses a different approach? Soft Matter. 2010;6(20):4976–87.

31. Mentaverri R, Yano S, Chattopadhyay N, Petit L, Kifor O, Kamel S, et al. The calcium sensing receptor is directly involved in both osteoclast differentiation and apoptosis. FASEB J. 2006;20(14):2562–4.

32. Fariña NM, Guzón FM, Peña ML, Cantalapiedra AG. In vivo behaviour of two different biphasic ceramic implanted in mandibular bone of dogs. J Mater Sci Mater Med. 2008;19(4):1565–73.

33. Zhu XD, Fan HS, Xiao YM, Li DX, Zhang HJ, Luxbacher T, et al. Effect of surface structure on protein adsorption to biphasic calcium-phosphate ceramics in vitro and in vivo. Acta Biomater. 2009;5(4):1311–8.

34. Sager M, Ferrari D, Wieland M, Dard M, Becker J, Schwarz F. Immunohistochemical characterization of wound healing at two different bone graft substitutes. Int J Oral Maxillofac Surg. 2012;41(5):657–66.

35. Kim K, Yeatts A, Dean D, Fisher JP. Stereolithographic bone scaffold design parameters: osteogenic differentiation and signal expression. Tissue Eng Part B Rev. 2010;16(5):523–39.

36. Hulbert SF, Young FA, Mathews RS, Klawitter JJ, Talbert CD, Stelling FH. Potential of ceramic materials as permanently implantable skeletal prostheses. J Biomed Mater Res. 1970;4(3):433–56.

37. Wilson CE, de Bruijn JD, van Blitterswijk CA, Verbout AJ, Dhert WJA. Design and fabrication of standardized hydroxyapatite scaffolds with a defined macro-architecture by rapid prototyping for bone-tissue-engineering research. J Biomed Mater Res A. 2004;68(1):123–32.

38. Trombetta R, Inzana JA, Schwarz EM, Kates SL, Awad HA. 3D printing of calcium phosphate ceramics for bone tissue engineering and drug delivery. Ann Biomed Eng. 2017;45(1):23–44.

Gwénael Raoul, Ludovic Lauwers, and Joël Ferri

3.1 Introduction

In completely resorbed maxilla, there is poor outcome with conventional implants in both the premaxillary and the posterior region of the maxilla. In case of patients with extremely resorbed maxilla, if removable prosthesis do not meet patient's expectations, several possibilities of implant-supported rehabilitation could be available [1], among them the zygomatic implants are an alternative based in the concept of the lack of resorption at the level of the zygomatic bone which allows the fixation of long implants at this anatomic level [2, 3]. Use of special fixtures such as short implants if enough bone height is available, subperiosteal implants, or longer implants inserted in the pterygoid process [4] can also avoid bone grafting procedures but frequently cannot be used in extremely atrophic maxilla. Standard implants (cylindrical and screwed) could need previous alveolar regeneration or reconstruction by means of biomaterials [5, 6] or

autologous bone [7], Le Fort I osteotomy may also be considered [8, 9].

After developing the concept of osteointegration with conventional implants, Bränemark developed the "zygomaticus fixture" [2], also called zygomatic implants, as an alternative approach to avoid alveolar bone reconstruction in severely resorbed maxilla. The biomechanical concept is based on obtaining anchorage in both zygomatic bones by using two long fixtures called "zygomatic implants." In the original description of this technique, two posterior zygomatic implants were linked to two or four conventional implants in the anterior region of the maxilla supporting a full arch prosthetic restoration. Some authors also placed two implants on each side ("Zygoma quad") [10] (Fig. 3.1) or three zygomatic implants bilaterally in order to get a six zygomatic implants restoration [3]. An asymmetric positioning of the implants is also possible (Fig. 3.2).

Zygomatic implants are not conventional implants and need specific skills in order to achieve good result. As for every treatment planning dealing with implants, three major points are to be considered: the expertise in the management of the paranasal sinus, the knowledge of the specific anatomical obstacles and of the management of their potential complications, and the feasibility of immediate prosthetic loading.

G. Raoul · J. Ferri (✉)
Departement of Stomatology and Oral and
Maxillofacial, Roger Salengro Hospital, INSERM U 1008,
CHRU, Lille Cedex, France
e-mail: joel.ferri@univ-lille.fr

L. Lauwers
Department of Stomatology, Oral and Maxillo-facial
Surgery, Roger Salengro-CHRU, Lille Cedex, France

© Springer Nature Switzerland AG 2021
J. Acero (ed.), *Innovations and New Developments in Craniomaxillofacial Reconstruction*,
https://doi.org/10.1007/978-3-030-74322-2_3

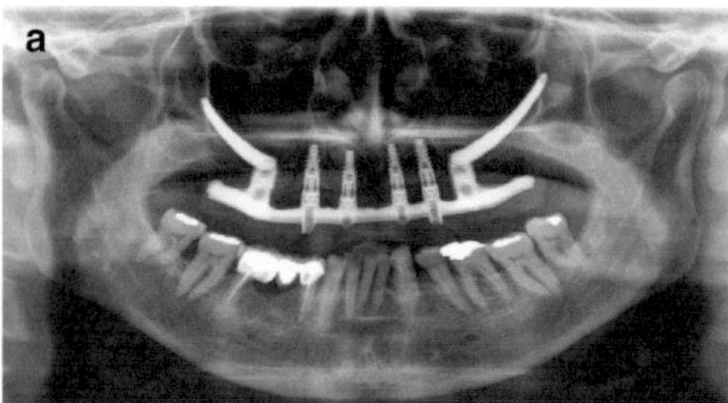
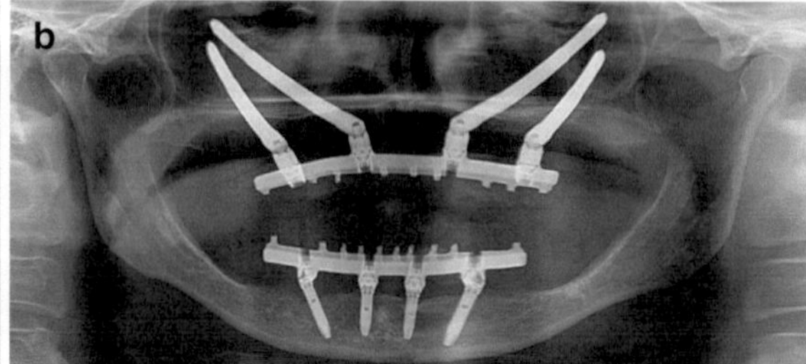

Fig. 3.1 (**a**) Association of two zygomatic implants associated with four standard implants in the anterior maxilla. (**b**) Two posterior zygomatic implants or quad four

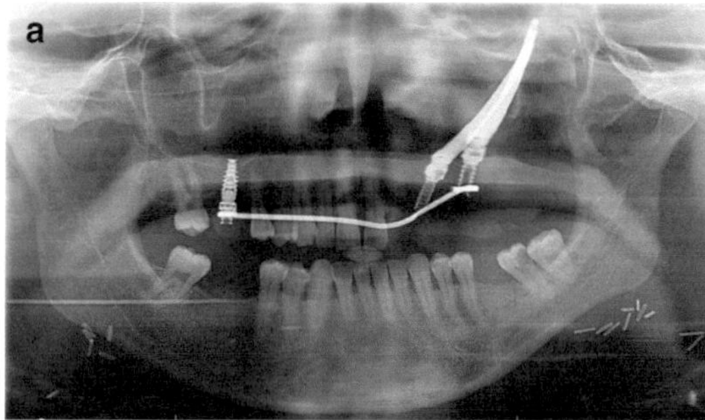
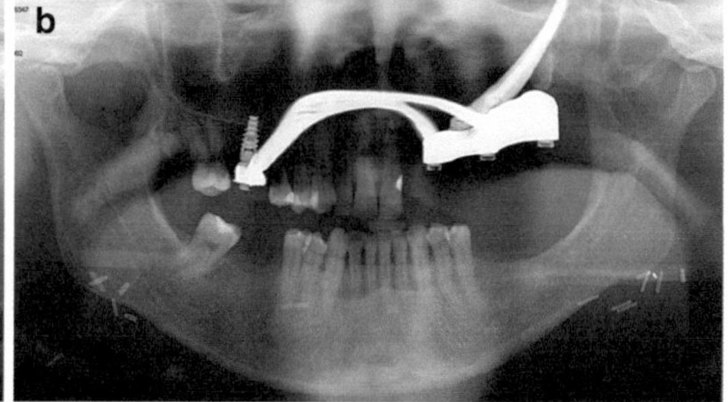

Fig. 3.2 (**a**) Use of two left zygomatic implants and a right conventional implant after left maxillectomy. (**b**) Final result: a framework for removable prosthesis has been designed allowing for visual control of the resected maxilla

Introduction of the zygomatic implants has opened a new field in the implant treatment of the severely resorbed upper jaw. This type of fixations may be used in different situations to get a quick and reliable prosthetic rehabilitation, from the edentulous patients to the absence of maxillae after tumor resection [11].

3.2 Indications of Zygomatic Implants

Zygomatic implants are indicated in atrophic maxilla or after maxillary resection in order to perform implant-supported dental rehabilitation while avoiding bone grafting.

Indications of zygomatic implants need to be fixed after a complete analysis of the patient's situation as a multidisciplinary approach including the medical, prosthetic, and dental point of view and taking into account the patient's desire. It is important to keep in mind that the patient is asking for a prosthetic rehabilitation and not for a technique. For each individual patient when dealing with the indications for the treatment of the abovementioned situations, the different options such as the use of zygomatic implants, short implants, bone regeneration or bone grafts (vascularized or not) including Le Fort I osteotomy technique have to be evaluated and presented to the patient [8, 9].

Zygomatic implants can be indicated in every situation of edentulous maxilla allowing a fixed dental rehabilitation with immediate loading without using any grafting technique. Prosthetic rehabilitation in this type of implants includes two steps: the first is a temporary immediate prosthesis, followed by a new final prosthesis 6 months after the implant placement. Zygomatic implants can be also very useful for dental rehabilitation after maxillectomy. Asymmetric placement of the implants is possible in case of implant-supported rehabilitation after hemi-maxillectomy (Fig. 3.2) [11–13].

The use of zygomatic implants, as mentioned above, allows for the immediate loading of the prosthesis by connecting the implants (conventional and zygomatic) with a splinted prosthetic framework. Primary stability of the implants inserted with a *torque* of at *least 35* N cm is necessary for an immediate loading protocol. Even with high implant angulation, immediate loading with zygomatic implants shows long-term good results [2, 14–18] with high patient satisfaction [19, 20]. However, certain situations may require secondary loading. In that case, the implants will remain unloaded until complete osteointegration is achieved and any contact or pressure over the implants has to be avoided.

3.3 Treatment with Zygomatic Implants: Planning of the Surgical Technique

3.3.1 Surgical Technique: Preoperative Planning

Pre-surgical planning is currently widely used for conventional implants placement. In case of indication of zygomatic implants, a correct planning is mandatory in order to evaluate the bone anatomy in malar region. Zygomatic implants planning requires a complete DICOM acquisition of the zygomatic volume including the orbital roof and the entire maxilla. CT scan will help to evaluate the anatomy of the malar bone and to check the absence of paranasal sinus pathology such as chronic sinusitis, sinus retention cysts, polyposis, or foreign body in the paranasal sinuses. Prior to implant placement in the zygomatic region, any anomaly of the paranasal sinuses must be excluded and eventually treated if needed. Paranasal sinus infection is the most frequent complication of zygomatic implants [21].

Preoperative planning will set the position, length, size, and direction of the implants (Fig. 3.3). Implants placement design needs to avoid damaging of important anatomic areas such as the orbit or the infraorbital nerve. Usually the landmarks for positioning the zygomatic implants at the mucosal side are the canine and first molar sites. The apex of the implant should be placed in direction to the zygomatic bone through the paranasal sinuses ending at a vertical line passing on the zygomatic buttress and the ascending branch of the zygoma. Nowadays, a variety of software including zygomatic implants virtual planning tools are available. This is not aim of this chapter to compare different software. They should offer every possibility of allowing for virtual planning of the reconstruction including a virtual panoramic view in order to check the final position of the quad zygoma design (Figs. 3.4 and 3.5).

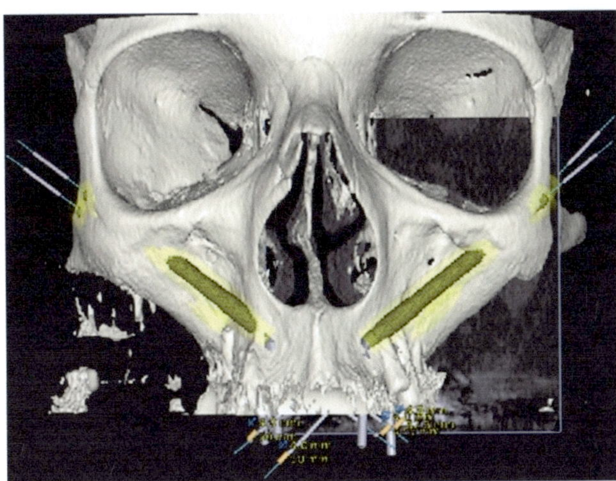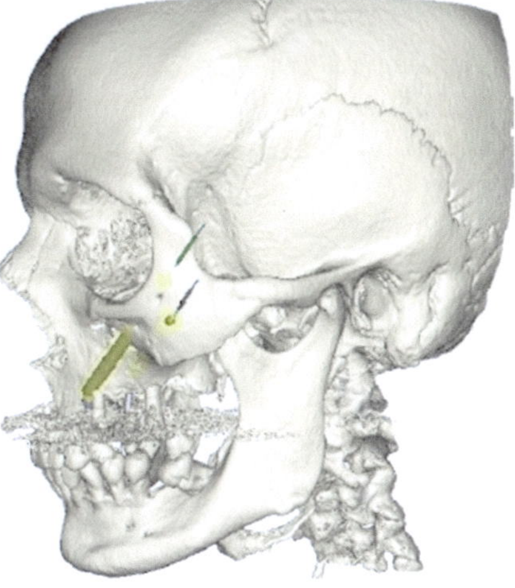

Fig. 3.3 Virtual planning of zygoma quad

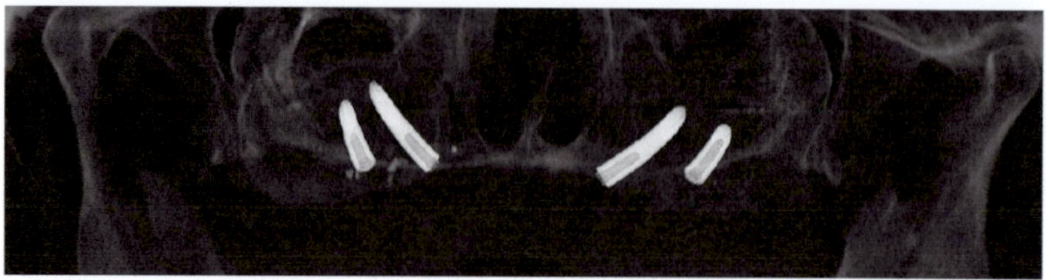

Fig. 3.4 Virtual position of the planned zygomatic implants

planned position of the abutments. A hybrid alternative (both extra- and trans-sinusal implant placement) could be indicated (Fig. 3.6).

3.3.2 Surgical Guides

In order to transfer the preoperative virtual planning aiming to get a perfect position of the implants, surgical guides may be designed [23, 24]. These splints may either be manufactured by the industry or "in house" by the department itself by using a 3D printer.

Limitations of the guides can be the absence of remaining teeth to get a precise position in case of mucosal supported surgical guides. The volume of the guide could be also a problem for drilling, even using angulated handpieces and short drills. The available space for the instruments depends on the mouth opening, the presence or absence of lower teeth, and the possibility to stretch the lips. Sometimes, only the visual landmarks are available to the surgeon (position at the maxillary crest and position of the apex at the zygomatic bone as set on the virtual planification). It may be tricky to get a precise position of the implants and to avoid the anatomical obstacles such as the infraorbital nerve and the orbit.

Surgical navigation and robot-assisted technology is under research although still have not been introduced as a routine procedure in zygomatic implants surgery [25].

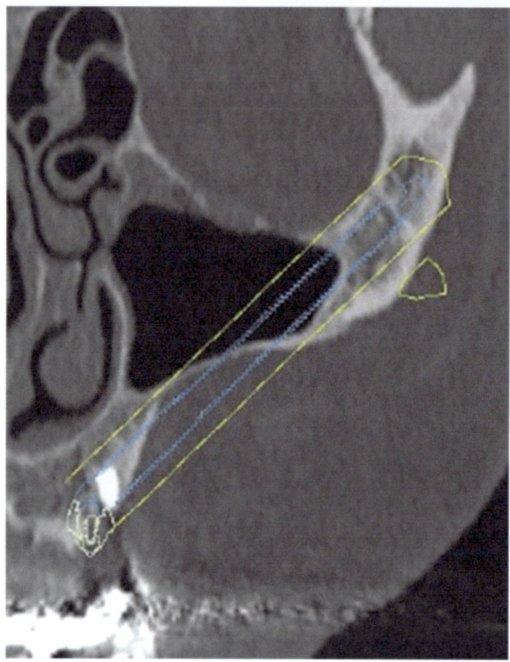

Fig. 3.5 Virtual planning of a zygomatic implant in canine position. Coronal. Note the distance between the implant and the orbit and the strong anchorage in the zygoma

The correct anchorage of the implant in the zygomatic bone is a condition for implant placement. Insufficient zygomatic bone volume may require additional grafting procedures. Originally Brånemark described the trans-sinus tilted zygomatic implants placement opening a window at the maxillary sinus antero-lateral wall with palatal position of the abutments, leading to a large palatal prosthetic extension. Later, many authors moved to place the prosthetic abutments in a most crestal position with extra-sinusal placement of the implants (sinus slot technique) [22]. Selection of the technique depends on the severity of the resorption, the bone anatomy, and the

3.3.3 Prosthodontic Procedure

After implant placement at the end of the surgery, specific abutments with adequate height and angulation are placed on the coronal end of

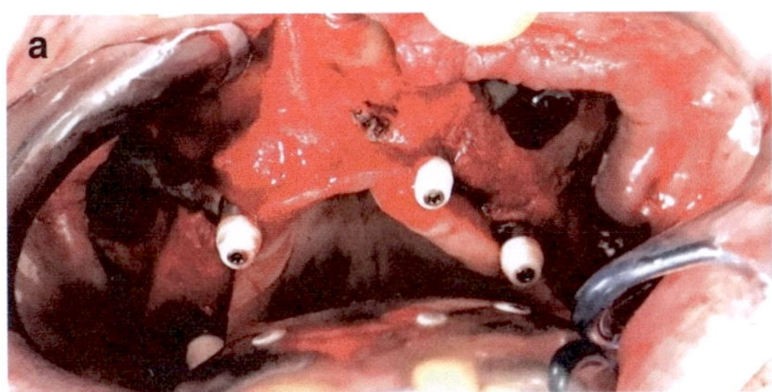
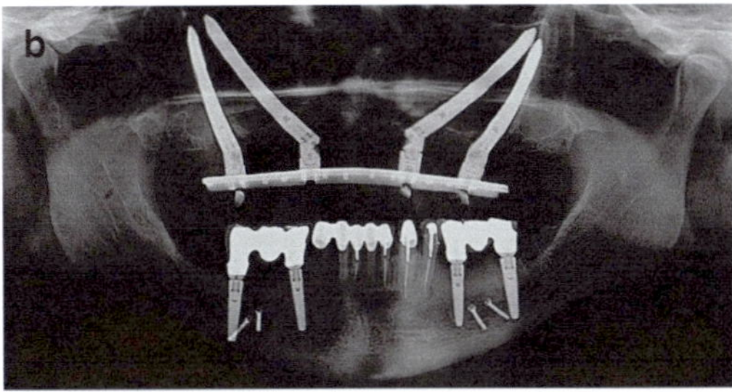

Fig. 3.6 (**a**) Association of a quad four zygomatic implant at the maxilla with a bilateral inferior alveolar nerve lateralization at the mandible in a 56-year-old man. Intraoperative surgical view. Combination of the slot and the window technique for trans-sinusal implant placement. Note the crestal position of the abutments. (**b**) Final restoration. Panoramic view

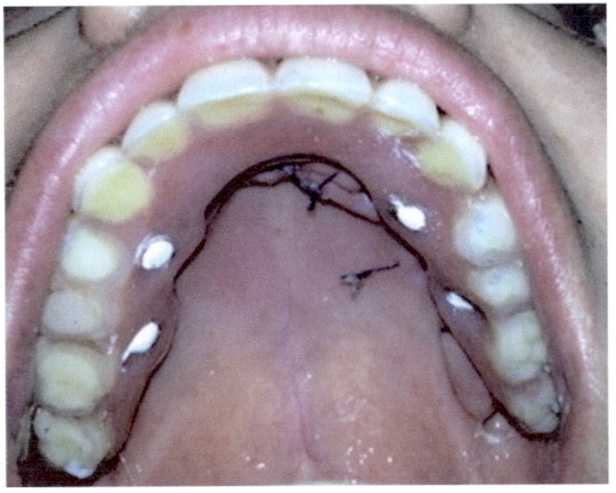

Fig. 3.7 Screw-retained temporary fixed dental prosthesis, note the palatal position of the abutments

each implant in order to facilitate paralleling emergence of the implants. After wound closure, an impression is made using the pick-up technique. A screw-retained temporary or provisional fixed prosthesis allowing for immediate loading can be immediately made and attached to the abutments (Fig. 3.7). It is also possible to place the provisional prosthesis one day after the surgery checking the dynamic occlusion. This procedure is a safety measure in order to avoid any imbalance.

Six months after zygomatic implants insertion, the temporary rehabilitation is removed and a definitive new screw-retained prosthesis is created following the conventional prosthetic procedures. The new prosthesis can be a full arch restoration made of porcelain or acrylic resin teeth fused with a titanium framework connecting all the implants (Figs. 3.8 and 3.9).

3.4 Contraindications

Potential contraindications must be investigated before inserting zygomatic implants in order to ensure a good outcome of the technique. Most important contraindications are listed as follows:

3.4.1 Paranasal Sinuses Infection or Chronic Sinusitis

Despite precise imaging examination before zygomatic implant placement, paranasal sinuses pathologies may not be always diagnosed. Zygomatic implant placement must be avoided until any paranasal sinus opacity will be investigated. Infection of the paranasal sinuses can be related to a dental origin or to sino-nasal obstruction which needs to be excluded or solved in case of sinusitis. Examination of the sinus mucosa to exclude any disease or inflammation may require endoscopic exploration and ENT consultation. Paranasal sinuses must be completely clean before implant placement thus treatment of any paranasal sinus infection has to be proposed to the patient, not being recommended the use of trans-sinusal zygomatic implants in case of sinus mucosa pathology even after a correct treatment. If sinusitis occurs in contact to a zygomatic implant, beside inflammation an oro-nasal fistula can be developed leading frequently to implant's lost.

Some authors try to avoid sinus-related complications by using the extra-sinusal way to place

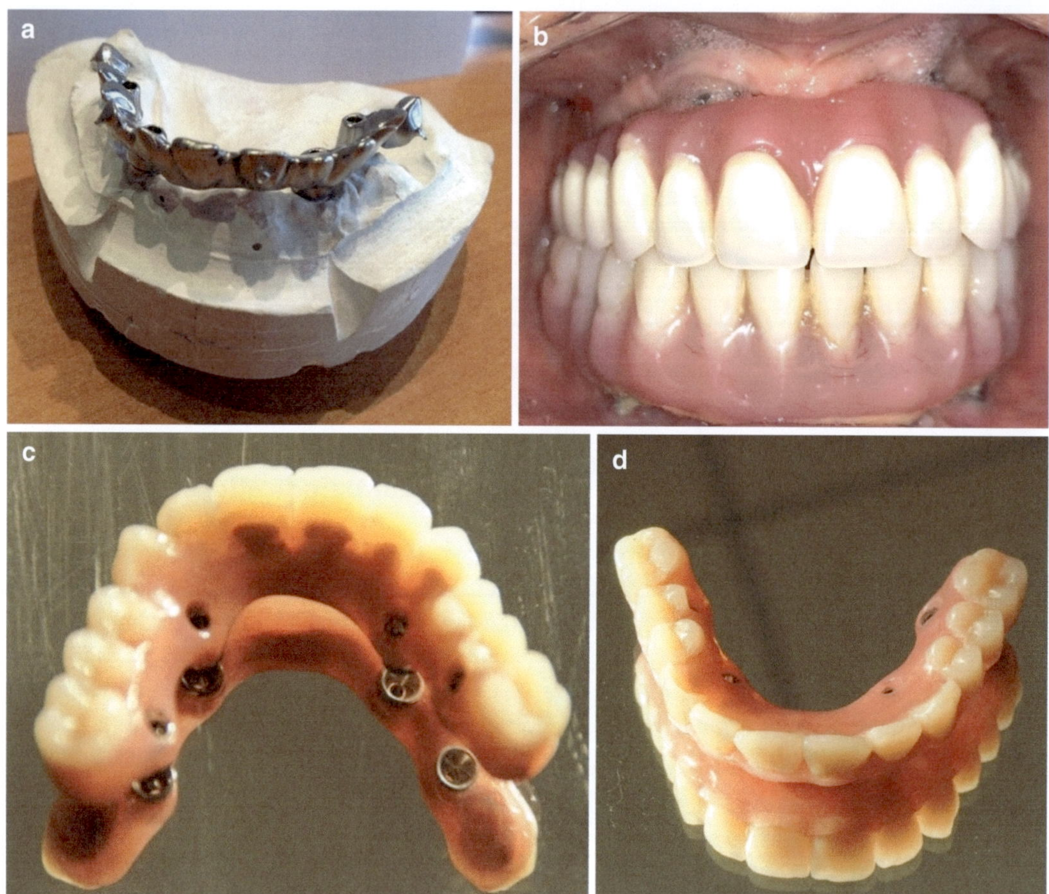

Fig. 3.8 (**a–d**) Full arch final prosthesis. Titanium framework

the implant, thus avoiding any contact of the implant with the sinuses [26]. However even in an initial extra-sinusal position, the bone resorption may lead to contact between zygomatic implants and the sinus mucosa. Both practitioner and patient must be aware of this situation.

and checked during the whole osteointegration period in order to avoid any implant loss. Lower and upper full arches rehabilitation is possible at both levels (mandibulae and maxillae); however, a proper occlusion needs to establish an adequate previous or simultaneous preparation of the lower arch (Fig. 3.9).

3.4.2 Incorrect Dental or Prosthetic Rehabilitation at the Mandible

Concept of the zygomatic implants is usually related to immediate loading with full connection of all the maxillary implants. To avoid any implant loss of integration, the correct occlusion must be set at the time of the implants loading

3.4.3 Insufficient Zygomatic Bone Volume

Virtual planning of the treatment will help to check the possibility of inserting one or two zygomatic implants on each side. Some authors propose to insert six zygomatic implants, three on each side, depending on the available bone volume [3].

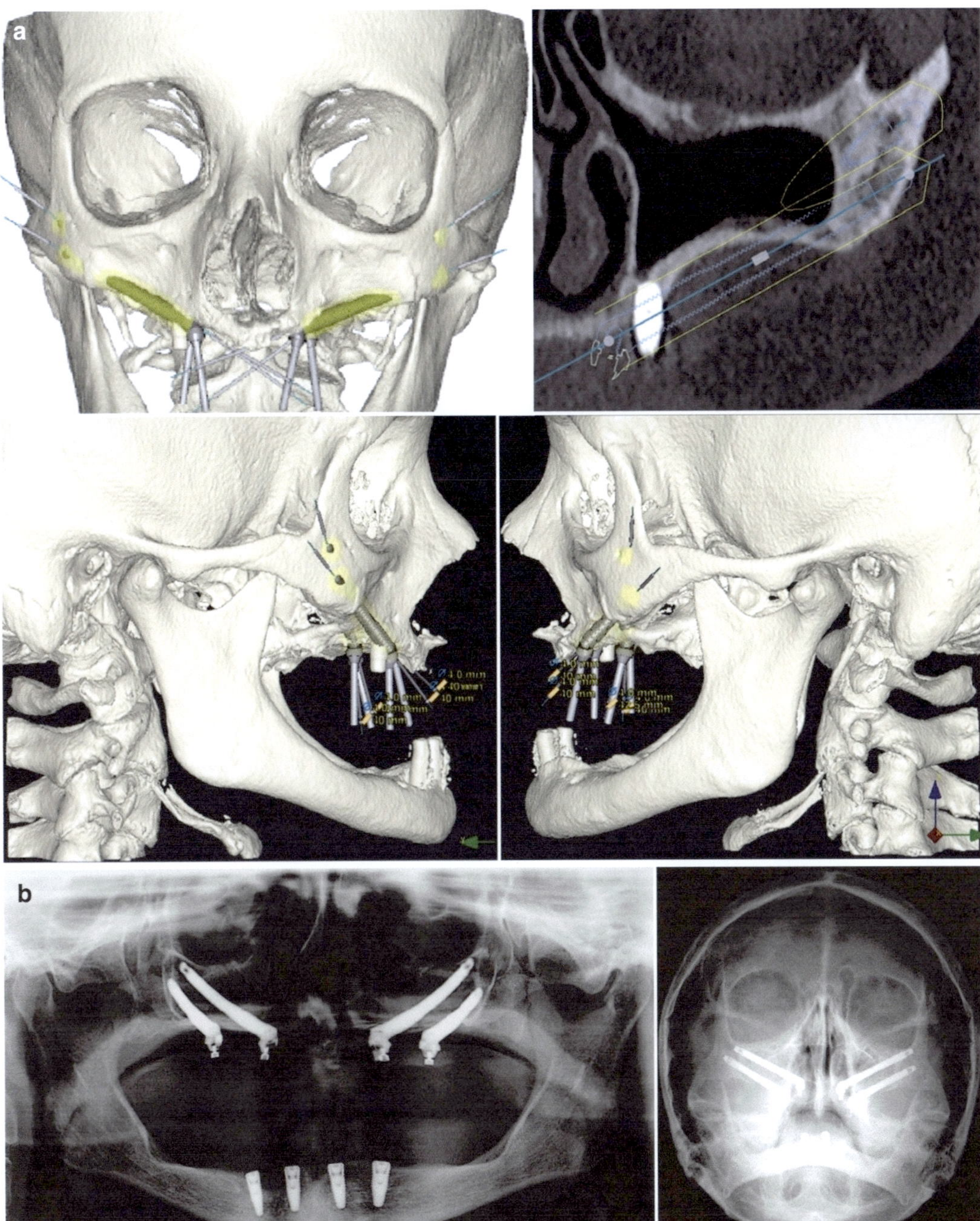

Fig. 3.9 (**a–f**) Full mouth implant-supported rehabilitation. Sixty-four years old women after conventional implants loss. Quad zygoma at the upper jaw. (**a**) Initial planning with palatal position of the abutments. (**b**) X-ray control after surgery. (**c**) Intrabuccal view with temporary coping abutments in place. (**d**) Use of the temporary prosthesis for impression by a pick-up technique. (**e**) Screw-retained prosthesis. (**f**) Final restoration. X-ray panoramic control and intrabuccal view

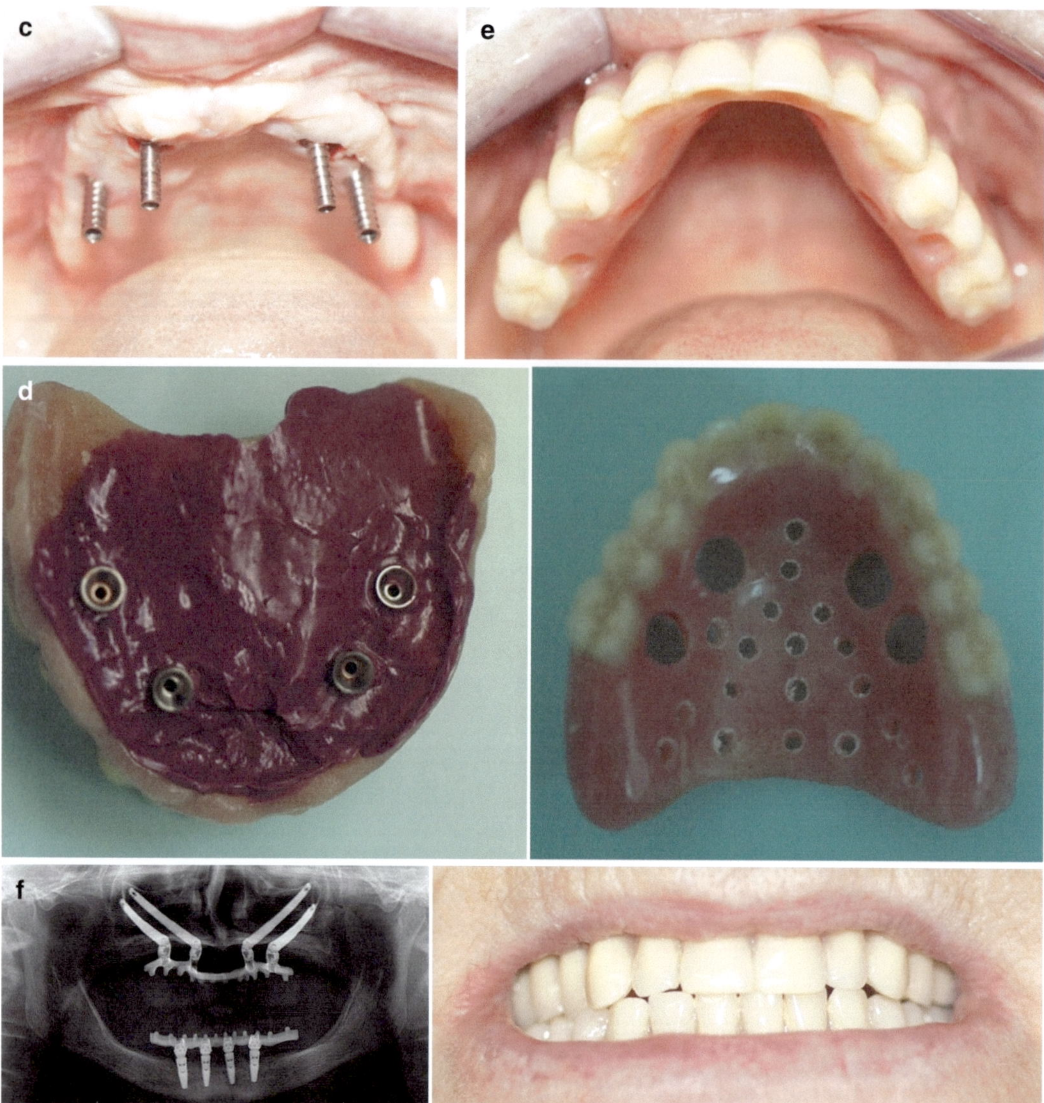

Fig. 3.9 (continued)

The zygomatic bone volume could be limited in some situations like malformations with dental agenesis [27] or after tumor resection. Virtual planning will help to evaluate these situations and can lead to exclude the zygomatic implants technique or to graft the zygoma bone in order to get enough bone volume (Fig. 3.10). A new evaluation of the zygomatic bone has to be performed at least 6 months after the grafting procedure in order to confirm if bone graft integration allowing for zygomatic implants placement has been obtained.

3.5 Complications

3.5.1 Paranasal Sinusitis and Oral Fistula

Sinusitis is both a contraindication and a potential complication of the zygomatic implants. When sinusitis is present, implant removal and fistula closure are mandatory. Before considering removal of the zygomatic implants, the sinusitis needs to be treated. As mentioned before, it may be related to the presence of den-

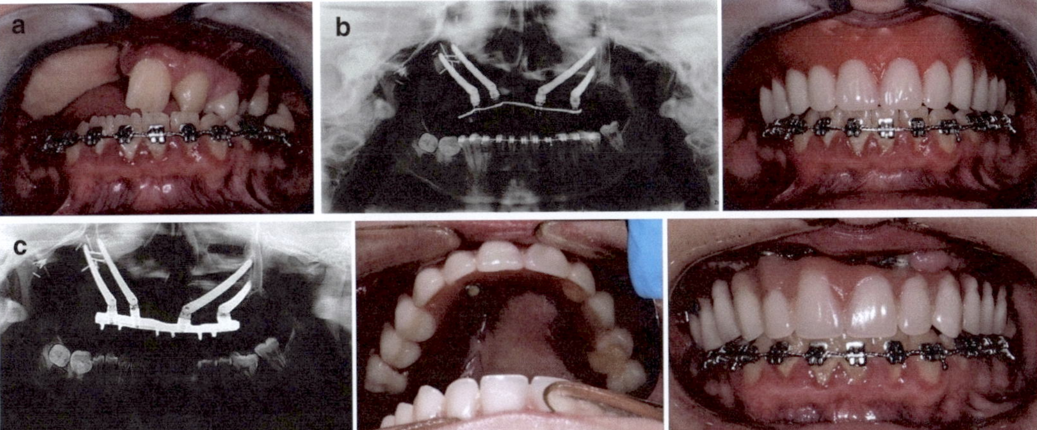

Fig. 3.10 Grafting the zygomatic bone with posterior insertion of zygomatic implants in a 17-year-old girl 10 years after maxillary resection including part of the zygomatic bone. (**a**) Initial situation before implant insertion. Primary reconstruction was achieved by a latissimus dorsi free flap without bone defect repair. At the end of the growth, four zygomatic implants were inserted after calvarial grafting of the right zygomatic bone. (**b**) Zygomatic implants after grafting the right zygomatic body. Temporary restoration with immediate loading. Note the screws left in place to avoid wound opening. (**c**) Final result

tal infection, pathologic dental roots or cysts which have to be removed. The sinus ventilation must also be checked and require endoscopic investigation [26].

3.5.2 Fracture of the Zygomatic Bone

This complication may occur in multi-operated patients and/or use of too large diameter zygomatic implants. In this situation, primary stability of the implant is impaired making necessary to remove the implants and to repair the zygomatic bone. For zygomatic bone fracture repair, osteosynthesis may be necessary, with or without additional bone grafting depending on the bony volume and the planning of a second implant insertion. In every situation of fractured zygomatic bone, immediate loading cannot be considered.

3.5.3 Ocular Complications

Penetration in the orbit may occur during drilling or implant placement. This situation may lead to intra-orbital lesions, hemorrhage, or diplopia [28]. In this case, the implant must be removed and the orbital walls repaired immediately. This complication must be absolutely prevented by a precise planning establishing accurate landmarks for implant placement. In case of any doubt during the drilling procedure, the integrity of the orbital walls must be checked before the procedure is continued.

3.5.4 Cutaneous Fistula

This condition may be associated with paranasal sinusitis and is usually related to an infection of the zygomatic implant at the level of the zygomatic bone [29]. This complication is not frequent but may lead to implant loss.

3.6 Conclusions

Zygomatic implants are a useful technique allowing to get a fixed rehabilitation at the maxilla without using conventional grafting procedures in the atrophic maxilla. This technique can be used at any age after the end of the growth to solve complex cases in different situations including oral and maxillofacial cancer.

A multidisciplinary team approach with detailed virtual planning, advanced surgical skills, and knowledge of the prosthetic procedure are necessary in order to obtain adequate results and to prevent and treat potential complications.

References

1. Hoefler VJ, Al-Sabbagh M. Are there alternatives to invasive site development for dental implants? Part II. Dent Clin North Am. 2019;63(3):489–98.
2. Malevez C. [Zygomatic anchorage concept in full edentulism]. Rev Stomatol Chir Maxillofac. 2012;113(4):299–306.
3. Bothur S, Jonsson G, Sandahl L. Modified technique using multiple zygomatic implants in reconstruction of the atrophic maxilla: a technical note. Int J Oral Maxillofac Implants. 2003;18(6):902–4.
4. Balaji VR, Lambodharan R, Manikandan D, Deenadayalan S. Pterygoid implant for atrophic posterior maxilla. J Pharm Bioallied Sci. 2017;9(Suppl 1):S261–S3.
5. Chai F, Raoul G, Wiss A, Ferri J, Hildebrand HF. [Bone substitutes: classification and concerns]. Rev Stomatol Chir Maxillofac. 2011;112(4):212–21.
6. Myon L, Ferri J, Chai F, Blanchemain N, Raoul G. [Oro-maxillofacial bone tissue engineering combining biomaterials, stem cells, and gene therapy]. Rev Stomatol Chir Maxillofac. 2011;112(4):201–11.
7. Torres Y, Raoul G, Lauwers L, Ferri J. The use of onlay bone grafting for implant restoration in the extremely atrophic anterior maxilla. A case series. Swiss Dent J. 2019;129(4):274–85.
8. Ferri J, Lauwers L, Jeblaoui Y, Genay A, Raoul G. Le Fort I osteotomy and calvarial bone grafting for dental implants. Rev Stomatol Chir Maxillofac. 2010;111(2):63–7.
9. Schlund M, Nicot R, Lauwers L, Raoul G, Ferri J. Le Fort 1 osteotomy and calvarial bone grafting for severely resorbed maxillae. J Craniomaxillofac Surg. 2016;44(7):859–67.
10. Davó R, David L. Quad zygoma: technique and realities. Oral Maxillofac Surg Clin North Am. 2019;31(2):285–97.
11. Butterworth CJ, Rogers SN. The zygomatic implant perforated (ZIP) flap: a new technique for combined surgical reconstruction and rapid fixed dental rehabilitation following low-level maxillectomy. Int J Implant Dent. 2017;3(1):37.
12. Butterworth CJ. Primary vs secondary zygomatic implant placement in patients with head and neck cancer—a 10-year prospective study. Head Neck. 2019;41(6):1687–95.
13. Dattani A, Richardson D, Butterworth CJ. A novel report on the use of an oncology zygomatic implant-retained maxillary obturator in a paediatric patient. Int J Implant Dent. 2017;3(1):9.
14. Davó R, Malevez C, Pons O. Immediately loaded zygomatic implants: a 5-year prospective study. Eur J Oral Implantol. 2013;6(1):39–47.
15. Degidi M, Nardi D, Piattelli A, Malevez C. Immediate loading of zygomatic implants using the intraoral welding technique: a 12-month case series. Int J Periodontics Restorative Dent. 2012;32(5):e154–61.
16. Kahnberg KE, Henry PJ, Hirsch JM, Ohrnell LO, Andreasson L, Brånemark PI, et al. Clinical evaluation of the zygoma implant: 3-year follow-up at 16 clinics. J Oral Maxillofac Surg. 2007;65(10):2033–8.
17. Malevez C, Daelemans P, Adriaenssens P, Durdu F. Use of zygomatic implants to deal with resorbed posterior maxillae. Periodontol 2000. 2003;33:82–9.
18. Malevez C, Abarca M, Durdu F, Daelemans P. Clinical outcome of 103 consecutive zygomatic implants: a 6-48 months follow-up study. Clin Oral Implants Res. 2004;15(1):18–22.
19. Pineau M, Nicot R, Lauwers L, Ferri J, Raoul G. Zygomatic implants in our daily practice. Part I: treatment plan and surgical technique. Swiss Dent J. 2018;128(9):689–93.
20. Pineau M, Nicot R, Lauwers L, Ferri J, Raoul G. Zygomatic implants in our daily practice. Part II: prosthetic rehabilitation and effect on quality of life. Swiss Dent J. 2018;128(9):694–700.
21. Davó R, Malevez C, López-Orellana C, Pastor-Beviá F, Rojas J. Sinus reactions to immediately loaded zygoma implants: a clinical and radiological study. Eur J Oral Implantol. 2008;1(1):53–60.
22. Araújo PP, Sousa SA, Diniz VB, Gomes PP, da Silva JS, Germano AR. Evaluation of patients undergoing placement of zygomatic implants using sinus slot technique. Int J Implant Dent. 2016;2(1):2.
23. Rinaldi M, Ganz SD. Computer-guided approach for placement of zygomatic implants: novel protocol and surgical guide. Compend Contin Educ Dent. 2019;40(3):e1–4.
24. Wang CI, Cho SH, Cho D, Ducote C, Reddy LV, Sinada N. A 3D-printed guide to assist in sinus slot preparation for the optimization of zygomatic implant axis trajectory. J Prosthodont. 2020;29(2):179–84.
25. Cao Z, Qin C, Fan S, Yu D, Wu Y, Qin J, et al. Pilot study of a surgical robot system for zygomatic implant placement. Med Eng Phys. 2020;75:72–8.
26. Aleksandrowicz P, Kusa-Podkańska M, Grabowska K, Kotuła L, Szkatuła-Łupina A, Wysokińska-Miszczuk J. Extra-sinus zygomatic implants to avoid chronic sinusitis and prosthetic arch malposition: 12 years of experience. J Oral Implantol. 2019;45(1):73–8.
27. Wang H, Hung K, Zhao K, Wang Y, Wang F, Wu Y. Anatomical analysis of zygomatic bone in ectodermal dysplasia patients with oligodontia. Clin Implant Dent Relat Res. 2019;21(2):310–6.
28. Tran AQ, Reyes-Capó DP, Patel NA, Pasol J, Capó H, Wester ST. Zygomatic dental implant induced orbital fracture and inferior oblique trauma. Orbit. 2019;38(3):236–9.
29. Garcia Garcia B, Ruiz Masera JJ, Zafra Camacho FM. Bilateral cutaneous fistula after the placement of zygomatic implants. Int J Oral Maxillofac Implants. 2016;31(2):e11–4.

Principles of Navigation

4

Luis Ley

4.1 Introduction

Surgeons need to know exactly where we are in the course of a surgical act. This location is easy in case of having clear anatomical references, being more complicated in complex anatomical areas, especially in cases in which surgery is performed on a solid organ, where it is more difficult, if not impossible, to find obvious anatomical references. This limitation is even more critical in the case that all organ tissue is functionally effective, as in the case of the brain and that is why neurosurgery has been a pioneer in the development of surgical navigation systems that allow neurosurgeons to know with high accuracy the real-time location of the surgical action. This development is carried out based on the advances made in stereotaxy systems, which are designed to create an exact coordinate system that allows to locate with high precision any point within the referenced system [1].

Classically, stereotactic systems required rigid and bulky frames of reference attached to the skull of the patient that, while offering extraordinary accuracy, they limit both patient placement and surgical work. The progressive technological evolution led to the development of frameless stereotactic systems with which a much greater freedom of work is achieved, as no rigid systems or solid frames that could limit surgical mobility or the patient's position are needed.

Modern navigation systems allow preoperative planning to be carried out, which can be also extremely useful when creating 3D models that allow a preoperative study of the case, as well as the ability to create images and to upload them into surgical vision systems in order to facilitate the surgery: augmented reality by injection of microscope images, surgical glasses,... [2–4] (Fig. 4.1). The evolution of these systems has expanded the scope of this technology beyond the frontiers of neurosurgery, being currently of common use in specialties such as Maxillofacial Surgery (CMF), Orthopedics or Otolaryngology (ENT), allowing not only to accurately locate the limits of a tumor or to find a deep lesion but also to program exact cutting areas. Moreover, use of navigation systems can be combined with "Computer Aided Design/Computer Aided Manufacturing" (CAD/CAM) techniques in order to transfer into the operative field previously designed customized 3D implants to repair complex defects achieving an exact fit of the implant in the intraoperative defect. Finally, these systems allow comparing the postoperative results with the preoperative studies in order to check the results of the procedure in tumor patients.

The purpose of this chapter is to review the operational basis of these systems in order to

L. Ley (✉)
Department of Neurosurgery, Ramon y Cajal University Hospital, Madrid, Spain
e-mail: luis.ley@salud.madrid.org

© Springer Nature Switzerland AG 2021
J. Acero (ed.), *Innovations and New Developments in Craniomaxillofacial Reconstruction*,
https://doi.org/10.1007/978-3-030-74322-2_4

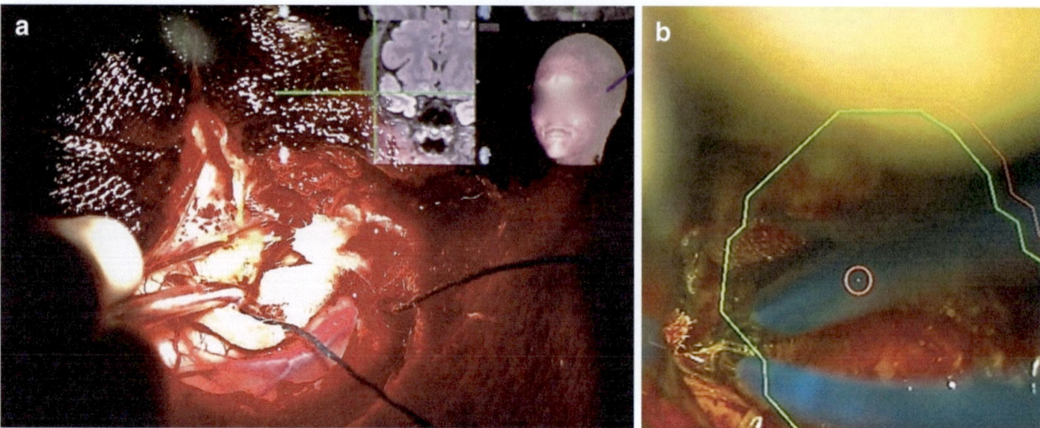

Fig. 4.1 (**a**) Augmented reality: The objective focused under the microscope is precisely located by the navigation system, showing its location on the preoperative magnetic resonance image. This image is injected on the surgeon's objective, allowing the surgeon greater precision and facilitating the surgical workflow. (**b**) Augmented reality: The contour of the tumor is injected into the surgeon's view

allow the surgeon to understand the procedure and to choose the type of navigation depending on the type of procedure and which one best suit his needs.

4.2   History

The exact location of structures or objectives within a solid organ is a challenge that neurosurgery has faced almost since its inception. The first stereotactic guide dates from the early twentieth century, developed by Sir Victor Horsley and Robert Clarke [5]. Its functional limitations were mainly due to the technological deficiencies of the time, especially in matters of neuroimaging. With the improvement of radiodiagnosis systems new developments appear, the best known, by Leksell and Talairach [6–9]. These guidelines were mainly intended to perform more or less punctiform lesions in certain brain areas for the treatment of psychiatric pathology (psychosurgery) and more frequently, movement disorders (Parkinson's disease, tremor, etc.) and their use declined with the arrival of effective medical treatments for these diseases [10, 11].

Stereotaxy allows the surgeon to locate a structure inside the skull and guide him through it, but it was necessary to do the opposite process, that is: mark a point, a resection boundary or a tumoral volume and the system shows us where that point is exactly, this is image-guided surgery. In the late twentieth century, there were numerous advances in techniques that allowed the surgeon to accurately locate a structure inside the skull. Initially, they started studying the performances of ultrasonic location systems [12, 13] and articulated arms that served as pointers to locate the point we wanted inside the skull [14–16] although the limitations of this type of technology based on mechanical systems were quickly established, so the interest and research moved the focus to systems based on magnetic tracking [17] and optical tracking [18] of different types of probes, avoiding systems based on rigid structures that limit the functionality of the navigation system (mechanical pointers).

One more step was the introduction on clinical use of the Magnetic Resonance Imaging (MRI), very useful for the study of the soft tissue, and the possibility of fusing this MR images with computer tomography imaging studies (CT), that have lesser spatial deformities and offer better resolution for bone and calcium structures. This new capability improved the options of stereotactic presurgical planification while, in parallel, technological advances allow working with three-dimensional structures based on these imaging studies, thus improving the ability to locate intracranial structures and the development of techniques that allowed volumetric resections of intracranial structures and not simply to locate a point in space [11, 19]. At the beginning of the twenty-first century, these systems were generalized within neurosurgery and started to be developed in other specialties, such as ENT, orthopedics, and CMF. The combination of the use of navigation and CAD/CAM three-dimensional models allows the surgeon not only to perform surgeries with topographic and spatial accuracy but also to visualize the structures preoperatively, to perform virtual surgeries, calculate resections, design prostheses in three dimensions that will correct the defects caused by surgery and finally including intraoperative imaging techniques such as intraoperative CT, to compare the surgical results with those expected in preoperative planning.

4.3　Technology

Although, as mentioned in the historic review, at first the technology used was based on mechanical systems that calculated the position by changing the position of a rigid articulated lever system, the development of systems based on optical tracking and magnetic tracking avoids the need for hardware that limit the freedom of movement or position of the patient. Both optical and magnetic systems coincide in the creation of a virtual space that includes the entire cranial volume.

In the case of optical tracking, the skull must be fixed directly or indirectly to a reference visible by the cameras that will track. At the present time a passive follow-up is used, which means that the patient and the instruments that are going to be tracked must have couplings that reflect the light emitted by a distant emitter (generally reflective spheres) that is collected by a specific camera system (transmitter/receiver). The tracking is done by two fixed infrared light emitters coupled with two fixed cameras. The infrared light is reflected by the spheres fixed both in a reference system and in the spheres fixed in the instrument to be tracked. The cameras must "see" both: the reference system and the instrument. Spheres are used because they improve the reflec-

tion capacity from a wider range of angles. The main advantage of this type of systems is that there are no cables that hinder the surgical work and the main limitation is that at all times there must be a free line of sight between the light emitter/receiver, the fixed references to the patient and the probes and instruments that are being used. Its accuracy and tracking speed is greater than that achieved by magnetic systems (Fig. 4.2).

The magnetic tracking system is based on the creation of a magnetic field in which the cranial volume is introduced. A device that creates a magnetic field is placed near the head of the patient (Fig. 4.3). The introduction of active probes within this magnetic field causes changes in it that are recognized by the system calculating their position. This system presents as main limitations that the probes or instruments must be wired, since they are active. However, the magnetic systems are slightly less accurate and slower than systems based on optical tracking and are affected by the presence of ferromagnetic instruments within the surgical field [20–22]. On the other hand, magnetic tracking systems allow malleable instruments to be used (Table 4.1).

Although nowadays it is advisable to have a mixed system, adaptable to both types of monitoring, in general, optical systems are more used in neurosurgery, where the surgical field remains fixed, and magnetic systems are used with higher frequency in ENT and CMF, where the surgical field moves frequently. To allow mobility of the skull, different devices have been developed in both magnetic tracking and optical tracking systems, which are based on attaching the reference directly on the patient's skull, screwing it or adhering it [23].

4.4　Indications

The main usefulness of these systems are the planning and execution of personalized surgeries in complex cases in which it is important to know the exact position of the surgeon in the surgical field at any given time. Navigation-assisted surgery is especially useful in complex

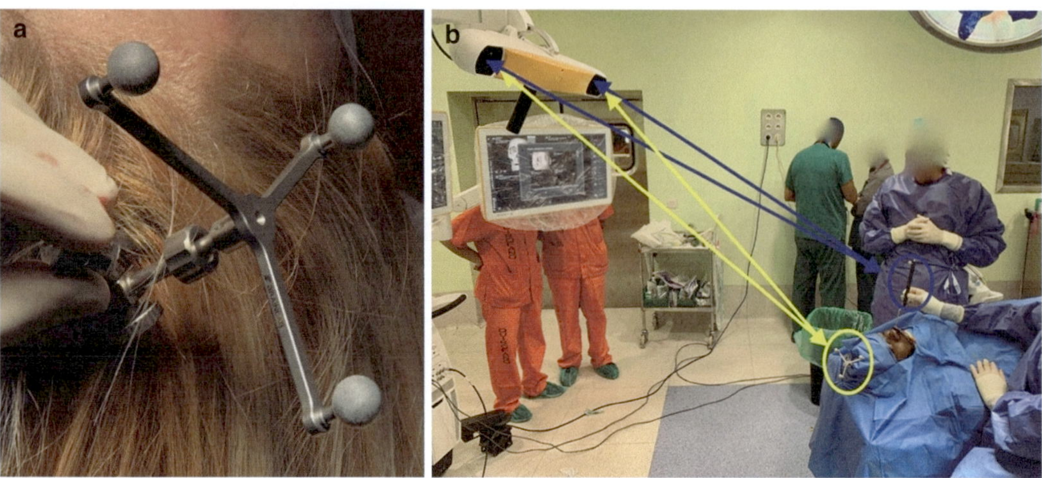

Fig. 4.2 (**a**) In CMF surgery with optical tracking navigation, the reference star is attached to the patient's skull in order to provide more freedom of movement. (**b**) Optical tracking: This picture shows the "lines of view" that cannot be interrupted during surgical navigation. The emitter/receptor must be able to see at once the reference star (yellow lines) and the pointer device (blue lines). It is of the upmost importance to define before the start of the surgical procedure the placement of the reference star and the emitter/receptor in order to have a good surgical navigation procedure

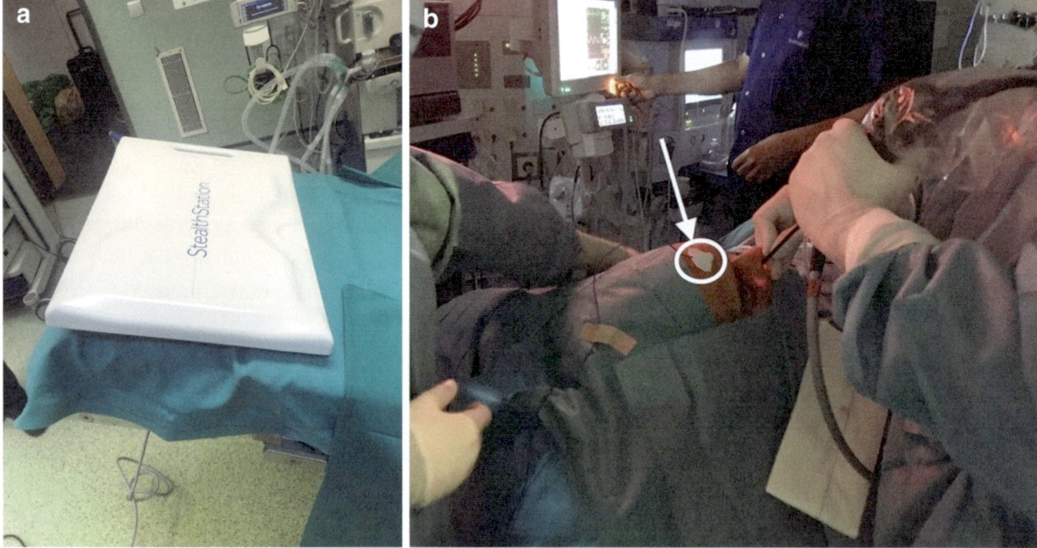

Fig. 4.3 (**a**) Magnetic tracking: This "pillow like" device is the emitter that creates the magnetic field. (**b**) Magnetic tracking: The reference (arrow) is attached to the patient's skull, either through an adhesive or through screws

Table 4.1 Pros and cons of optical and magnetic tracked systems

Optical tracked	Magnetic tracked
PRO: higher accuracy	PRO: freedom of movement
PRO: faster tracking	PRO: malleable instruments available for navigation
PRO: wireless	CON: smaller referred surgical field
CON: line of sight	CON: sensitivity to ferromagnetic instruments

anatomical regions such as the cranial and maxillofacial regions, being especially useful in cases of loss of anatomical landmarks in those patients who have undergone previous surgeries, in order to avoid injury to critical anatomical structures, or to remove accurately and completely a tumoral lesion. Furthermore, navigation can also aid to transfer to the surgical field the preoperative planning of the tumor resection, thus contributing to the exact reconstruction in patients who need the placement of a previously designed and 3D manufactured individualized prosthesis.

4.5 Workflow

The workflow with navigation systems is (Fig. 4.4):

Preoperative planning: acquisition of images and creation of three-dimensional models with definition of the target structures of and the structures to be avoided and performance of a virtual surgery in which both the placement of the patient and the steps to be followed during the intervention will be assessed, being possible to simulate different approaches in order to avoid surrounding critical structures (Table 4.2).

At least one data set (from CT or from MRI) must be acquired under a navigation protocol:

1. Must include the whole skull (including nose and ears).
2. With no gap or 1 mm between slices.
3. No tilt allowed.
4. There are different protocols in different commercial systems that must be known.

CT images have better spatial accuracy, can better define the bone tissue (more useful for planning lines of resection) and are easier to

Table 4.2 Checklist

Preop:
Acquisition of images (CT and MRI).
Transfer images to planification station.
Anatomic segmentation:
Target: tumor, design of the line of cut, etc.
Other critical structures.
Creation of the 3D model.
Surgical simulation.
Intraop:
Placement of the reference system.
Placement of the emitter/register system.
Surface registration of the face/cranium of the patient.
Check accuracy.
Navigate.
Check accuracy.
Postop:
Acquire MRI/CT images.
Compare with preop sets of images.

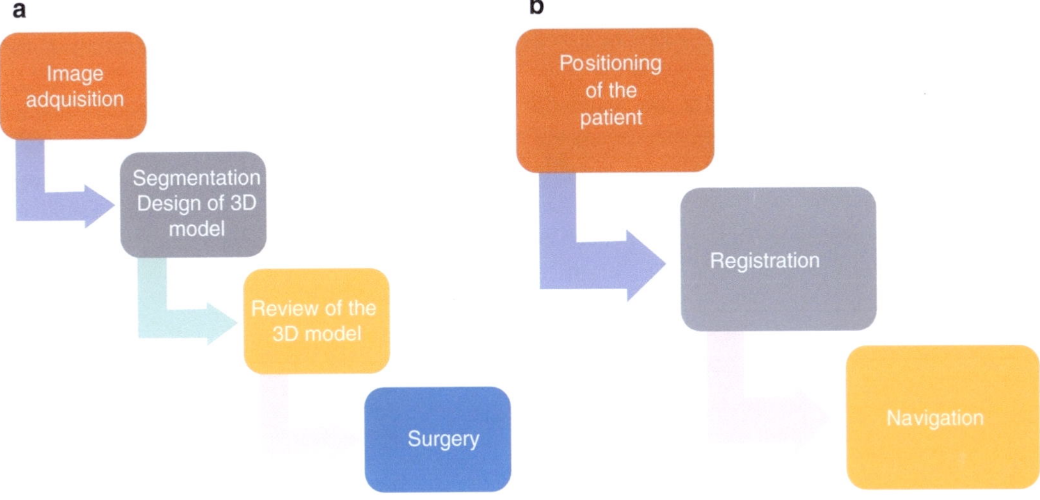

Fig. 4.4 (**a**) General workflow. (**b**) Intraoperative workflow in navigation

obtain in clinical daily basis. It is common to use a basic MRI data set not designed for navigation together with a CT data set obtained under the navigation protocol. These data set can be fused and the model obtained will have a good spatial accuracy (CT) and a good anatomic sensitivity (MRI). If we select to use this strategy, we have to use MR images in the three spatial planes. Obviously, it is possible to use only MRI data sets, only CT data sets or to combine MRI and CT data sets.

Once the data set are transferred to the planification system, the next steps are to:

1. Segment all the structures that we consider critical (tumor, critical surrounding organs like optical nerves, carotid artery, etc.).
2. Delineate lines of cut in order to plan a resection. This would contribute to design a customized 3D prosthesis if necessary to repair a postsurgical defect.
3. Create a 3D model.
4. Simulate surgery (patient position, position of the reference attached to the skull, approach, location of surrounding critical structures, etc).

Performing surgery: A correct placement of the reference system is crucial taking into account the position of the patient, cameras, and emitter. In case of optical tracked systems, it must be placed in a location easily to be seen by the emitter and out of the line of work of the scrub personnel. The operating room staff should be asked not to obstruct the line of sight between the components of the system. In case of magnetic tracked system, any ferromagnetic instruments in the surgical field (for example, any metallic device for holding the head) or any instrument that can cause interferences in the system such as mobile phones must be avoided. It is important to remark that the closer the reference with the target, the better accuracy, but the reference never can be an obstacle during surgery (never can be placed inside or very close to the surgical field in order to avoid an accidental displacement).

Once secured the reference on the skull of the patient (directly or indirectly), the next step is to register the surface of the face and cranium of the patient in order to create the navigational space. This step is different in the different commercial navigation systems but is crucial in order to avoid mistakes during the procedure. Once the navigation space has been created and before starting the surgical procedure, it is mandatory to check the precision of the generated model by touching different visible and recognizable points of the surgical field with the probe. It is important to know that accuracy is not constant into all the navigational space and it is not infrequent to have a good superficial accuracy but not a good accuracy in the deeper planes. In order to avoid this problem, it is very useful to obtain the more superficial points as well to obtain points close to the target but also at the contralateral side.

It is important to check the spatial accuracy of the system regularly and periodically during the intervention. In case of doubt, visible anatomical references will always have a greater value than the position given by the system. During the surgical procedure, it is mandatory to continue checking accuracy by touching the anatomical landmarks. Beside the anatomical references, artificial landmarks can be useful in cases in which could be difficult to have an easily identifiable landmark. Simply some screws placed into the surgical field and marked as references can serve as artificial landmarks.

4.6 Postoperative

Postoperative comparison of preoperative and postoperative images are very useful in oncologic cases in order to check the extent of resection and the effectiveness of postoperative therapies (radio- and chemotherapy). Intraoperative imaging systems combined with the navigation system are available and can contribute to the immediate control of the results of the procedure.

References

1. Dorward NL. Neuronavigation—the surgeon's sextant. Br J Neurosurg. 1997;11(2):101–3. https://doi.org/10.1080/02688699746429.
2. Putze F, Vourvopoulos A, Lécuyer A, et al. Editorial: brain-computer interfaces and augmented/virtual

reality. Front Hum Neurosci. 2020;14:144. https://doi.org/10.3389/fnhum.2020.00144. Published 2020 May 12.

3. Carl B, Bopp M, Saß B, Pojskic M, Voellger B, Nimsky C. Spine surgery supported by augmented reality. Global Spine J. 2020;10(2 Suppl):41S–55S. https://doi.org/10.1177/2192568219868217.

4. Fiani B, De Stefano F, Kondilis A, Covarrubias C, Reier L, Sarhadi KJ. Virtual reality in neurosurgery: "can you see it?" A review of the current applications and future potential. World Neurosurg. 2020;141:291–8. https://doi.org/10.1016/j.wneu.2020.06.066.

5. Horsley V, Clarke RH. The structure and functions of the cerebellum examined by a new method. Brain. 1908;31:45–124.

6. Spiegel EA, Wycis HT, Marks M, Lee A. Stereotactic apparatus for operations on the human brain. Science. 1947;106:349–50.

7. Leksell L. Stereotaxic apparatus for intracerebral surgery. Acta Chir Scand. 1949;99:229–33.

8. Talairach J, Hecaen M, David M, Monnier M, Ajuriaguerra J. Recherches sur la coagulation therapeutique des structures sous-corticales chez l'homme. Rev Neurol. 1949;81:4–24.

9. Riechert T, Wolff M. Ueber ein neues Zielgeraet zur intrakraniellen elektrischen Abteilung und Ausschaltung. Arch Pyschiatr Z Neurol. 1951;186:225–30.

10. Gildenberg PL. Whatever happened to stereotactic surgery? Neurosurgery. 1987;20(6):983–7.

11. Galloway RL Jr. Introduction and historical on perspectives on image-guided surgery. In: Golby AJ, editor. Image-guided neurosurgery. Cambridge: Academic Press; 2015.

12. Roberts DW, Strohbehn JW, Hatch JF, Murray W, Kettenberger H. A frameless stereotaxic integration of computerized tomographic imaging and the operating microscope. J Neurosurg. 1986;65:545–9.

13. Koivukangas J, Louhisalmi Y, Alakuijala J, Oikarinen J. Ultrasound-controlled neuronavigator-guided brain surgery. J Neurosurg. 1993;79(1):36–42. https://doi.org/10.3171/jns.1993.79.1.0036.

14. Watanabe E, Watanabe T, Manaka S, Mayanagi Y, Takakura K. Three-dimensional digitizer (neuronavigator): new equipment for computed tomography-guided stereotaxic surgery. Surg Neurol. 1987;27:543–7.

15. Galloway RL, Edwards C, Haden GL, Maciunas RJ. An interactive, image-guided articulated arm for laser surgery. In: Proceedings of the strategic defense initiative organization's fourth annual meeting on medical free-electron lasers, Dallas, TX, September 22–24, 1989, vol. 15.

16. Schlöndroff G, Mösges R, Meyer-Ebrecht D, et al. CAS (computer assisted surgery) Ein neuartiges Verfahren in der Kopfund Halschirurgie. HNO. 1989;37:187–9.

17. Kato A, Yoshimine T, Hayakawa T, et al. A frameless, armless navigational system for computer assisted neurosurgery. J Neurosurg. 1991;74(5):845–9.

18. Zamorano LJ, Nolte L, Kadi AM, Jiang Z. Interactive intraoperative localization using an infrared based system. Neurol Res. 1993;15(5):290–8.

19. Brown RA. A computerized tomography-computer graphics approach to stereotaxic localization. J Neurosurg. 1979;50(6):715–20.

20. Ricci WM, Russell TA, Kahler DM, Terrill-Grisoni L, Culley P. A comparison of optical and electromagnetic computer-assisted navigation systems for fluoroscopic targeting. J Orthop Trauma. 2008;22(3):190–4. https://doi.org/10.1097/BOT.0b013e31816731c7.

21. Mascott CR. Comparison of magnetic tracking and optical tracking by simultaneous use of two independent frameless stereotactic systems. Neurosurgery. 2005;57(4 Suppl):295–301. https://doi.org/10.1227/01.neu.0000176411.55324.1e; discussion 295–301.

22. Kral F, Puschban EJ, Riechelmann H, Pedross F, Freysinger W. Optical and electromagnetic tracking for navigated surgery of the sinuses and frontal skull base. Rhinology. 2011;49(3):364–8. https://doi.org/10.4193/Rhino10.177.

23. Koivukangas T, Katisko JP, Koivukangas JP. Technical accuracy of optical and the electromagnetic tracking systems. Springerplus. 2013;2(1):90–7. https://doi.org/10.1186/2193-1801-2-90.

Computer-Assisted Surgery and Intraoperative Navigation in Acute Maxillofacial Trauma Repair

5

Frank Wilde and Alexander Schramm

5.1 Introduction

Detailed knowledge of the anatomical structures and their relationships are essential for surgical reconstructions of the facial skeleton, because functionally important structures are located in very close proximity and biologically inadequate reconstructions are inevitably leading to unsatisfactory functional and/or cosmetic results [1]. For this reason, both the clinical evaluation of patients and the imaging techniques that are used for diagnosis and treatment planning must meet the highest standards. Furthermore, however, the surgical techniques and adjuncts such as navigation systems, intraoperative imaging, patient-specific implants, and surgical guides that are used in reconstructive procedures play an important role in the outcome of reconstruction [2–5].

F. Wilde (✉) · A. Schramm
Department of Oral, Maxillofacial and Plastic Surgery, German Armed Forces Hospital of Ulm, Ulm, Germany

Department of Oral and Maxillofacial Surgery, University Hospital, Ulm University, Ulm, Germany
e-mail: frank.wilde@uni-ulm.de; alexander.schramm@uni-ulm.de

5.2 The Algorithm of Computer-Assisted Reconstruction of the Facial Skeleton

In computer-assisted maxillofacial reconstructions, the algorithm >*diagnosis → planning and simulation → surgical procedure → validation and quality control*< has been established (Fig. 5.1).

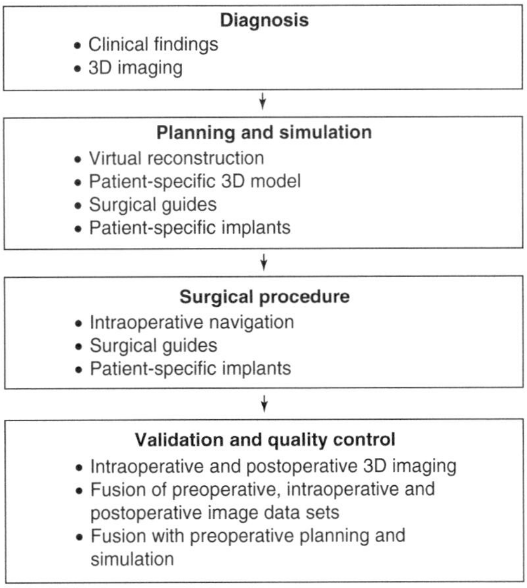

Diagnosis
- Clinical findings
- 3D imaging

↓

Planning and simulation
- Virtual reconstruction
- Patient-specific 3D model
- Surgical guides
- Patient-specific implants

↓

Surgical procedure
- Intraoperative navigation
- Surgical guides
- Patient-specific implants

↓

Validation and quality control
- Intraoperative and postoperative 3D imaging
- Fusion of preoperative, intraoperative and postoperative image data sets
- Fusion with preoperative planning and simulation

Fig. 5.1 Algorithm of computer-assisted maxillofacial reconstruction

© Springer Nature Switzerland AG 2021
J. Acero (ed.), *Innovations and New Developments in Craniomaxillofacial Reconstruction*,
https://doi.org/10.1007/978-3-030-74322-2_5

5.2.1 Diagnosis and Analysis

Diagnosis precedes the computer-assisted reconstruction of the facial skeleton and is based on clinical findings and 3D imaging since the usefulness of conventional two-dimensional radiographs is considerably limited as a result of superimposition [6–10]. With the exception of panoramic radiographs, which provide a good overview of major anatomical structures and are therefore still useful, two-dimensional images of the facial skeleton (images of the paranasal sinuses, posterior-anterior or lateral images of the skull, etc.) are no longer required.

Computed tomography (CT), magnetic resonance imaging (MRI), and cone-beam computed tomography (CBCT) are high-resolution imaging modalities that provide three-dimensional morphological information. Since the reconstruction of the facial skeleton requires the visualization of bone structures in great detail, CT and CBCT are currently the only imaging modalities that provide a resolution that is high enough to meet the requirements of facial bone reconstruction [9, 10]. MRI is particularly suitable for imaging soft tissues and is therefore useful for detecting soft-tissue processes such as soft-tissue tumors or soft-tissue inflammation and for planning the surgical management of these conditions [9, 10]. A comparison of CT and CBCT reveals that both modalities provide excellent resolution of bone structures and that the effective radiation dose delivered to a patient during a CT examination is generally higher than that resulting from a CBCT scan [11–17]. In spite of this, CT must be regarded as the gold standard for primary diagnosis preceding facial skeleton and orbital reconstruction and should be preferred to CBCT as the standard imaging modality for the assessment of bone structures since it not only provides excellent resolution of bone structures but, unlike CBCT, also allows soft-tissue structures to be evaluated, especially with the use of contrast agent [9, 10]. This additional information is of decisive importance especially in the diagnosis of facial fractures since it provides a basis for assessing concomitant injuries to soft-tissue structures such as the globe or the muscles of the eye and the optic nerve. Retrobulbar hemorrhage too can usually not be identified by CBCT alone [18].

> Computed tomography is the gold standard for the assessment and planning of maxillofacial reconstructions.

As a rule, not only axial but also coronal and sagittal reconstructions should be generated in order to obtain multiplanar views [10, 19]. Data sets should be reconstructed with a slice thickness not exceeding 2 mm. Nevertheless, a slice thickness of 1 mm or less is recommended since important details may otherwise be visualized with insufficient resolution and accuracy may be compromised by the segmentation of virtually generated three-dimensional objects (orbit, zygomatic bone, mandible, etc.) and the interpolation of slices [4, 10, 20]. This can in particular adversely affect the accuracy of fit of patient-specific implants and guides and can thus have negative effects on the entire reconstruction.

5.2.2 Planning and Simulation

Virtual computer-assisted planning and simulation of a maxillofacial reconstruction is performed on the basis of preoperative 3D data sets in order to increase the predictability of the desired outcome and the safety of the surgical procedure. Reconstruction is planned using appropriate planning software that allows any number and many different types of simulations to be performed without a loss of information and allows two-dimensional and three-dimensional images to be displayed in any plane [1, 3–5]. Different data sets can be combined by semi-automatic fusion and can then be used for a precise preoperative analysis of images from different imaging modalities and for reliable intraoperative and postoperative quality control [2, 4, 19, 21]. The objective of surgical planning is to create a virtual model that matches the desired outcome of surgery [1, 2, 19, 21–24].

Planning software that has been developed for this purpose allows for threshold-based segmentation and/or even atlas-based automatic segmentation during the process of creating such a virtual model [2, 21, 25]. In addition, it should enable users to mirror parts of a data set and to freely move, rotate, and modify the generated virtual models in a rapid and easy way [2–4, 19–21, 26].

In the future, atlas-based automatic molding and deformation will more and more replace the procedures like mirroring, rotation, and manual deformation of virtual objects and will lead to more precise and especially quicker planning procedures.

During computer-assisted planning and simulation, a virtual 3D model of the desired result is created.

STL ("Standard Tessellation Language" or "Standard Triangle Language") data sets of three-dimensional bodies (titanium mesh structures, dental implants, etc.) can be imported into planning software so that standard implants, anatomically preformed implants, and patient-specific implants can be virtually positioned in the patient data set preoperatively and their shape, size, and fit can be assessed [2, 4, 21, 27].

STL data sets can be exported so that virtually generated models or reconstructions can be produced by a 3D printer and thus allow patient-specific models to be manufactured. Such models can be used to adapt and preoperatively bend patient-specific titanium implants such as titanium mesh for midface reconstruction (Fig. 5.2a) [1–4, 20, 28, 29].

The next step on the ladder of computer-assisted maxillofacial reconstruction is to process virtual reconstruction STL data sets using computer-aided design (CAD) software for planning patient-specific implants and to directly produce these implants using computer-aided manufacturing (CAM) techniques, e.g., selective laser melting (Fig. 5.2b).

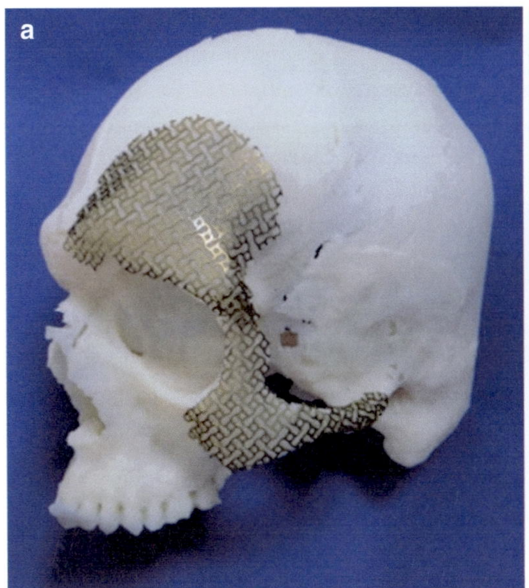
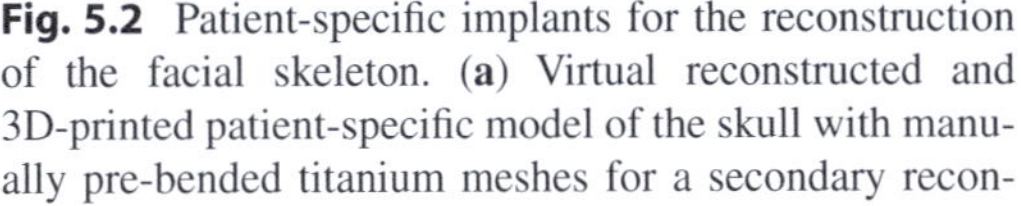
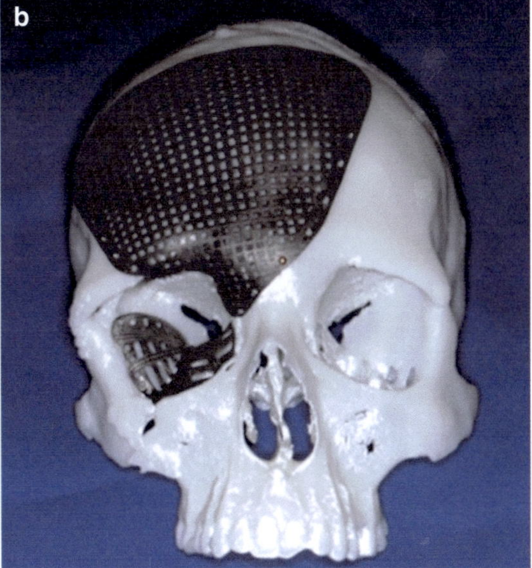

Fig. 5.2 Patient-specific implants for the reconstruction of the facial skeleton. (**a**) Virtual reconstructed and 3D-printed patient-specific model of the skull with manually pre-bended titanium meshes for a secondary reconstruction of the facial skeleton. (**b**) Via selective laser melting (SLM) manufactured patient-specific CAD/CAM-titanium-implant for the reconstruction of the frontal bone and the right orbit

5.2.3   Surgery

During the surgical procedure, surgeons have the difficult task of transferring the result of virtual computer-assisted planning to the surgical site as accurately as possible. For this purpose, they can use or combine a variety of different methods and devices, depending on the complexity of the task.

5.2.3.1 Intraoperative Navigation

Nowadays, intraoperative navigation with modern infrared-based navigation systems is an integral part of computer-assisted maxillofacial reconstruction (Fig. 5.3) [1, 19, 27, 30–37]. At the beginning of the surgical procedure, the patient on the operating table must be "fused" with the image data set that is displayed on the screen. This process is known as referencing and is based on reference points that must be clearly identifiable and reproducible both on the patient and in the image data set.

Furthermore, the patient's position must be permanently registered since patient movements during surgery cannot be prevented or may even

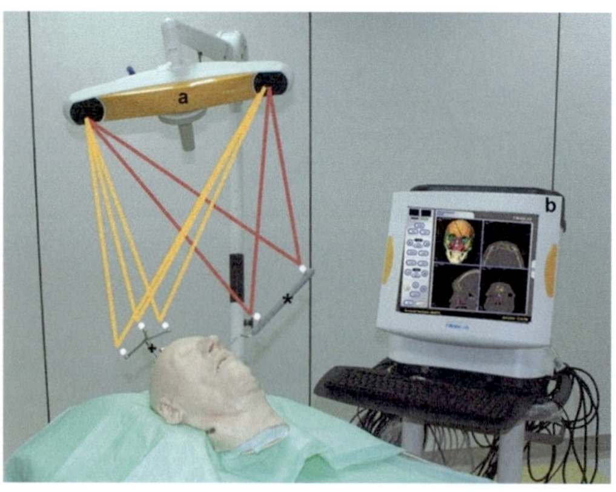

Fig. 5.3 Intraoperative setup of an indirect navigation system (a = camera with integrated LEDs, b = screen, * = pointer with two reflective spheres, + = reference array with three reflective spheres attached to the calvaria). The yellow lines represent the light waves that are emitted by the camera system and reflected back to the camera system by the reflective spheres of the referencing system (patient tracking). The red lines represent the light waves that are emitted by the camera system and reflected back to the camera system by the reflective spheres of the pointer (instrument tracking)

be necessary during the procedure. This is best accomplished by using a reference array that is attached to the patient's head and allows the navigation system to register all patient movements without limiting head mobility [1, 4, 19].

Once the technical requirements are met, the position of the pointer or tip of the pointer can be visualized in the data set on the screen of the navigation system. This enables surgeons to verify the realignment of bone fragments and the position and fit of inserted implants during surgery and to make any necessary changes without patient exposure to ionizing radiation. In this process, the virtual reconstruction that has been made during the planning phase serves as an intraoperative template that helps surgeons align bone fragments and/or place implants [1, 2, 19, 22, 23].

5.2.3.2 Patient-Specific Surgical Implants

Patient-specific CAD/CAM-fabricated implants are increasingly used for midface and orbital reconstructions [38]. Apart from polyether ether ketone (PEEK) and ceramics, which are particularly suitable for reconstructing calvarial defects, titanium mesh structures or patient-specific titanium plates are recommended for maxillofacial reconstructions. Selective laser melting (SLM) of titanium powder allows high-precision titanium mesh structures of any complexity and geometry to be manufactured [39, 40]. These implants are superior to conventional implants in particular for complex reconstructions and/or secondary reconstructions.

In the beginning, such implants were only available for secondary reconstructions due to long production times and logistics. However, since it is now possible to obtain such patient-specific implants within five working days from planning to delivery, it has also become possible to use such implants more and more for primary reconstructions.

Accurate positioning of patient-specific implants at the surgical site in accordance with preoperative planning is achieved either by an exact fit (Fig. 5.2b), which allows the placement of an implant in only one possible position, or by the use of surgical guides. In addition, intraoperative navigation can be used to position these implants.

> Navigation and/or patient-specific guides and implants are used to transfer preoperative planning and simulation to the surgical field.

5.2.4 Validation and Quality Control

5.2.4.1 Intraoperative imaging

Following the completion of a reconstruction procedure, surgical outcome should be validated in three dimensions. If possible, such a validation should be performed during the surgical procedure immediately after reconstruction.

This allows necessary modifications such as incorrect positions of bone fragments and implants to be made during the surgical procedure [2, 4, 8, 41–44].

Intraoperative imaging for facial skeleton reconstruction must meet a number of special requirements [4]:

- Sufficient resolution, especially for imaging the thin bone structures of the midface and orbits and the inserted implants
- Rapid availability in the operating room
- Short scan time
- Fast and safe use by surgeons and assistant personnel
- Multiplanar imaging (in the axial, coronal, and sagittal planes)
- Export of Digital Imaging and Communications in Medicine (DICOM) data for the fusion of intraoperative images with preoperative images or preoperative planning
- Data storage on the Picture Archiving and Communication System (PACS) of the medi-

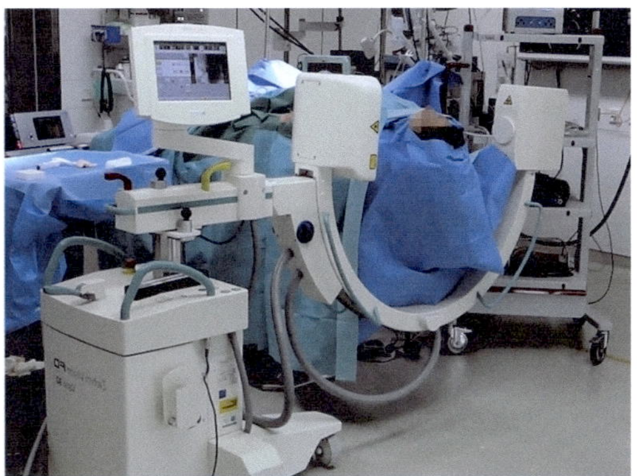

Fig. 5.4 Mobile 3D C-arm device for intraoperative imaging in action. Ziehm® Vario (FD) 3D with a flat panel detector

cal facility for meeting the requirement of archiving intraoperative image data sets

Cone-beam computed tomography (CBCT) offers a number of advantages that make this modality superior to others in meeting the aforementioned requirements. CBCT systems are available as mobile, ceiling-suspended or floor-mounted 3D C-arm systems for use in the operating room [4, 45] or as small compact CBCT systems for intraoperative use (Fig. 5.4).

The systems produce image series for multiplanar imaging in the axial, coronal, and sagittal planes and thus allow hard tissues to be imaged during surgery. Soft tissues, however, cannot be assessed. The applied radiation dose is lower than that from a comparable conventional CT scan of the facial skeleton, but depends on the system used, and in particular on tube output, image repetition rate, and exposure time.

> Mobile CBCT systems can be recommended for intraoperative imaging. This allows visualization of the reduction already during the procedure. This enables minimally invasive access and prevents revision surgery.

The images that are produced by these systems are of such quality that additional postoperative imaging is usually not required anymore [8]. The use of a mobile 3D CBCT device can thus be regarded as the current standard intraoperative imaging modality in maxillofacial reconstruction [4].

5.2.4.2　Postoperative Imaging

Whereas intraoperative imaging with a 3D CBCT device makes postoperative imaging after maxillofacial reconstruction unnecessary in many cases, postoperative 3D imaging in addition to intraoperative imaging may still be required especially after panfacial and complex reconstructions of the facial skeleton.

In these cases, CBCT may theoretically be preferred to CT because it is associated with a lower effective radiation dose. Clinically, however, care must be taken to ensure that the field of view of the CBCT system is large enough to provide the necessary information. Since postoperative images of both bone and soft tissues may be required, a suitable imaging modality must be chosen after surgery. This applies, for example, to entrapped muscle tissue after orbital wall reconstruction and to the presence of intracerebral free air after a surgical procedure that involves the posterior wall of the frontal sinus or the region of the skull base. Despite a higher radiation dose, CT should therefore be preferred to CBCT in complex cases.

> - Quality control requires postoperative 3D imaging.
> - Mobile CBCT systems offer a number of advantages and can be recommended, therefore, for intraoperative imaging.

5.2.4.3　Image Fusion and Outcome Evaluation

The purpose of intraoperative and postoperative 3D imaging is not only to perform a surgical procedure under radiological control but also to provide data sets for computer-assisted fusion with preoperative image data sets and especially with preoperative computer planning. Image fusion allows differences between preoperative planning and surgical outcome to be visualized and, if required, to be quantitatively evaluated within the scope of quality assurance.

5.3　Examples of Computer-Assisted Surgery in Acute Maxillofacial Trauma Repair

5.3.1　Isolated Fractures of the Zygomatic Arch (Fig. 5.5)

Computer-assisted surgery with intraoperative imaging allows surgeons to increasingly use or to revive the use of minimally invasive techniques without decreasing the predictability of the outcome of reduction procedures. This, for example, applies to the closed reduction of zygomatic arch fractures. Immediately after the surgical intervention, reduction is verified using a 3D C-arm in the operating room. If necessary, reduction can be directly corrected and unstable fractures can be managed by open reduction and internal fixation.

5.3.2　Fractures of the Zygomatico-orbital Complex (Fig. 5.6)

Fractures of the zygomatico-orbital complex are associated not only with zygomatic bone fractures but often also with displaced fractures in the region of the orbital floor. In such cases, the question is what degree of orbital floor displacement requires surgical reconstruction in addition to a reduction of the zygomatic bone fracture. Surgical reconstruction involves an intraorbital procedure with increased morbidity. For this reason, a surgical reconstruction of the orbital floor should only be performed if absolutely necessary. Since the zygomatic bone forms part of the orbital floor, a reduction of the zygomatic bone—including a closed reduction of the orbital floor—is sufficient in many cases. After zygomatic bone reduction and especially after a closed reduction,

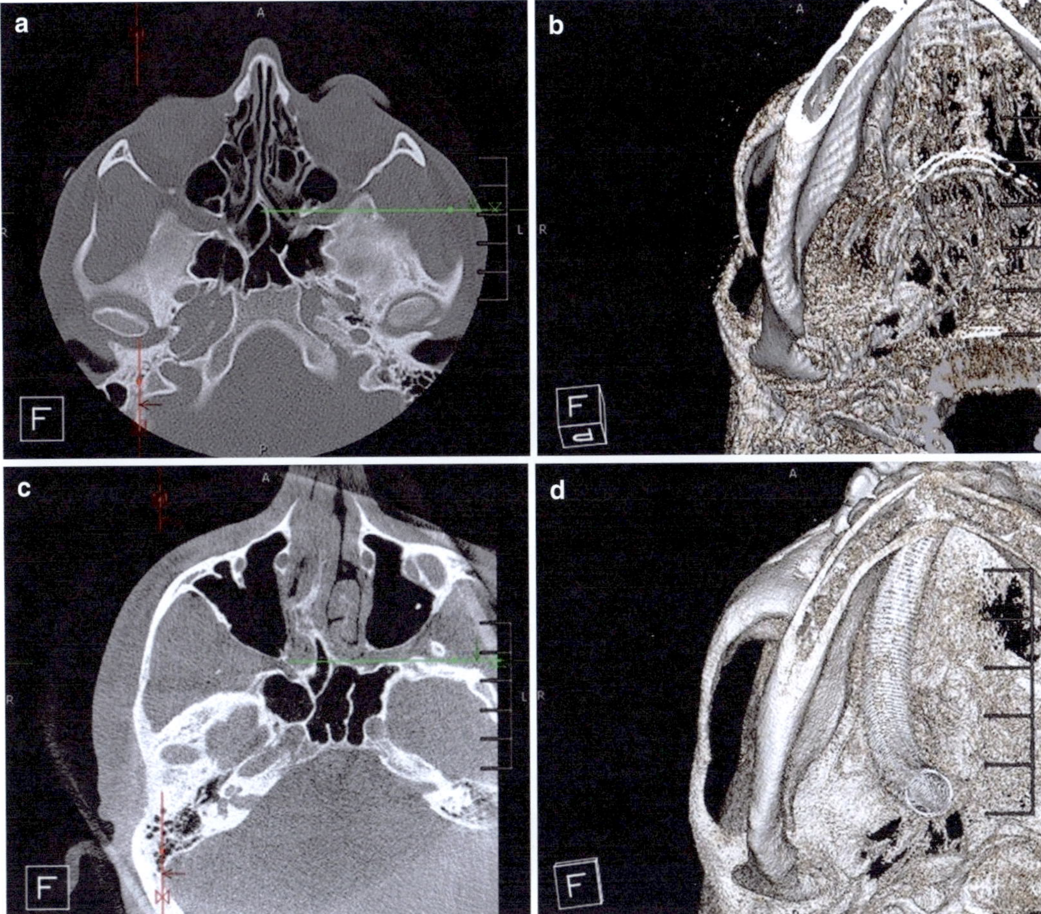

Fig. 5.5 Axial view (**a**) and 3D bottom view (**b**) of a preoperative CT scan with isolated zygomatic arch fracture. Axial view (**c**) and 3D bottom view (**d**) of an intraoperative 3D C-arm scan after closed reduction of the zygomatic arch fracture

it is still unclear during surgery whether zygomatic bone reduction has also resulted in a sufficient reduction of the orbital floor or whether additional orbital reconstruction is required. Intraoperative 3D imaging allows surgeons to rapidly assess the condition of the orbit and to avoid unnecessary explorations and orbital reconstructions [8].

5.3.3 Orbital Wall Fractures (Figs. 5.7 and 5.8)

Especially orbital wall fractures with involvement of the junction between the posterior orbital floor and the medial orbital wall and blow-out fractures of the orbital wall are associated with an increased risk of malposition of reconstruction material [1, 2]. The first step in the management of complex orbital wall fractures is virtual reconstruction by automatic segmentation of the CT data set into anatomical and surgical structures. Before surgery, a virtual template for reconstruction can be created either by mirroring the unaffected side in the case of unilateral fractures or by using free-form segments in the case of bilateral fractures with subsequent alignment of segmentation. Anatomically preformed titanium implants or patient-specific titanium implants, e.g., manufactured by selective laser melting can be virtually

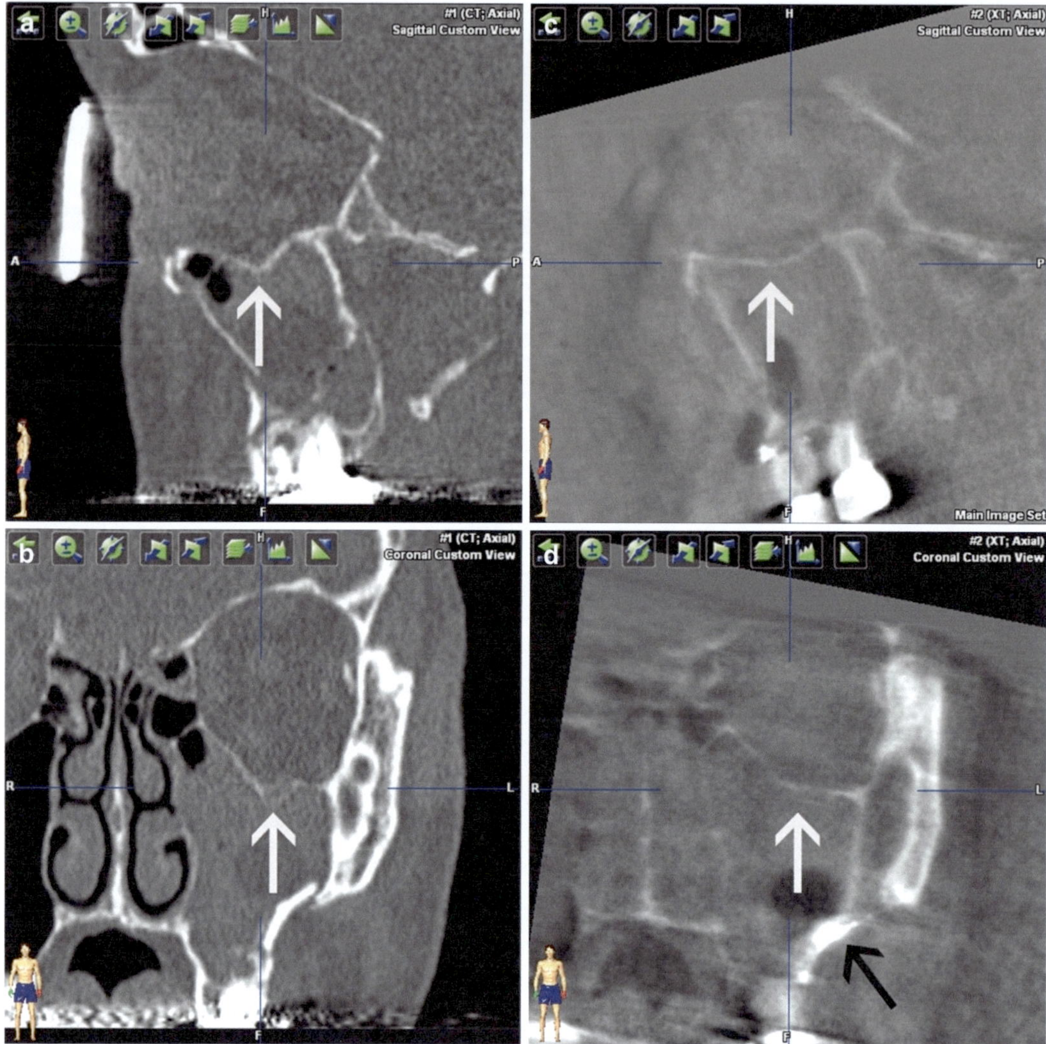

Fig. 5.6 Fusion of preoperative CT scans and intraoperative 3D C-arm images after the reduction of a zygomatico-orbital complex fracture. (**a, b**) Preoperative CT scans of a displaced fracture of the orbital floor (white arrows). (**c, d**) Intraoperative images after zygomatic bone reduction and fixation on the zygomatico-alveolar crest (black arrow). The images show an anatomically correct position of the orbital floor (white arrows). There is no need for open exploration and further management of the orbital floor

placed before surgery in order to assess the accuracy of fit. A navigation system can then be used to verify the alignment of bone fragments after reduction and the position and shape of the inserted implants. The tip of the pointer is placed on the implant or bone and the position of the pointer tip shows the current position of the structure of interest. This enables surgeons to verify reduction as well as the position and accuracy of fit of implants and to make any necessary corrections. Intraoperative 3D imaging is then performed as a final assessment of the procedure. Details of radiological images are sufficient to allow reconstruction results to be accurately validated on the basis of intraoperative data sets that are fused with preoperative data sets and simulations. Whereas previously orbital floor and medial orbital wall reconstructions required a coronal incision, the combined use of patient-specific or anatomically preformed implants,

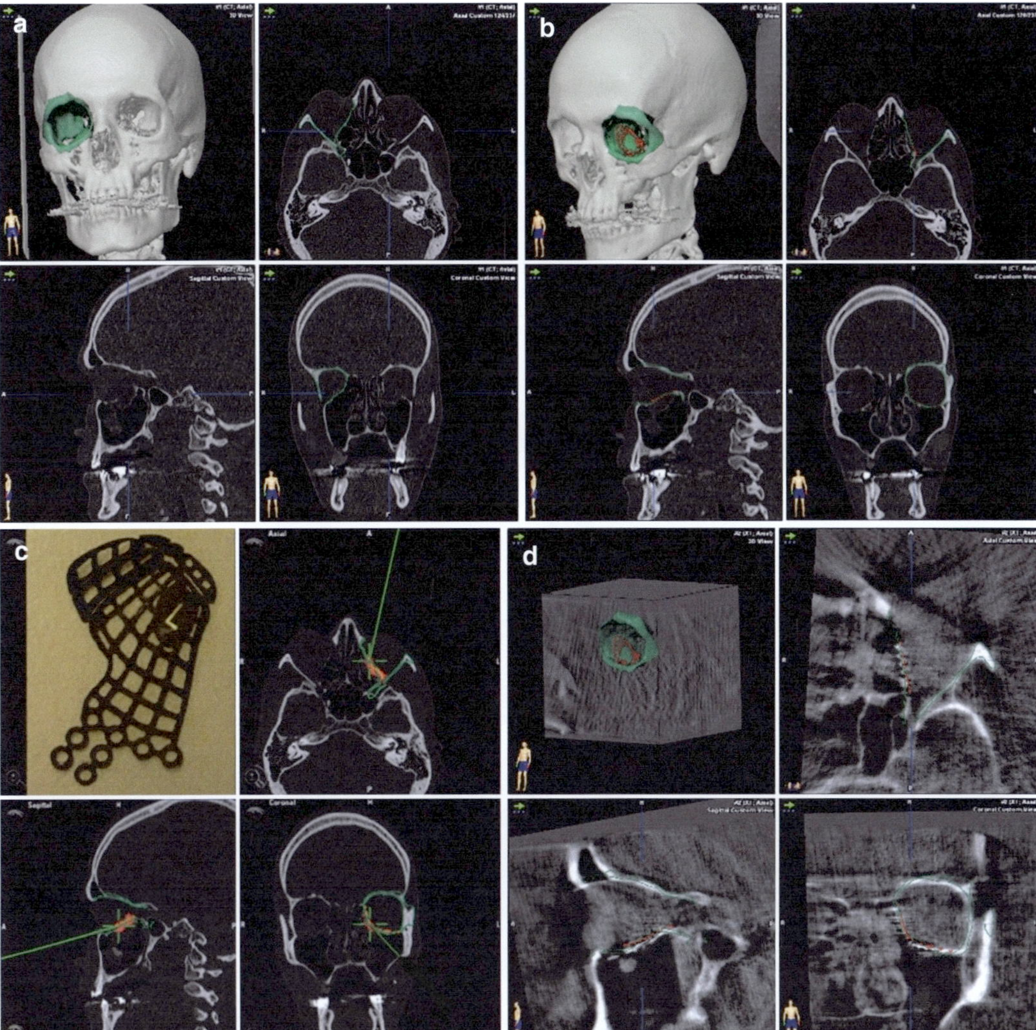

Fig. 5.7 Computer-assisted primary reconstruction of the left orbit using an anatomically preformed implant. (**a**) Multiplanar view of the virtual planning and creation of a template for orbital wall reconstruction by means of automatic segmentation of the unaffected right orbit using iPlan CMF 3.0 (BrainLAB®) (green contour lines). (**b**) Multiplanar view of the virtual reconstruction of the left orbit by means of mirroring the segmentation of the unaffected side (green contour lines) and virtual placement of an anatomically preformed orbital implant (red contour lines). The virtual placement of the anatomically preformed titanium implant allows surgeons to verify the size and accuracy of fit of the orbital implant. During surgery, implant placement (red contour lines) is performed according to the virtual reconstruction of the orbit (green contour lines) or the virtual placement of the implant. (**c**) Multiplanar view of the navigation-assisted placement of an anatomically preformed orbital implant (**c**: top left) (DePuySynthes®). The green contour line shows the virtual reconstruction of the orbit (analogous to the green contour line in **b, d**). During the surgical procedure, the red contour line displays the surface of the orbital implant inserted on the basis of implant surface data provided by the navigation tool. The orange contour line shows the virtually planned orbital implant on the screen of the navigation system (analogous to the red contour line in **b, d**). (**d**) Multiplanar view of intraoperative 3D imaging with superimposition of virtual planning. The green contour line represents the virtual reconstruction (analogous to **b, c**) and the red contour line shows the virtually placed orbital implant (analogous to **b**). The image shows good fit of the radio-opaque implant in accordance with virtual planning

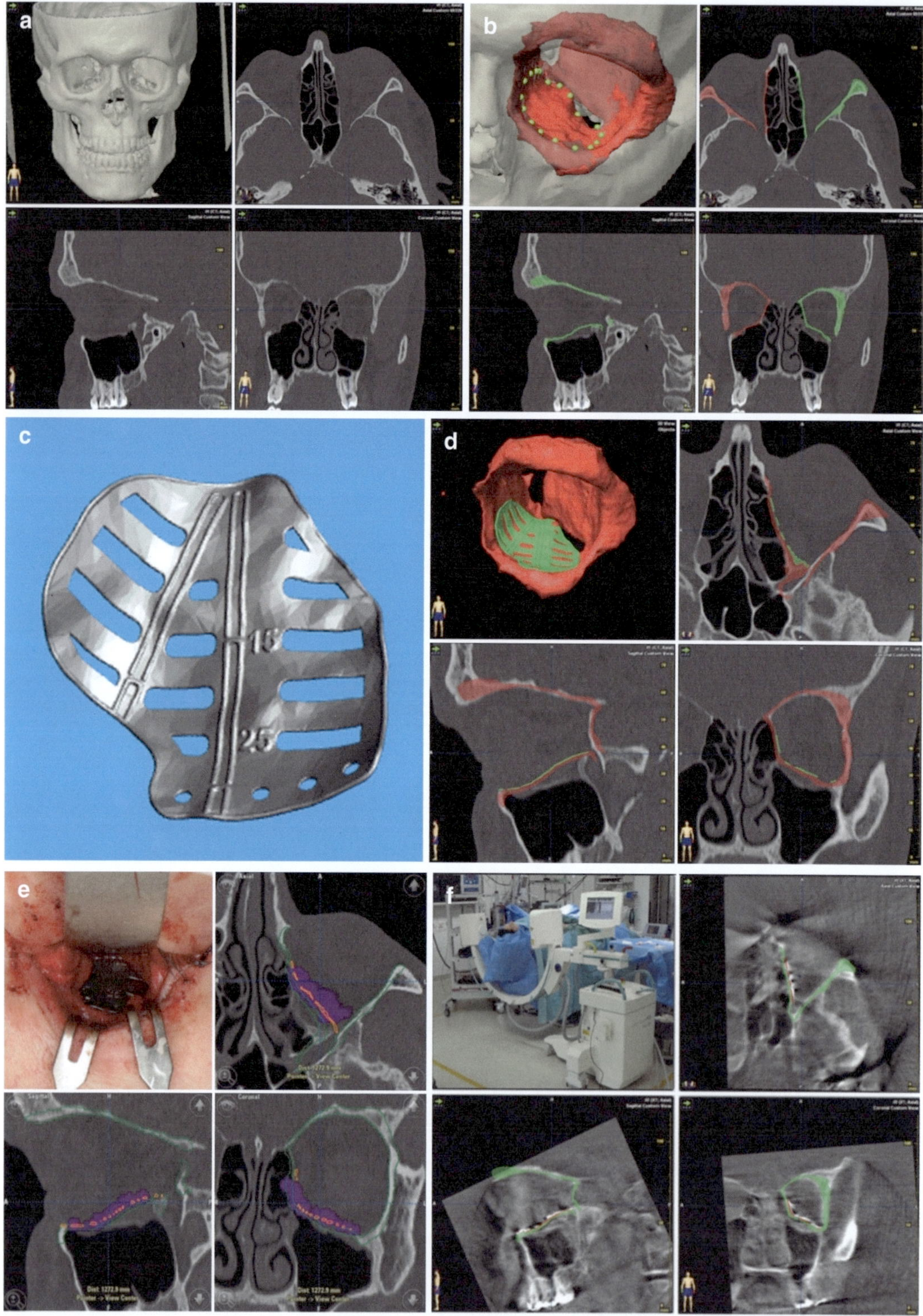

Fig. 5.8 Computer-assisted reconstruction of the left orbit with a patient-specific implant manufactured by selective laser melting (KLS Martin®). (**a**) Multiplanar view of an orbital wall fracture of left orbit with an enlargement of orbital volume resulting in an enophthalmos and diplopia. (**b**) Virtual planning and creation of a template for orbital wall reconstruction of the left orbit (green contour lines) by means of automatic segmentation and mirroring of the unaffected right orbit (red contour lines) using iPlan CMF 3.0 (BrainLAB®). Top left: Determination of the size of the patient-specific implant (yellow dots). (**c**) Computer-aided design of the patient-specific implant. The implant corresponds to the implant that is virtually placed as an STL data set in **d**. (**d**) Multiplanar view of the virtual reconstruction with a virtually placed patient-specific implant that was imported into the left orbit as an STL data set after industrial planning (green contour line). Virtual implant placement allows the accuracy of fit to be verified before the implant is manufactured. (**e**) Multiplanar view of the navigation-assisted placement of the orbital implant. The green contour line shows the virtual reconstruction of the orbit (analogous to the green contour line in **b** and the red contour line **d**). During the surgical procedure, the purple contour line displays the surface of the orbital implant inserted on the basis of implant surface data provided by the navigation tool. The orange contour line shows the virtually planned orbital implant on the screen of the navigation system (analogous to the green contour line in **d**). (**f**) Multiplanar view of intraoperative 3D imaging with superimposition of virtual planning. The green contour line shows the virtual reconstruction (analogous to **b, d,** and **e**). The image shows good fit of the radio-opaque implant in accordance with virtual planning (red contour line analogous to the green contour line in **d**)

intraoperative navigation and intraoperative imaging now enables surgeons to perform even extensive reconstructions of the orbital floor and medial orbital wall via a transconjunctival approach and thus to avoid visible scars [2, 4, 21].

5.3.4 Complex Midface Fractures (Fig. 5.9)

In complex midfacial fractures, the treatment follows the described algorithm of computer-assisted surgery as well. After data acquisition using computer tomography, virtual 3D planning is also carried out here with the creation of a virtual model of the reconstruction as described above. In the case of acute trauma repair, the reconstruction result is then checked using intraoperative navigation and/or intraoperative 3D imaging. Immediate image fusion between preoperative virtual plan and intraoperative 3D dataset facilitates intraoperative control of the achieved result and, if necessary, immediate correction.

5.3.5 Fractures of the Mandible: Condyle Fracture (Fig. 5.10)

Currently the use of navigation in the treatment of fractures of the mandible is limited because of the mobility of this area. Intraoperative imaging can be a valuable tool in order to check the result of the treatment especially in fractures of the condyle. The treatment of mandibular condyle fractures is a challenge for the surgeon in the large number of cases. Due to the intraoperatively limited view of the reduction result, independent of the surgical approach (extraoral or intraoral), malpositions of the condyle cannot always be excluded intraoperatively. For this reason, intraoperative imaging with a mobile 3D C-arm device can be recommended to avoid malpositioning. This allows the intraoperative radiologic control and documentation of the reduced fracture and of the position of the plates in a multiplanar view and enables an immediate intraoperative correction when the result of the procedure is not satisfactory. This reduces the risk for revision surgeries considerably [2, 4].

5.4 Summary

As a result of advances in 3D imaging, 3D printing, intraoperative visualization, and intraoperative navigation at the end of the last century and further improvements in these techniques in recent years, computer-assisted reconstruction of the facial skeleton has become an integral part of oral and maxillofacial surgery. In recent years, an algorithm has been established which involves

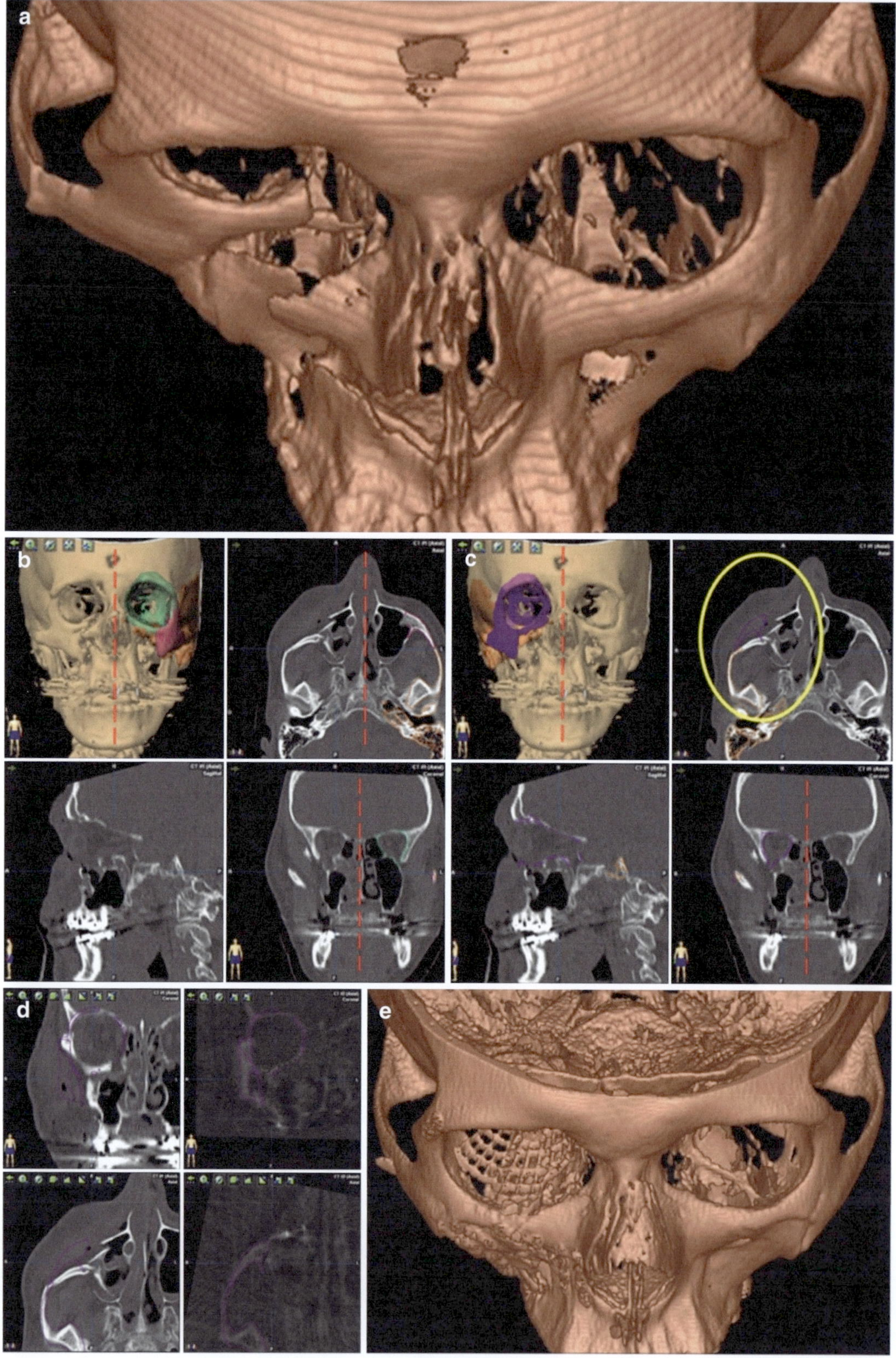

Fig. 5.9 Computer-assisted reconstruction of lateral complex midface fracture. (**a**) 3D reconstruction of the preoperative CT scan showing the dislocated right lateral midface. (**b**, **c**) Multiplanar views of the virtual planning and creation of a virtual model of the desired reconstruction result by means of automatic segmentation and mirroring of (**b**) the unaffected left site (green, red, orange contour lines) to the (**c**) affected right site (purple and orange contour lines) by using iPlan CMF 3.0 (BrainLAB®). (**d**) Intraoperative comparison of the preoperative (left) and intraoperative (right) findings after the scan with a 3D C-arm device and fusion with the virtual planning (purple contour lines). (**e**) 3D reconstruction of the postoperative CT scan

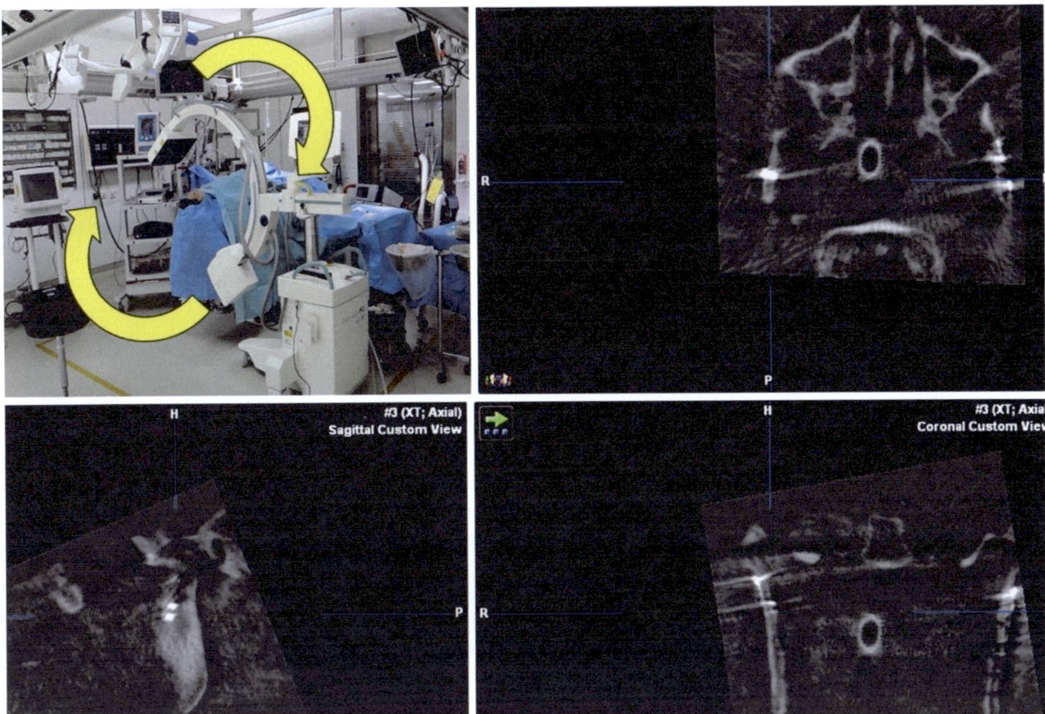

Fig. 5.10 Multiplanar view of intraoperative imaging with a 3D C-arm device (Ziehm, Erlangen, Germany) after endoscopic assisted open reduction and internal fixation of a bilateral condyle fracture via an intraoral approach

the following steps: >diagnosis → planning and simulation → surgical procedure → validation and quality control<.

The focus of diagnosis is on 3D imaging especially on computed tomography and clinical findings. Planning and simulation involve the creation of a virtual model of the desired surgical outcome. Apart from the fusion of different data sets, planning software allows the virtual models to be segmented in a user-friendly manner and to be manipulated (e.g., to be mirrored, shifted, rotated, and modified) in an easy way. In addition, surface tessellation language (STL) data sets can be imported and exported. When STL data sets are imported, the accuracy of implant fit can be virtually verified before surgery. When STL data sets are exported, patient-specific 3D models and virtual reconstructions can be directly printed and can be used for manufacturing patient-specific implants. STL data sets that are imported into computer-aided design (CAD) software are helpful in planning patient-specific implants and in manufacturing them using computer-aided manufacturing (CAM) techniques. During the surgical procedure, planning must be transferred to the surgical site as accurately as possible. A number of techniques are available for this purpose, e.g., closed reduction, open reduction with the placement of anatomically preformed or patient-specific implants in combination with surgical guides, and the additional use of navigation and intraoperative imaging. After reconstructions, three-dimensional imaging should be performed even before surgery is completed. Malpositions can thus be directly corrected and unnecessary open reconstructions or explorations—for example of the orbital walls—can be avoided. Mobile 3D C-arms are particularly useful for intraoperative 3D imaging. Validation and quality control require postprocedural 3D imaging. Whereas intraoperative imaging with a 3D C-arm makes postoperative imaging after midface reconstruction unnecessary in many cases, postoperative 3D imaging in addition to intraoperative imaging may still be required after complex reconstructions of the facial skeleton and mandible.

References

1. Schramm A, Gellrich NC. Intraoperative Navigation und computerassistierte Chirurgie. In: Schwenzer N, Ehrenfeld M, editors. Zahn-Mund-Kieferheilkunde, Mund-Kiefer-Gesichtschirurgie, vol. 2011. 4th ed. Stuttgart: Thieme; 2011. p. 479–99.
2. Schramm A, Wilde F. Die computergestützte Gesichtsschädelrekonstruktion. HNO 2011;59:800–6.
3. Markiewicz MR, Bell RB. Modern concepts in computer-assisted craniomaxillofacial reconstruction. Curr Opin Otolaryngol Head Neck Surg. 2011;19:295–301.
4. Wilde F, Schramm A. Intraoperative imaging in orbital and midface reconstruction. Facial Plast Surg. 2014;30:545–53.
5. Parthasarathy J. 3D modeling, custom implants and its future perspectives in craniofacial surgery. Ann Maxillofac Surg. 2014;4:9–18.
6. Manson PN, Markowitz B, Mirvis S, Dunham M, Yaremchuk M. Toward CT-based facial fracture treatment. Plast Reconstr Surg. 1990;85:202–12.
7. Tanrikulu R, Erol B. Comparison of computed tomography with conventional radiography for midfacial fractures. Dentomaxillofac Radiol. 2001;30:141–6.
8. Wilde F, Lorenz K, Ebner AK, Krauss O, Mascha F, Schramm A. Intraoperative imaging with a 3D-C-arm system after zygomatico-orbital complex fracture reduction. J Oral Maxillofac Surg. 2013;71:894–910.
9. Wikner J, Riecke B, Gröbe A, Heiland M, Hanken H. Imaging of the midfacial and orbital trauma. Facial Plast Surg. 2014;30:528–36.
10. Cornelius C-P, Gellrich N-C, Hillerup S, Kusumoto K, Schubert W. AO foundation; midface-diagnosis, AO surgery reference. 2014. http://www.aocmf.org/surgeryref.aspx. Accessed 5 Oct 2019.
11. Schulze D, Heiland M, Thurmann H, Adam G. Radiation exposure during midfacial imaging using 4- and 16-slice computed tomography, cone beam computed tomography systems and conventional radiography. Dentomaxillofac Radiol. 2004;33:83–6.
12. Ludlow JB, Ivanovic M. Comparative dosimetry of dental CBCT devices and 64-slice CT for oral and maxillofacial radiology. Oral Surg Oral Med Oral Pathol Oral Radiol Endod. 2008;106:106–14.
13. Loubele M, Bogaerts R, Van Dijck E, Pauwels R, Vanheusden S, Suetens P, Marchal G, Sanderink G, Jacobs R. Comparison between effective radiation dose of CBCT and MSCT scanners for dentomaxillofacial applications. Eur J Radiol. 2009;71:461–8.
14. Suomalainen A, Kiljunen T, Käser Y, Peltola J, Kortesniemi M. Dosimetry and image quality of four dental cone beam computed tomography scanners compared with multislice computed tomography scanners. Dentomaxillofac Radiol. 2009;38:367–78.
15. Chau AC, Fung K. Comparison of radiation dose for implant imaging using conventional spiral tomography, computed tomography, and cone-beam computed tomography. Oral Surg Oral Med Oral Pathol Oral Radiol Endod. 2009;107:559–65.
16. Geibel M-A. DVT – Indikationen und Strahlenbelastung. 2013. http://www.zwp-online.info/de/fachgebiete/digitale-zahnmedizin/digitale-bildgebung/dvt-indikationen-und-strahlenbelastung. Accessed 10 Dec 2019.
17. Deman P, Atwal P, Duzenli C, Thakur Y, Ford NL. Dose measurements for dental cone-beam CT: a comparison with MSCT and panoramic imaging. Phys Med Biol. 2014;59:3201–22.
18. Brisco J, Fuller K, Lee N, Andrew D. Cone beam computed tomography for imaging orbital trauma—image quality and radiation dose compared with conventional multislice computed tomography. Br J Oral Maxillofac Surg. 2014;52:76–80.
19. Schramm A, Gellrich NC, Schmelzeisen R. Navigational surgery of the facial skeleton. Berlin: Springer; 2007.
20. Markiewicz MR, Bell RB. The use of 3D imaging tools in facial plastic surgery. Facial Plast Surg Clin North Am. 2011;19:655–82.
21. Wilde F, Hilbert J, Kamer L, Hammer B, Metzger M, Schmelzeisen R, Gellrich N-C, Schramm A. The combination of automatic segmentation, preformed implants, intraoperative imaging in primary orbital wall reconstruction: description of a new method. Int J Comput Assist Radiol Surg. 2009;4(Suppl 1):134.
22. Schramm A, Gellrich NC, Schön R, Gutwald R, Schmelzeisen R. Navigational maxillofacial surgery using virtual models. In: Tachibana E, Furukawa T, Mukai Y, Ma H, editors. Proceedings of the international symposium modelling applications, Daegu, Korea, 2002. p. 71–6.
23. Hohlweg-Majert B, Schön R, Schmelzeisen R, Gellrich NC, Schramm A. Navigational maxillofacial surgery using virtual models. World J Surg. 2005;29:1530–8.

24. Schipper J, Klenzner T, Berlis A, Maier W, Offergeld C, Schramm A, Gellrich NC. Objektivierung von Therapieergebnissen in der Schädelbasischirurgie durch virtuelle Modellanalyse. HNO. 2006;54:677–83.
25. Metzger MC, Bittermann G, Dannenberg L, Schmelzeisen R, Gellrich NC, Hohlweg-Majert B, Scheifele C. Design and development of a virtual anatomic atlas of the human skull for automatic segmentation in computer-assisted surgery, preoperative planning, and navigation. Int J Comput Assist Radiol Surg. 2013;8:691–702.
26. Gellrich N-C, Schramm A, Hammer B, Schmelzeisen R. The value of computer-aided planning and intraoperative navigation in orbital reconstruction. Int J Oral Maxillofac Surg. 1999;28:52–3a.
27. Essig H, Dressel L, Rana M, Rana M, Kokemueller H, Ruecker M, Gellrich NC. Precision of posttraumatic primary orbital reconstruction using individually bent titanium mesh with and without navigation: a retrospective study. Head Face Med. 2013;9:18.
28. Kernan BT, Wimsatt JA 3rd. Use of a stereolithography model for accurate, preoperative adaptation of a reconstruction plate. J Oral Maxillofac Surg. 2000;58:349–51.
29. Hallermann W, Olsen S, Bardyn T, Taghizadeh F, Banic A, Iizuka T. A new method for computer-aided operation planning for extensive mandibular reconstruction. Plast Reconstr Surg. 2006;117:2431–7.
30. Schmelzeisen R, Gellrich NC, Schoen R, Gutwald R, Zizelmann C, Schramm A. Navigation-aided reconstruction of medial orbital wall and floor contour in cranio-maxillofacial reconstruction. Injury. 2004;35:955–62.
31. Fuller SC, Strong EB. Computer applications in facial plastic and reconstructive surgery. Curr Opin Otolaryngol Head Neck Surg. 2007;15:233–7.
32. Bell RB, Markiewicz MR. Computer-assisted planning, stereolithographic modeling, and intraoperative navigation for complex orbital reconstruction: a descriptive study in a preliminary cohort. J Oral Maxillofac Surg. 2009;67:2559–70.
33. Beumer HW, Puscas L. Computer modeling and navigation in maxillofacial surgery. Curr Opin Otolaryngol Head Neck Surg. 2009;17:270–3.
34. Markiewicz MR, Dierks EJ, Potter BE, Bell RB. Reliability of intraoperative navigation in restoring normal orbital dimensions. J Oral Maxillofac Surg. 2011;69:2833–40.
35. Austin RE, Antonyshyn OM. Current applications of 3-D intraoperative navigation in craniomaxillofacial surgery: a retrospective clinical review. Ann Plast Surg. 2012;69:271–8.
36. Yu H, Shen SG, Wang X, Zhang L, Zhang S. The indication and application of computer-assisted navigation in oral and maxillofacial surgery—Shanghai's experience based on 104 cases. J Craniomaxillofac Surg. 2013;41:770–4.
37. Novelli G, Tonellini G, Mazzoleni F, Bozzetti A, Sozzi D. Virtual surgery simulation in orbital wall reconstruction: integration of surgical navigation and stereolithographic models. J Craniomaxillofac Surg. 2014;42:2025–34.
38. Gander T, Essig H, Metzler P, Lindhorst D, Dubois L, Rücker M, Schumann P. Patient specific implants (PSI) in reconstruction of orbital floor and wall fractures. J Craniomaxillofac Surg. 2015;43:319–22.
39. Vandenbroucke B, Kruth JP. Selective laser melting of biocompatible metals for rapid manufacturing of medical parts. Rapid Prototyp J. 2007;13:196–203.
40. Bilz M, Uhlmann E. Generative manufacturing methods: selective laser melting. 2014. http://www.ipk.fraunhofer.de/fileadmin/user_upload/IPK_FHG/publikationen/themenblaetter/ps_ft_selective_laser_melting_en.pdf. Accessed 10 Oct 2019.
41. Heiland M, Schmelzle R, Hebecker A, Schulze D. Intraoperative 3D imaging of the facial skeleton using the SIREMOBIL Iso-C3D. Dentomaxillofac Radiol. 2004;33:130–2.
42. Heiland M, Schulze D, Blake F, Schmelzle R. Intraoperative imaging of zygomaticomaxillary complex fractures using a 3D-C-arm system. Int J Oral Maxillofac Surg. 2005;34:369–75.
43. Klatt J, Heiland M, Blessmann M, Blake F, Schmelzle R, Pohlenz P. Clinical indication for intraoperative 3D imaging during open reduction of fractures of the neck and head of the mandibular condyle. J Craniomaxillofac Surg. 2011;39:244–8.
44. Hanken H, Christian L, Assaf AT, Heiland M. Intraoperative Bildgebung in der Mund-, Kiefer- und Gesichtschirurgie. Intraoperative imaging of the facial skeleton. OP J. 2013;29:130–5.
45. Gebhard F, Riepl C, Richter P, Liebold A, Gorki H, Wirtz R, König R, Wilde F, Schramm A, Kraus M. Der Hybridopertionssaal. Zentrum intraoperativer Bildgebung. Unfallchirurg. 2012;115:107–20.

Secondary Post-traumatic Orbital Reconstruction

6

Joseph Lopez, Shannath L. Merbs, and Michael P. Grant

6.1 Introduction

Diplopia, dystopia, and enophthalmos are complications that can persist after primary orbital traumatic reconstruction [1, 2]. Unfortunately, these complications can lead to unsatisfactory functional and aesthetic outcomes. Recent studies suggest that approximately 13–37% of patients have persistent diplopia after primary orbital fracture repair [3, 4]. Similarly, clinically significant enophthalmos has been found to persist in 27% of patients [5]. These complications can also be induced after repair of orbital fractures. A recent well-designed study by Ramphul et al. found that diplopia can be induced in 10% of patients after primary orbital fracture repair [6]. Many factors have been reported to contribute to post-operative complications after primary orbital repair including delayed surgical repair, poor or inaccurate fracture repair, fracture type

(i.e., fracture compromising the inferonasal bony strut), extraocular muscle damage, orbital content adherence issues (e.g., inferior oblique muscle adherence syndrome, peri-muscular scarring), or patient age [7–9]. Addressing some of these factors with secondary orbital reconstruction can be quite challenging. In fact, a comprehensive clinical and radiologic evaluation is critical to determine which of these factors can be addressed with secondary orbital reconstruction, and therefore improve on primary orbital fracture repair results.

6.2 Anatomy

A thorough understanding of orbital anatomy is critical to properly manage complications secondary to inaccurate orbital fracture repair. Additionally, a complete understanding of the ocular motility muscles and nerves is necessary to determine the etiology of complications after primary orbital fracture repair.

The orbit is composed of seven bones: frontal, maxillary, zygoma, sphenoid, ethmoid, palatine, and lacrimal; it's shaped like a four-sided pyramid which is approximately 30 mL in volume and 35–40 mm in length (Fig. 6.1). The orbit is composed of orbital buttresses ("pillars") often used as reference points for orbital reconstruction. The medial transition zone, or also known as the inferonasal bony strut, has previously been

J. Lopez (✉) · M. P. Grant
Department of Plastic and Reconstructive Surgery, Johns Hopkins Hospital, Baltimore, MD, USA

Division of Plastic, Maxillofacial, and Reconstructive Surgery, R Adam Cowley Shock Trauma Center, Baltimore, MD, USA
e-mail: michael.grant@som.umaryland.edu

S. L. Merbs
Department of Ophthalmology and Visual Sciences, University of Maryland Medical Center, Baltimore, MD, USA
e-mail: smerbs@som.umaryland.edu

© Springer Nature Switzerland AG 2021
J. Acero (ed.), *Innovations and New Developments in Craniomaxillofacial Reconstruction*,
https://doi.org/10.1007/978-3-030-74322-2_6

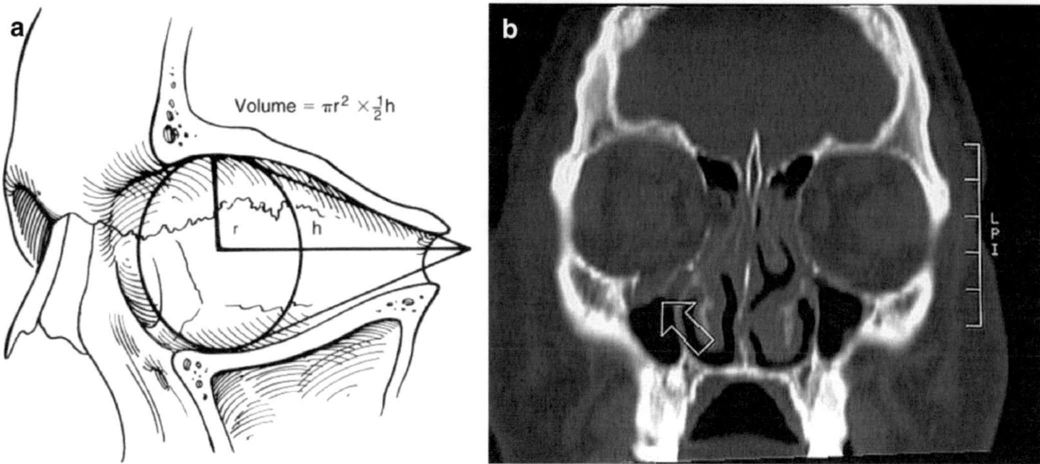

Fig. 6.1 (a) Illustration representation of the orbital cone volume; (b) thin-cut coronal CT demonstrating a right orbital floor with herniation of orbital content including the inferior rectus muscle

reported to be of anatomical significance since when this buttress is missing, one loses a critical anatomical reference point necessary for optimal implant placement in combined medial and orbital floor fractures [10]. When this buttress is fractured and not adequately repaired, unstable reconstruction of this area can lead to undesirable secondary changes such as dystopia, enophthalmos, or diplopia [11].

The orbit also includes seven muscles responsible for extraocular movements. The annulus of zin serves as the origin of four of these extraocular muscles (inferior rectus, medial rectus, lateral rectus, and superior rectus), forming a tendinous ring on the anterior end of the optic canal and middle third of the superior orbital fissure. The three other extraocular muscles (inferior oblique, levator palpebrae, and superior oblique) originate on the maxillary bone (just lateral to the nasolacrimal duct), lesser wing of sphenoid, and greater wing of sphenoid, respectively. Although all seven extraocular muscles can be damaged with trauma or during primary surgical repair, three muscles are more commonly encountered during surgical access: the lower rectus, inferior oblique, and superior oblique muscles. The lower rectus muscle runs along the orbital floor and attaches 6.5 mm inferior to the limbus, making it prone to entrapment. Therefore, an evaluation of the infe-

rior rectus muscle is critically important with computer tomography (CT) to assess for injury and preserve its function after orbital trauma. The inferior oblique muscle is commonly encountered during the dissection of combined medial and orbital floor fracture repairs [12]. Damage to this muscle can also lead to lasting orbital complications. Lastly, the superior oblique is often encountered during the dissection and repair of orbital roof fractures since it loops through the pulley-like structure (trochlea) on the medial orbital roof.

Cranial nerve III (oculomotor), IV (trochlear), VI (abducens) are the ocular motor nerves that innervate these extraocular muscles. Therefore, injury to these ocular motor nerves can impact orbital fracture repair outcomes as well. Although there is a paucity of data on the rate of ocular motor nerve injuries after orbital or maxillofacial trauma, studies in the neurosurgery literature have shown that head trauma can cause clinically significant injury to these cranial nerves [13, 14]. The abducens nerve is reported to be the most commonly injured ocular motor nerve after head trauma; it innervates the lateral rectus muscle. The trochlear nerve innervates the superior oblique muscle and head trauma has been shown to be the most common cause of trochlear nerve palsy [15]. The rest of the rectus muscles are innervated by the oculomotor nerve. Fortunately, isolated traumatic palsy to the oculomotor nerve from head trauma is very rare but more studies are necessary to determine its vulnerability to injury during orbital trauma or orbital fracture repair [16].

6.3 Goals of Secondary Reconstruction

The goals of secondary reconstruction are similar to those of primary repair:

1. Reposition herniated orbital contents (i.e., free incarcerated peri-muscle tissue).
2. Restore the premorbid orbital volume.

Placement of orbital implants in the incorrect position after inadequate dissection can lead to the incarceration or herniation of orbital contents outside of the orbital margins. Therefore, atrophy, contraction, and secondary undesirable clinical outcomes like diplopia can result from mal-reduction or incorrect placement of orbital implants. Therefore, performing a thorough clinical evaluation and radiologic assessment to address any issues with orbital implant positioning is important to determine whether secondary orbital fracture correction will improve patient symptoms. Additionally, a formal clinical and radiological evaluation of post-repair orbital volume is critical to determine whether secondary orbital implant repositioning can adequately restore the premorbid orbital volume.

6.4 Clinical Evaluation

A comprehensive patient history and physical examination should be performed in all patients presenting for secondary orbital reconstruction. A detailed history regarding the original trauma event, prior reconstructive procedures (especially those involving the orbit), and a timeline of pre-sentation and symptoms is important. In fact, operative reports containing prior surgical approaches, incisions, and implant type are important to device a sophisticated treatment plan. A complete understanding of the symptomatology timeline may lend clues to the etiology. For example, new onset symptoms of diplopia that have worsened since primary repair suggests a restrictive etiology while diplopia that is slowly improving over time suggests a neurogenic etiology.

In contrast to patients who are evaluated for primary orbital repairs, secondary orbital repair patients warrant a complete eye examination. A strabismus evaluation by an extraocular muscle specialist should be performed. Such an evaluation can help differentiate between restrictive and neurogenic symptoms, since a paralytic etiology is unlikely to improve with secondary orbital reconstruction (Fig. 6.2). In addition, an accurate exophthalmometer should be used to measure globe position relative to the lateral orbital rim to rule out hypoglobus or abnormal orbital volume.

6.5 Radiologic Evaluation

No secondary reconstruction should be performed without a recent, up-to-date, computed tomography (CT) scan. Like acute trauma evaluations, thin-cut CT imaging is the gold standard to evaluate the bony anatomy of the orbit. If there are contraindications to CT imaging, magnetic resonance imaging (MRI) can be utilized [17]. Recent imaging should be compared to prior studies with a focus on identifying potential abnormalities that are amenable to secondary correction (e.g., poor anatomical reduction, improper implant positioning) (Fig. 6.3). A focus on orbital volume assessment, comparing it to the injured side, if possible, is important. Lastly, one should also focus on evaluating orbital implant displacement or impingement in both soft tissue and bone windows, to look for herniation of orbital contents or peri-muscular implant impingement.

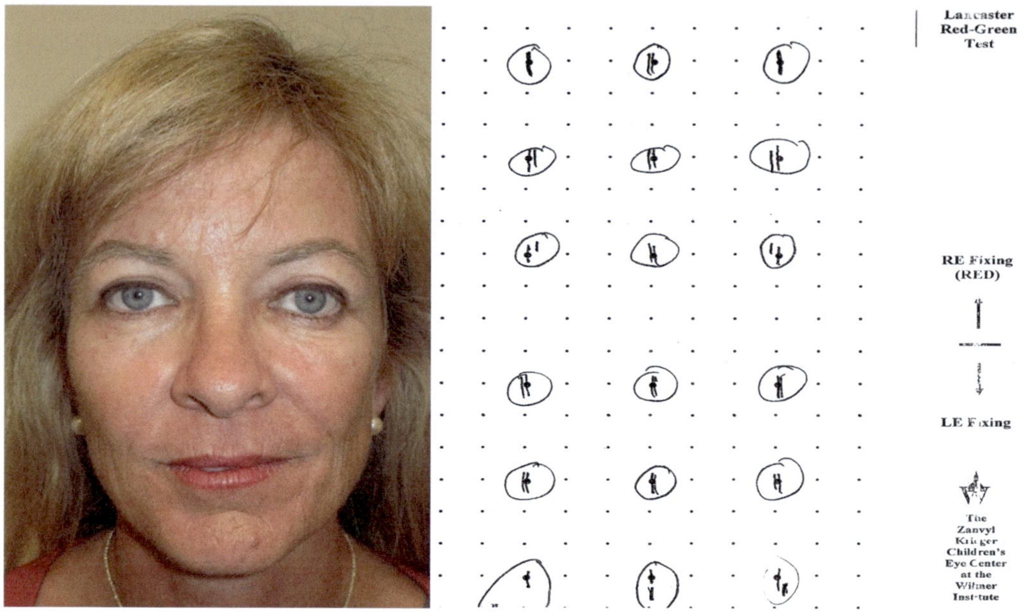

Fig. 6.2 (**a**) 54F who presents after a 2-month history of diplopia with downgaze. (**b**) Strabismus testing revealed restricted inferior rectus muscle. After removal of implant, diplopia resolved

6.6 Indication and Timing for Secondary Orbital Repair

Secondary surgical correction should be performed in patients with:

(a) Restrictive diplopia secondary to extraocular muscle impingement, enophthalmos secondary to orbital content herniation, or implant displacement or malposition. As described previously, neurogenic diplopia should be ruled out prior to secondary orbital surgery.

(b) Persistent symptoms of diplopia, enophthalmos, or dystopia attributable to an anatomically and surgically correctable defect. Most maxillofacial surgeons consider 2 mm or greater of enophthalmos as an indication for surgery [18].

Timing of secondary orbital repair should be thoroughly planned before embarking on revision surgery. Although delaying non-urgent, elective surgery for months can allow the periorbital soft tissue to heal and symptoms to stabilize, waiting too long after initial repair can result in significant bony or soft tissue remodeling (i.e., scarring) that can make revision surgery quite complicated. Therefore, most maxillofacial surgeons would agree that waiting 3–6 months after initial repair provides an adequate amount of time for symptoms to improve and not compromise secondary orbital surgery complexity [19]. However, acute symptoms suggestive of nerve or rectus muscle impingement (in addition to standard indications for acute repair of optic nerve impingement or orbital compartment syndrome) warrant more immediate intervention.

6.7 Surgical Approach

Standard surgical approaches used in primary orbital repair (transconjunctival, subciliary, or transcutaneous) apply for secondary orbital repair. Although scarring and abnormal anatomy may make revision surgery more challenging, the

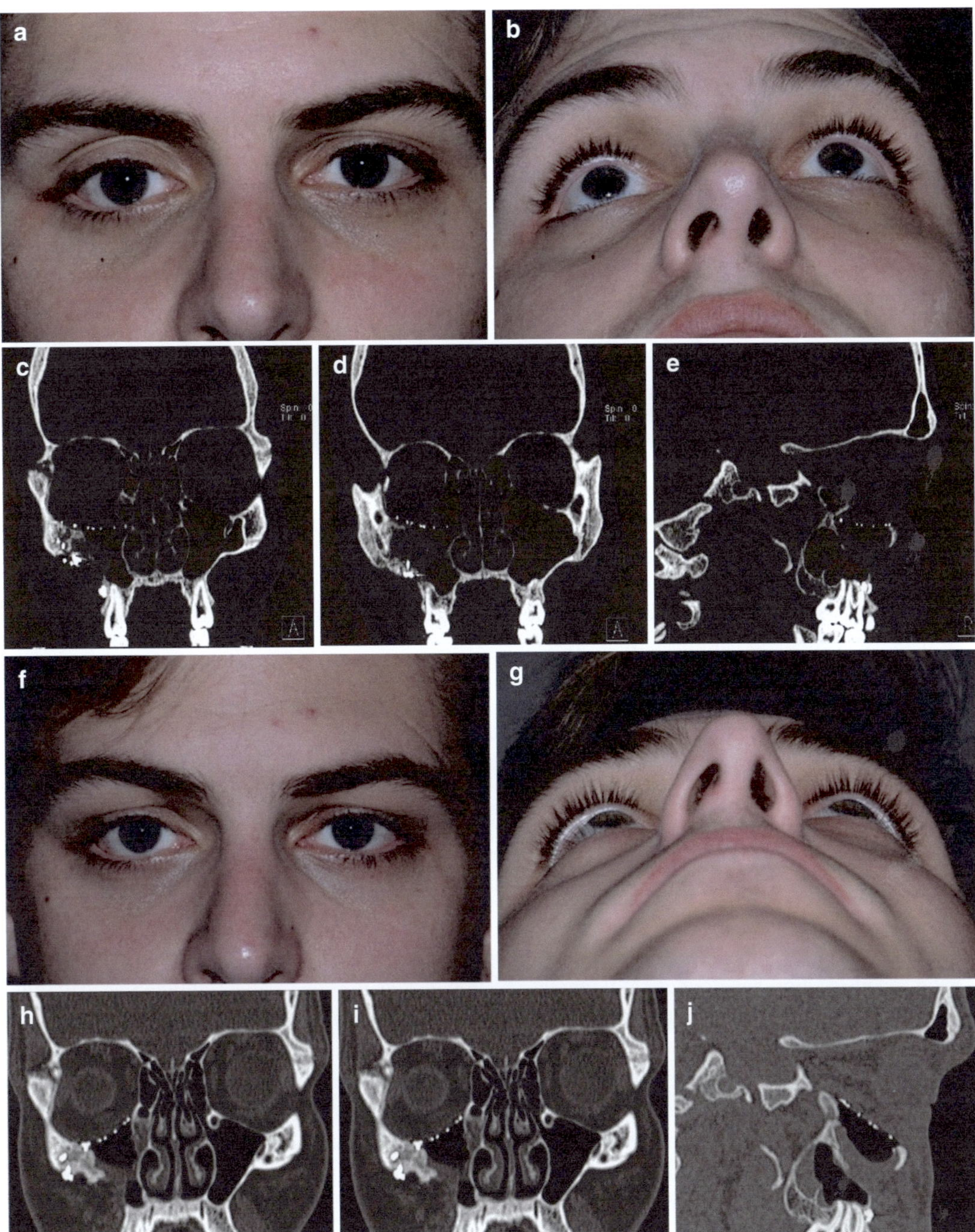

Fig. 6.3 (**a, b**) Young gentleman who presented 3 months following an orbito-zygomatico-maxillary complex (OZMC) repair complaining of diplopia with symptoms of enophthalmos on exam; (**c–e**) axial and sagittal CT scan showing improper implant position; (**f, g**) post-operative result showing resolution of enophthalmos; (**h–j**) axial and sagittal CT showing use of patient-specific implant with good position

surgical approach may be chosen independently of that used in primary repair. Surgeon-preference is critical to the success of any operation, but the maxillofacial surgeon should attempt to tailor the approach to specific pre-operative diagnoses and symptom etiologies. All prior implants should be removed and, ideally, replaced with pre-planned, pre-bent, or customized implants (more details below).

6.8 Surgical Technique: Computer-Assisted Surgical Planning

Recent studies and anecdotal evidence suggest that computer-assisted surgical (CAS) planning is essential for accurate and sophisticated secondary orbital reconstruction (Fig. 6.4) [20]. In order to perform CAS planning, updated orbital CT data is needed, in addition to proprietary software that can mirror the intricate orbital wall anatomy of the uninjured side onto the symptomatic orbit. Using this data, one can pre-bend implants to desired custom shapes or design customized patient-specific implants. As a result of the "customization" of the CAS planning process, accurate bony reconstruction is more common, reducing the need for bony revision surgery [21].

The utility of patient-specific implants in orbital reconstruction has dramatically increased recently, and its utility in secondary orbital repair is instrumental in achieving good outcomes. Because revision surgery is greatly complicated by prior surgical attempts and the delayed time-frame, accurately restoring the bony orbital anatomy is necessary to achieve good results. Additionally, the non-urgent nature of secondary orbital reconstruction affords the time to design such implants. In fact, all secondary orbital reconstructions at our institution are now exclusively performed with patient-specific implants. This technology has revolutionized a complex problem, now facilitating favorable results [22].

6.9 Surgical Technique: Intraoperative Navigation

Intraoperative navigation has only until recently been introduced, and it has already proven to be an invaluable resource for correction of secondary orbital abnormalities [23–27]. As previously discussed, accurate restoration of the orbital anatomy is critical for the success of secondary orbital repairs. However, abnormal bony anatomy, peri-orbital soft tissue scarring, and the presence of likely mal-positioned, old orbital implants make secondary operations quite difficult. The recent introduction of intraoperative navigation technology makes surgical access safer and ensures ideal bony reduction and implant placement [28]. In fact, a recent study by Hammer et al. found that intraoperative navigation led to implant repositioning 25% of the time, optimizing functional and aesthetic outcomes in patients [29].

6.10 Surgical Outcomes

CAS planning, pre-bent or custom implant fabrication, and intraoperative navigation have all emerged as sophisticated technologies that can assist the maxillofacial surgeon achieve good results in cases of complex secondary orbital reconstruction [30, 31]. However, patient selection is key to determine whether secondary orbital repair can improve patient symptoms. Although secondary orbital reconstruction has been tradiationally associated with higher rates of complications, these emerging technologies are leading to improved outcomes with more consistent results. That being said, patients should be cautioned regarding the possibility of persistent symptoms. Older studies suggest that some degree of improvement is achievable in 50% of patients with improvements in enophthalmos and hypo-globus after secondary correction without the use of these technologies [32]. Ongoing, long-term studies will determine the efficacy of these emerging technologies in improving patient results.

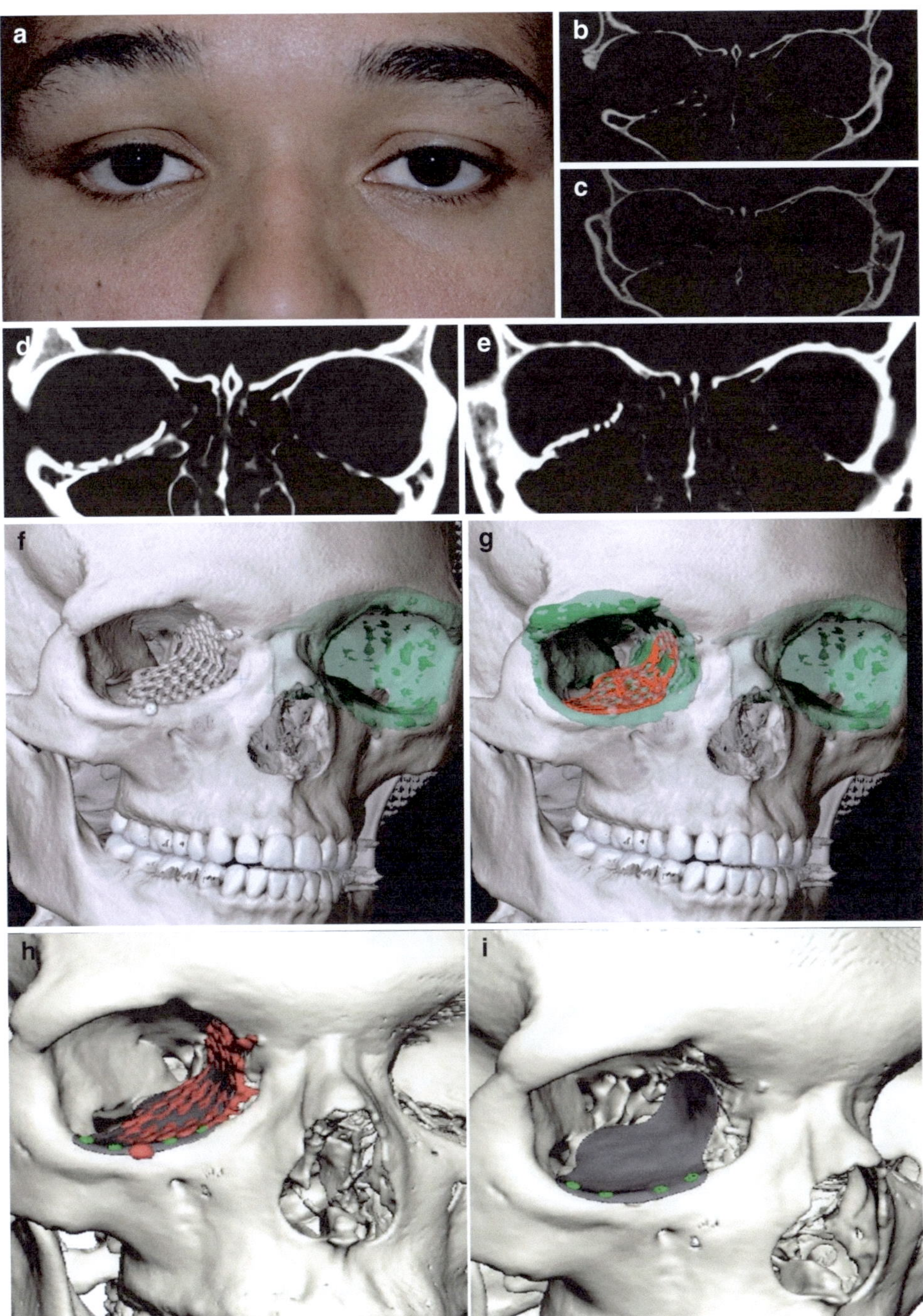

Fig. 6.4 (**a**) 24 year M with history of a two-wall fracture who presented with diplopia with extreme downgaze; (**b**, **c**) axial CT scans showing original medial and floor fractures including the medial transition zone; (**d**, **e**) postoperative axial CT scan showing implant malposition; (**f**, **g**) use of software to mirror the shape of the uninjured left orbit to create the shape of the right orbit; red figure designates the position of the original implant; (**h**) superimposed customized designed implant on old abnormally positioned implant; (**i**) patient-specific implant designed by mirroring from the opposite on injured side; (**j**, **k**) postoperative axial CT scan showing good anatomical positioning of patient-specific implant; (**l**) old orbital implant vs. new patient-specific implant; (**m**) intraoperative navigation showing the predicted and actual implant position showing accurate intraoperative placement of new implant

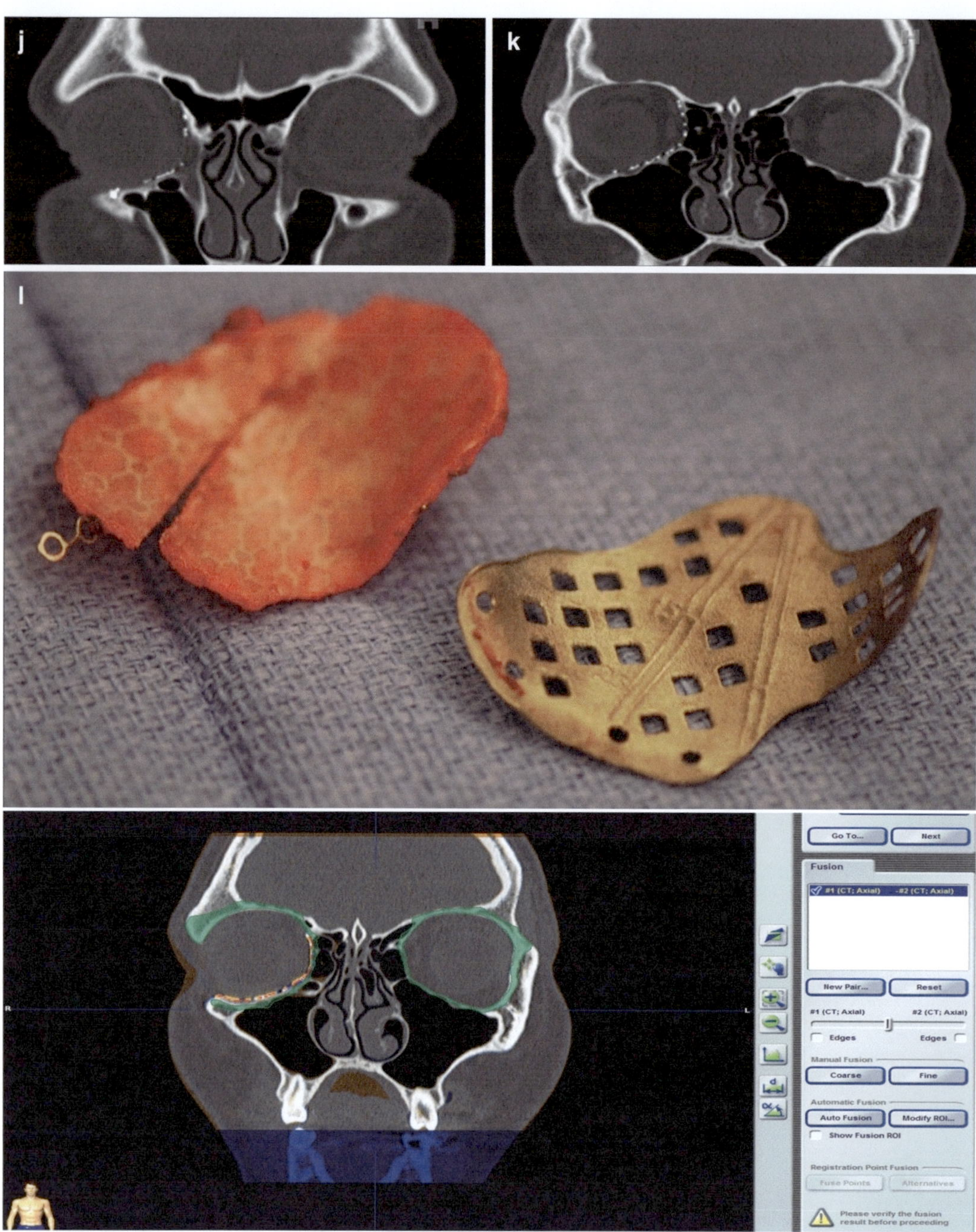

Fig. 6.4 (continued)

References

1. Brucoli M, Arcuri F, Cavenaghi R, Benech A. Analysis of complications after surgical repair of orbital fractures. J Craniofac Surg. 2011;22(4):1387–90.
2. Yim CK, Ferrandino R, Chelnis J, Leitman IM. Analysis of early outcomes after surgical repair of orbital floor fractures. JAMA Facial Plast Surg. 2018;20(2):173–5.
3. Biesman BS, Hornblass A, Lisman R, Kazlas M. Diplopia after surgical repair of orbital floor fractures. Ophthalmic Plast Reconstr Surg. 1996;12(1):9–16; discussion 17.
4. Harris GJ, Garcia GH, Logani SC, Murphy ML. Correlation of preoperative computed tomography

and postoperative ocular motility in orbital blowout fractures. Ophthalmic Plast Reconstr Surg. 2000;16(3):179–87.

5. Hosal BM, Beatty RL. Diplopia and enophthalmos after surgical repair of blowout fracture. Orbit. 2002;21(1):27–33.

6. Ramphul A, Hoffman G. Does preoperative diplopia determine the incidence of postoperative diplopia after repair of orbital floor fracture? An institutional review. J Oral Maxillofac Surg. 2017;75(3):565–75.

7. Tahiri Y, Lee J, Tahiri M, Sinno H, Williams BH, Lessard L, et al. Preoperative diplopia: the most important prognostic factor for diplopia after surgical repair of pure orbital blowout fracture. J Craniofac Surg. 2010;21(4):1038–41.

8. Brady SM, McMann MA, Mazzoli RA, Bushley DM, Ainbinder DJ, Carroll RB. The diagnosis and management of orbital blowout fractures: update 2001. Am J Emerg Med. 2001;19(2):147–54.

9. Silbert DI, Matta NS, Singman EL. Diplopia secondary to orbital surgery. Am Orthopt J. 2012;62:22–8.

10. Kempster R, Beigi B, Galloway GD. Use of enophthalmic implants in the repair of orbital floor fractures. Orbit. 2005;24(4):219–25.

11. Fan X, Li J, Zhu J, Li H, Zhang D. Computer-assisted orbital volume measurement in the surgical correction of late enophthalmos caused by blowout fractures. Ophthalmic Plast Reconstr Surg. 2003;19(3):207–11.

12. Alameddine RM, Tsao JZ, Ko AC, Lee BW, Kikkawa DO, Korn BS. Incidence of diplopia after division and reattachment of the inferior oblique muscle during orbital fracture repair. J Craniomaxillofac Surg. 2018;46(8):1247–51.

13. Coello AF, Canals AG, Gonzalez JM, Martin JJ. Cranial nerve injury after minor head trauma. J Neurosurg. 2010;113(3):547–55.

14. Dhaliwal A, West AL, Trobe JD, Musch DC. Third, fourth, and sixth cranial nerve palsies following closed head injury. J Neuroophthalmol. 2006;26(1):4–10.

15. Sydnor CF, Seaber JH, Buckley EG. Traumatic superior oblique palsies. Ophthalmology. 1982;89(2):134–8.

16. Lin C, Dong Y, Lv L, Yu M, Hou L. Clinical features and functional recovery of traumatic isolated oculomotor nerve palsy in mild head injury with sphenoid fracture. J Neurosurg. 2013;118(2):364–9.

17. Kolk A, Pautke C, Schott V, Ventrella E, Wiener E, Ploder O, et al. Secondary post-traumatic enophthalmos: high-resolution magnetic resonance imaging compared with multislice computed tomography in postoperative orbital volume measurement. J Oral Maxillofac Surg. 2007;65(10):1926–34.

18. Koo L, Hatton MP, Rubin PA. When is enophthalmos "significant"? Ophthalmic Plast Reconstr Surg. 2006;22(4):274–7.

19. Imola MJ, Ducic Y, Adelson RT. The secondary correction of post-traumatic craniofacial deformities. Otolaryngol Head Neck Surg. 2008;139(5):654–60.

20. Gellrich NC, Schramm A, Hammer B, Rojas S, Cufi D, Lagreze W, et al. Computer-assisted secondary reconstruction of unilateral posttraumatic orbital deformity. Plast Reconstr Surg. 2002;110(6):1417–29.

21. Lauer G, Pradel W, Schneider M, Eckelt U. Efficacy of computer-assited surgery in secondary orbital reconstruction. J Craniomaxillofac Surg. 2006;34(5):299–305.

22. Bly RA, Chang SH, Cudejkova M, Liu JJ, Moe KS. Computer-guided orbital reconstruction to improve outcomes. JAMA Facial Plast Surg. 2013;15(2):113–20.

23. Bell RB, Markiewicz MR. Computer-assisted planning, stereolithographic modeling, and intraoperative navigation for complex orbital reconstruction: a descriptive study in a preliminary cohort. J Oral Maxillofac Surg. 2009;67(12):2559–70.

24. Baumann A, Sinko K, Dorner G. Late reconstruction of the orbit with patient-specific implants using computer-aided planning and navigation. J Oral Maxillofac Surg. 2015;73(12 Suppl):S101–6.

25. Yang JR, Liao HT. Functional and aesthetic outcome of extensive orbital floor and medial wall fracture via navigation and endoscope-assisted reconstruction. Ann Plast Surg. 2019;82(1S):S77–85.

26. Wan KH, Chong KK, Young AL. The role of computer-assisted technology in post-traumatic orbital reconstruction: a PRISMA-driven systematic review. Sci Rep. 2015;5:17914.

27. Novelli G, Tonellini G, Mazzoleni F, Bozzetti A, Sozzi D. Virtual surgery simulation in orbital wall reconstruction: integration of surgical navigation and stereolithographic models. J Craniomaxillofac Surg. 2014;42(8):2025–34.

28. Azarmehr I, Stokbro K, Bell RB, Thygesen T. Surgical navigation: a systematic review of indications, treatments, and outcomes in oral and maxillofacial surgery. J Oral Maxillofac Surg. 2017;75(9):1987–2005.

29. Schmelzeisen R, Gellrich NC, Schoen R, Gutwald R, Zizelmann C, Schramm A. Navigation-aided reconstruction of medial orbital wall and floor contour in cranio-maxillofacial reconstruction. Injury. 2004;35(10):955–62.

30. Udhay P, Bhattacharjee K, Ananthnarayanan P, Sundar G. Computer-assisted navigation in orbitofacial surgery. Indian J Ophthalmol. 2019;67(7):995–1003.

31. Jansen J, Schreurs R, Dubois L, Maal TJJ, Gooris PJJ, Becking AG. The advantages of advanced computer-assisted diagnostics and three-dimensional preoperative planning on implant position in orbital reconstruction. J Craniomaxillofac Surg. 2018;46(4):715–21.

32. Freihofer HP. Effectiveness of secondary post-traumatic periorbital reconstruction. J Craniomaxillofac Surg. 1995;23(3):143–50.

Manuel Picón, Jorge Núñez,
and Fernando Almeida

7.1 Introduction

The mandible is a special U-shaped bone which constitutes the skeletal frame of the inferior third of the face. It may be affected by tumors, trauma, inflammatory diseases, and radiation or pharmacologically induced avascular necrosis. Mandible defects, frequently combined with soft tissue defects, can be complex and difficult to repair. Main objectives of mandibular reconstruction are the restoration of the mandibular continuity and facial contour, reconstruction of the soft tissues including oral mucosa and skin closure as well as to provide a functional dental rehabilitation [1]. The use of free vascularized fibula flap remains the gold standard for the restoration of large mandibular defects [2]. Other free vascularized flaps less frequently used are the iliac crest free flap for shorter bone defects [3] or the chimeric scapular free flap for complex combined osseous and soft tissues defects [4].

This surgical procedures are technically demanding because of the need to transform the long straight fibular bone into a three-dimensional (3D) structure that fits into the defect matching the original mandibular conformation as closely as possible, which requires the creation of specific angulations different for each patient. This process is accomplished by performing osteotomies in the fibular flap being difficult to determine the exact location and angulation of them. Even more, the fixation of the different mobile fibular fragments is also difficult and the whole process becomes tedious and time consuming.

The traditional approach as described in the literature [5–7] starts with the preplating procedure. The plate is molded on the buccal surface of the mandible. Then, it is placed across the entire defect and is secured to the bone on each side of the resection lines. The native mandible is used as a template while molding the titanium plate which ensures good three-dimensional (3D) reproduction of the preoperative conditions. The plate is placed along the inferior border of the mandible and is fixed with three or more bicortical screws in each mandible segment. Then the plate is removed and the mandibular resection is performed. Usually following a "two-team approach," the fibula flap is raised. The fibula is osteotomized at a back table in order to shape it properly to achieve matching the original mandibular conformation with maximal bone contact. Finally, the fibular bone fragments are fixed lingually to the reconstruction plate and inset between the mandible segments to fill the defect and the microvascular procedure is performed.

According to the literature [8], the preplating technique although being a highly subjective procedure, can be accurate when the external cortical bone of the mandible is not affected but in

M. Picón (✉) · J. Núñez · F. Almeida
Department of Maxillofacial Surgery, Ramon y Cajal
University Hospital, Madrid, Spain

© Springer Nature Switzerland AG 2021
J. Acero (ed.), *Innovations and New Developments in Craniomaxillofacial Reconstruction*,
https://doi.org/10.1007/978-3-030-74322-2_7

those cases when the vestibular cortical mandible is involved by the tumor or, even more, in secondary reconstruction cases when a mandibular segment is lacking, this vestibular preplating technique is not possible. Although there are different techniques that can be used like repositioning of the segments with intermaxillary fixation, they are difficult and very long time consuming. Furthermore, the traditional technique as previously reviewed, is experience-dependent, requires intraoperative trial and error and is difficult to carry out for the less-experienced surgeon. In these situations, computer-assisted surgery can help the surgeon to overcome the referred problems and pitfalls.

7.2 Computer-Assisted Surgery: Surgical Techniques

Computer-assisted surgery (CAS) refers to a process including virtual surgical planning, computer-aided design and modeling/rapid prototyping or computer-aided manufacturing (CAD/CAM) which can also be associated with intraoperative navigation.

7.2.1 Virtual Surgical Planning

High-resolutions computed tomographic scans (1-mm fine cuts) of the maxillofacial skeleton and donor site (lower extremities, iliac crest, or scapular bone) are obtained and shared with the biomedical engineer. Using any of the different software programs disposable at the market, three-dimensional reconstruction of both, maxillofacial skeleton and bone donor site, are obtained. A web-based teleconference is held between the biomedical engineer and the surgical team. Coordinating efforts for the planning is relatively simple, as each user is granted remote access to the planning session by means of conference-call and computer link-up. A typical planning session lasts approximately 30 min or less. Ideally, biomedical engineers could be part of the team in house.

Directed by the surgical team, virtual resection is performed to get appropriate surgical margins. Then, virtual reconstruction of the defect is performed by superimposing the patient's own three-dimensional fibula 3D images (or other donor bone: iliac crest or scapula) onto the mandibular defect performing the adequate osteotomies in order to recreate the mandibular original contour through a trial and error process, optimizing the number and cutting plane of the osteotomies and bone flap segments lengths while ensuring bone-to-bone contact. With these data, 3D models of the neomandible and cutting guides for the bone flap preparation and mandibular resection are manufactured. When this technique was firstly described, a standard mandibular titanium plate was prebent preoperatively over the manufactured neomandible model using a plate-bending template as a guide. Today, last generation software and 3D printing technology, allows to design in the virtual model a custom-made personalized plate perfectly adapted to the bone of the neomandible which can be directly manufactured from the virtual model as a patient-specific implant, thus avoiding the necessity of printing the mandibular models to shape the plate.

To increase the accuracy and facilitate the process, the same holes used to fix the cutting guides to the mandible and to the bone flap are later used to fix the personalized reconstruction plate. Personalized reconstruction plates avoid the risk of weakening the plate and early fracture at the bending sites.

The process previously described refers to primary reconstructive procedures when reconstruction is performed immediately after resection. In case of secondary procedures when the mandible is previously lacking and the remnant mandible is out of its normal position because of the fibrosis and scar retraction, the resected mandible cannot be used as a model. In these situations, the first step in the virtual planning process is to set the remnant mandible in its right place using the condyle fossa and maxillary arch as a reference. Then, mirroring the contralateral mandible, the new mandible is virtually created and the bone flap adapted to the defect.

As mentioned previously, the fibular flap is the work-horse in mandibular reconstruction, but in some circumstances, other bone flaps are used: iliac crest and scapular bone free flaps. The process described is the same for these three flaps with the only difference that the design of the bone flap cutting guides has to be adapted to the special anatomic conditions of any of them. Special mention has to be made to the necessity to take in account that the surgical guides cannot be fixed directly to the bone surface in the anatomical areas where the vascular pedicle lies in the soft tissues attached to the flap, which has to be considered in the design of the cutting guides.

7.2.2 Surgical Technique

Whenever it is possible, the surgery proceeds with a two-team approach. The cutting guides are secured to the mandible and the osteotomies are performed with a reciprocating saw guided by the cutting slots. It's advisable that the slots are manufactured in some metal material, so that the osteotomies effectively replicate the virtually planned mandibular osteotomies, avoiding wrong ways through the deformation of the soft material of the guides.

The fibula is concurrently dissected and isolated on its vascular pedicle. The cutting guide is secured to the fibula with unicortical screws. Guide placement can be adjusted according to perforator vessels location if a skin island is required. Orienting the vascular pedicle and lengthening the pedicle by subperiosteal dissection of the fibula is an important aspect of virtual planning in order to adequately design of the anastomosis to avoid the use of vein grafts in the neck. With the pedicle protected by a small malleable retractor, cutting guide-directed osteotomies are performed with a reciprocating or an oscillating sagittal saw, depending on the surgeon's preference. The fibular fragments are then fixed to the personalized reconstruction plate in situ, using the holes previously drilled for the cutting guides. The neomandible shape is confirmed and the vascular pedicle is divided. The neomandible/personalized reconstruction plate is transferred as a unit and secured to the mandibular remnant at its predetermined optimal position. This maneuver is greatly facilitated using again the holes already drilled to secure the mandibular cutting guides, once these are retrieved after the mandibular osteotomies have been performed. After bone fixation, microsurgical anastomosis is completed followed by soft-tissue insetting (Fig. 7.1).

The process is the same for iliac crest free flap (Fig. 7.2). If a scapular bone flap is used (Fig. 7.3), the two-team approach is frequently not possible, thus increasing the surgical time.

Once the surgical process is completed, the reconstruction is evaluated and compared with the virtual plan by superimposing the postoperative three-dimensional computed tomographic scans onto the virtual model.

7.3 Benefits and Disadvantages of VSP with CAD-CAM

The application of the most recent technological refinements including virtual surgical planning (VSP) with computer-aided design-computer-aided modeling (CAD-CAM) in the management of surgical ablative procedures of the craniofacial skeleton and subsequent reconstruction, represents a major advance in terms of shortening the operation time and achieving a precise bone-to-bone contact, as well as shows excellent functional and aesthetic results [9–11]. Unlike the traditional techniques of reconstruction based on the surgeons' clinical experience in which manual cutting and modeling of the free osseous flaps and bending the fixation plate was a laborious task with an unpredictable outcome, the use of preoperative surgical simulations with 3D technology, VSP and CAD-CAM with osteotomy guides and prebent or customized reconstruction plates increases operative efficiency and reduce total operative costs [12–15].

The introduction of the prefabricated surgical osteotomy guides based on 3D CT images of the

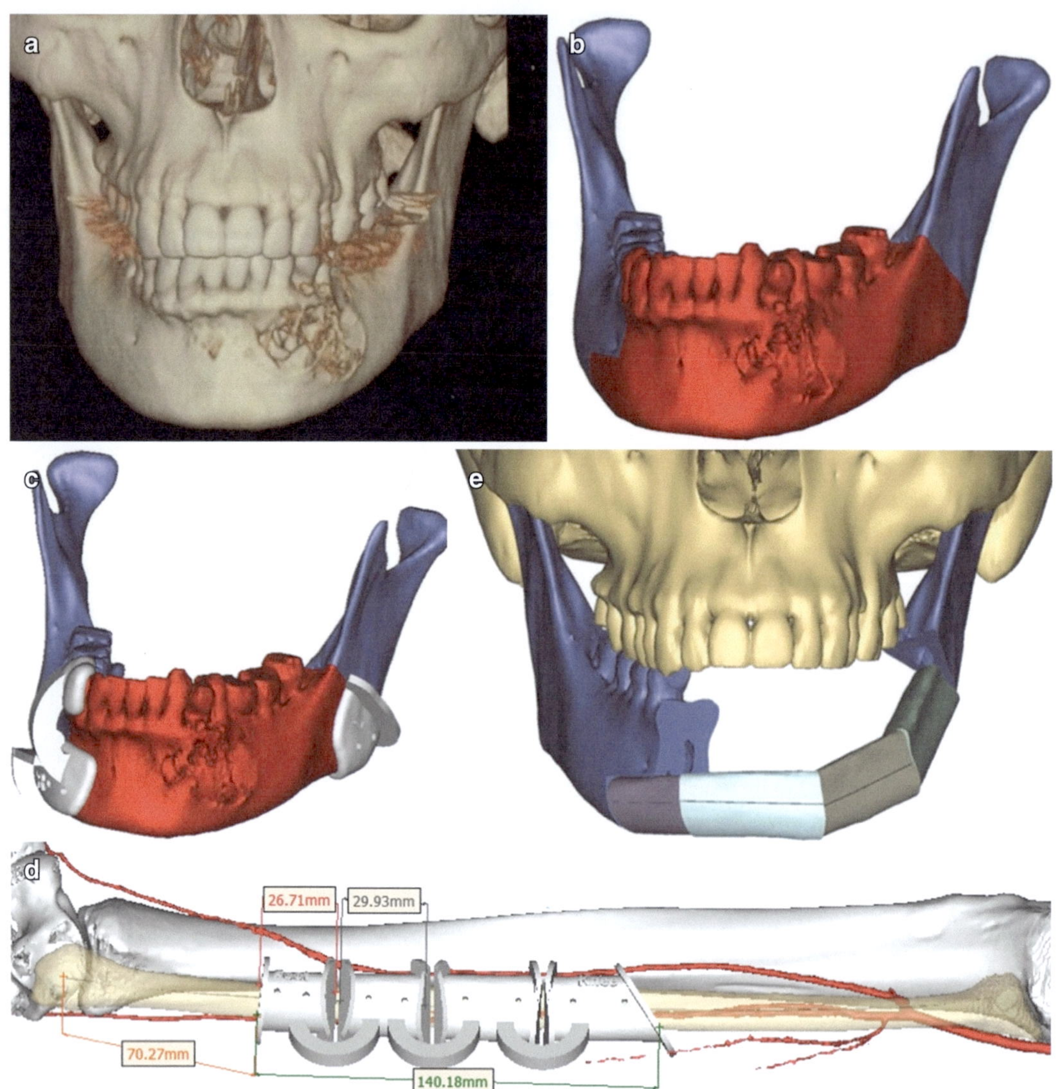

Fig. 7.1 Mandibular myxoma. Treatment with virtual surgical planning and reconstruction with microvascularized fibular flap. (**a**) Facial 3D CT. Multi-loculated left jaw image. (**b**) Facial 3D CT. Planned mandibular resection. (**c**) Facial 3D CT. Planned mandibular resection with cutting guides. (**d**) Leg 3D CT. Fibula cutting guides for jaw reconstruction. (**e**) Facial 3D CT. Planned final result. (**f**) Intraoperative image. Planned mandibular resection by intraoral approach. (**g**) Intraoperative image. Surgical specimen. (**h**) Intraoperative image. 3D model of cutting guides on fibula. (**i**) Intraoperative image. Fibula modeled as planned with the fixation plate. Pedicle still non-sectioned. (**j**) Facial 3D CT. Postoperative result with the fibula reconstructing the jaw. (**k**) Clinical image. Dental implants insetting for oral rehabilitation. (**l**) Clinical image. Vestibuloplasty and skin graft to improve periimplant tissue. (**m**) OPG. Final result. (**n**) Clinical image. Final result with prosthesis implant supported for oral rehabilitation

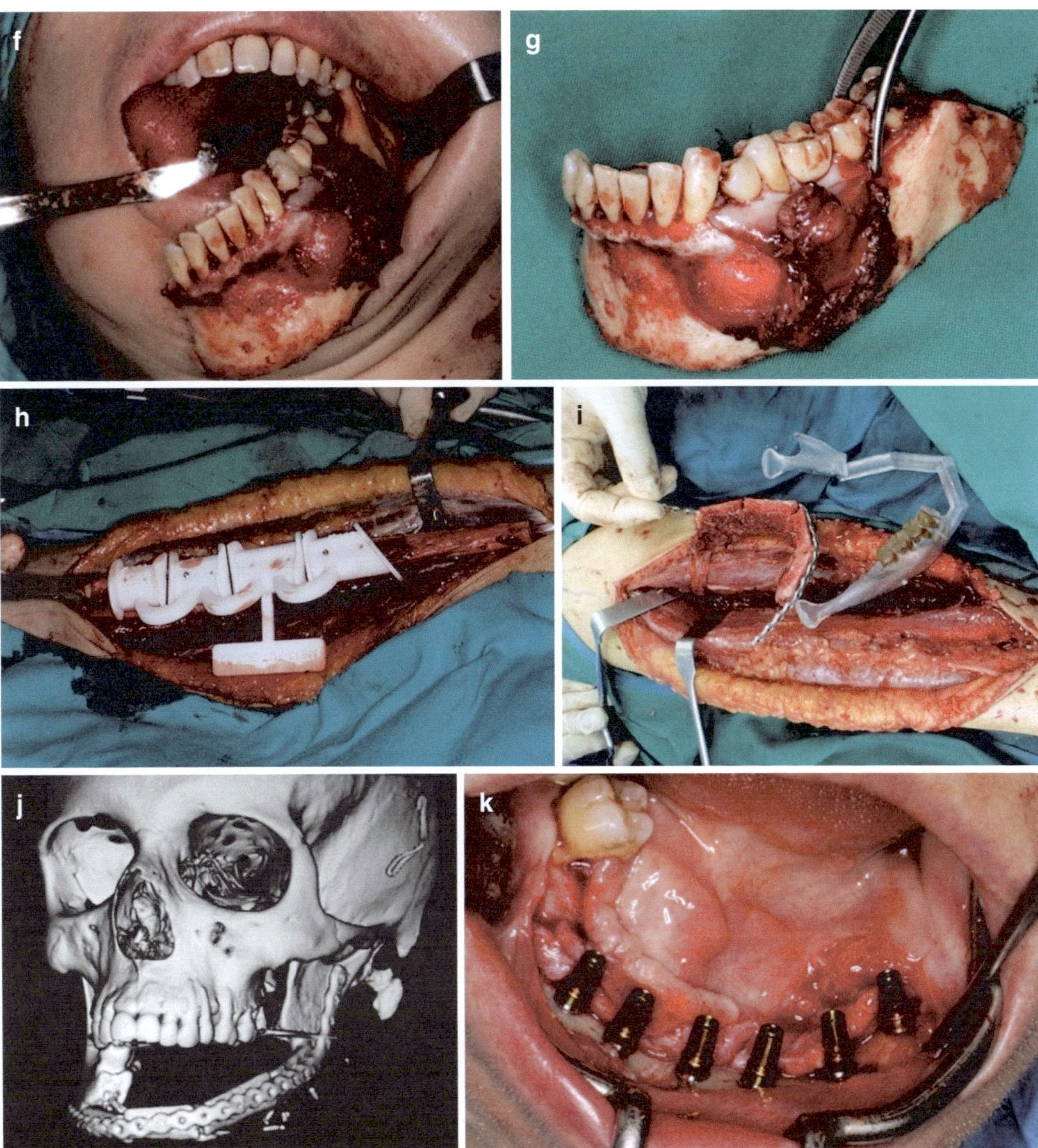

Fig. 7.1 (continued)

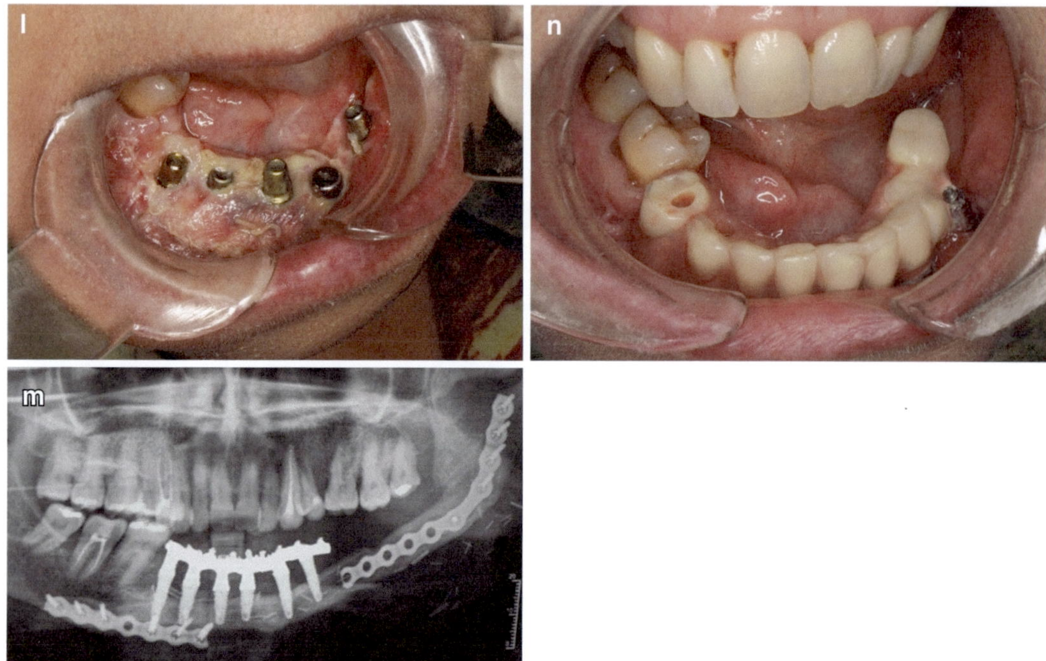

Fig. 7.1 (continued)

patient can be highlighted as one major advance related to the use of this technology. As described by Hirsch et al. [16], the cutting guides are designed for the mandibular resection and for the design and execution of the fibular osteotomies. After the virtual osteotomies are performed, the cutting guides are manufactured including slots delimiting the appropriate lengths along the mandible and the osseous flap in order to achieve an accurate bone alignment in the neomandible with minimal need for adjustments from the preoperative plan. Some articles have estimated the variability between the ablation phase and the bone reconstruction within the range of 1.5–2.5 mm in comparison with the preoperative surgical plan [17–19]. The accuracy of the reconstruction in terms of excellent apposition of bone segments and occlusion stability was confirmed by superimposing the preop CT scan with a postoperative CT scan.

Another major benefit of the preop VSP with CAD-CAM is the reduction in flap ischemia time attributed to the possibility of performing the shape of the fibula flap and fixing the reconstruction plate prior to pedicle división [20]. In a systematic review and meta-analysis accomplished by Tang et al. [21], VSP was associated with significantly decreased intraoperative time and ischemia of the flap reducing the number of overall complications. Kääriäinen et al. [22] reported a mean ischemic time using CAD-CAM technology of 99 min in contrast with the 120–180 min when using the conventional techniques. Therefore, lengthy ischemic procedures lead to negative implications on flap outcomes with increased rates of partial flap loss.

One of the major drawbacks with the CAD-CAM technology could potentially be if a necessity of changing the surgical plan arises

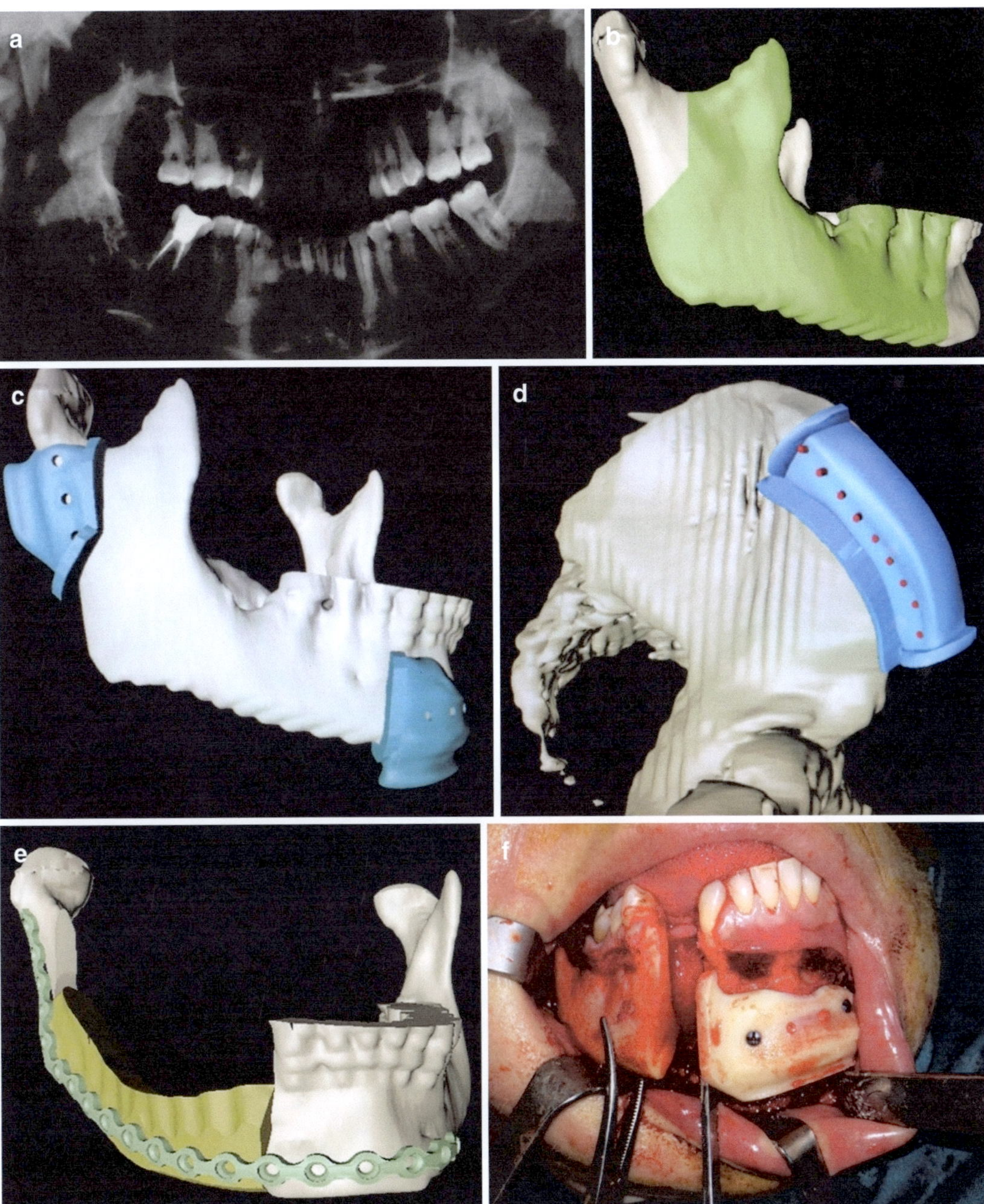

Fig. 7.2 Mandibular ameloblastoma. Treatment with virtual surgery planning and reconstruction with microvascularized iliac crest flap. (**a**) OPG. Ameloblastoma. Osteolytic right mandibular lesion. (**b**) Facial 3D CT. Planned jaw resection. (**c**) Facial 3D CT. Planned mandibular resection with cutting guides. (**d**) Iliac CT. Cutting guides designed in the iliac crest for mandibular reconstruction. (**e**) Planned final result. (**f**) Intraoperative image. Mandibular resection by a combined intraoral and conservative lateral cervicofacial approach. (**g**) Intraoperative image. Surgical specimen. (**h**) Intraoperative image. Cutting guides placed on iliac crest. (**i**) Intraoperative image. Iliac crest flap placed as planned for mandibular reconstruction. (**j**) Facial 3D CT. Postoperative result with the iliac crest flap reconstructing the jaw. (**k**) Clinical image. Dental implants insetting for oral rehabilitation. (**l**) OPG. Final result. (**m**) Clinical image. Final result. Oral rehabilitation with implant supported prosthesis. (**n**) Postoperative intraoral image. Patient occlusion

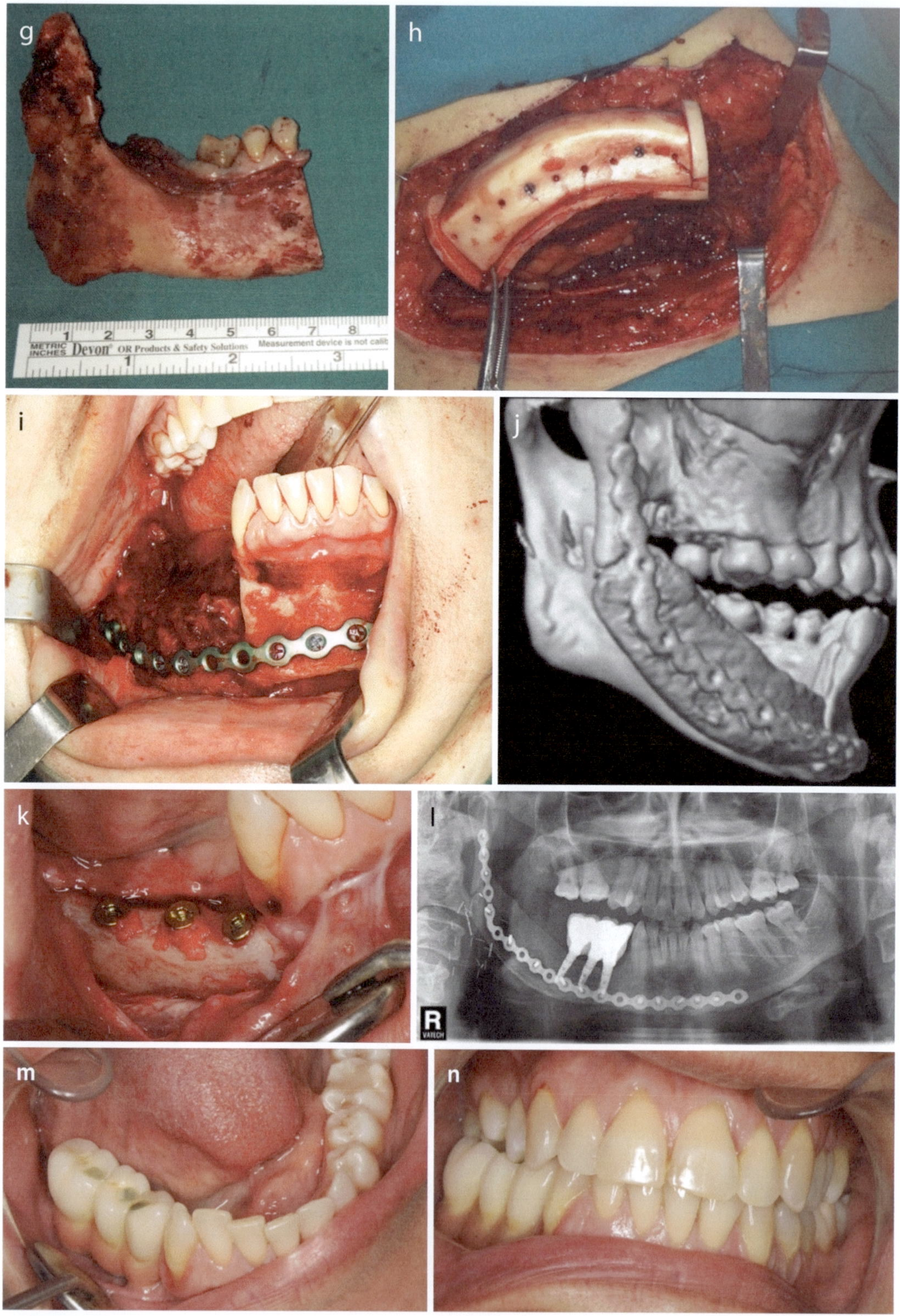

Fig. 7.2 (continued)

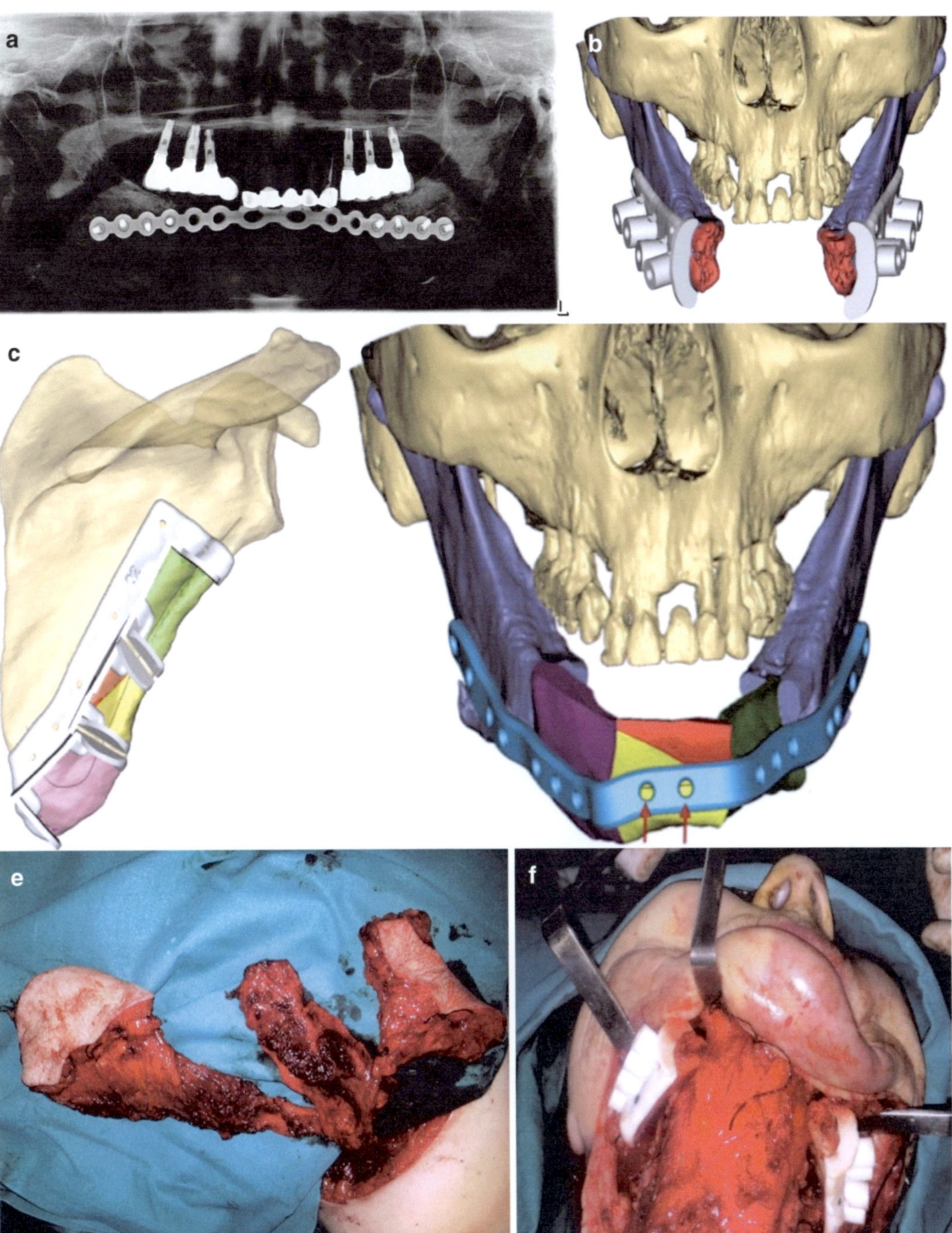

Fig. 7.3 Secondary mandibular reconstruction. Treatment with virtual surgical planning and reconstruction with microvascularized scapular flap. (**a**) OPG showing secondary anterior mandibular defect after squamous cell carcinoma resection. Bridging plate exposed. (**b**) Facial 3D CT. Planned mandibular preparation with cutting guides. (**c**) Scapular 3D CT. Cutting guides on scapula for mandibular reconstruction. (**d**) Facial 3D CT. Planned final result. (**e**) Intraoperative image. Scapular flap. (**f**) Intraoperative image. Mandibular stumps exposure through a cervical approach. (**g**) Intraoperative image. Scapular flap harvesting with stereolithographic cutting guides. (**h**) Intraoperative image. Mandibular reconstruction with scapula flap as planned. (**i**) Clinical image. Final result

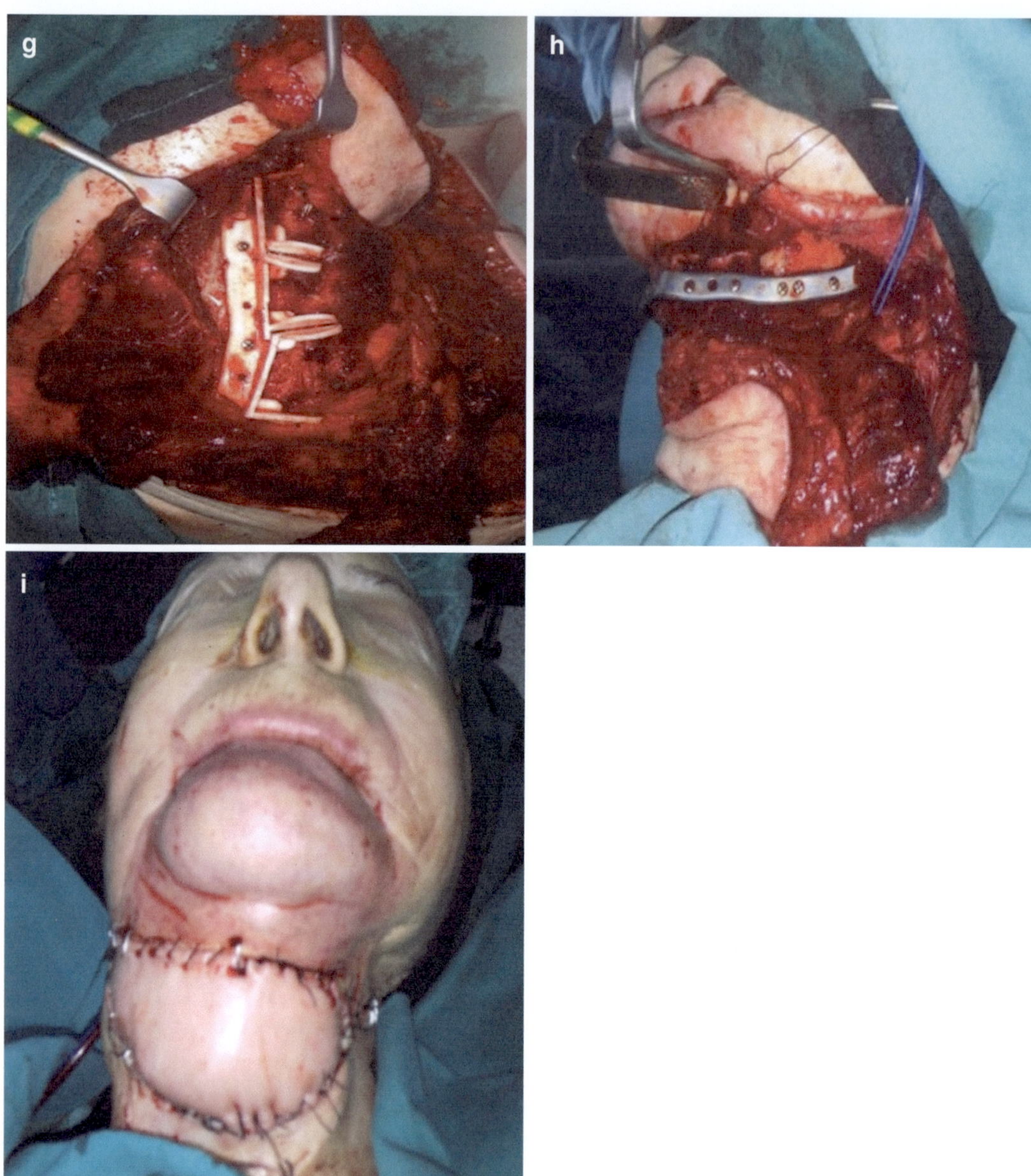

Fig. 7.3 (continued)

intraoperatively during the mandibular resection procedure. During VSP the limits of the tumor are visualized on the 3D model and the length of bone resection is planned [23]. The boundaries of mandibular involvement in cancer or osteoradio-necrosis (ORN) resection are estimated preoperatively by the clinical examination, CT and/or MRI and may differ during surgery. Also, due to a rapid cancer growth or a delay between the pre-operative diagnostic and planning procedures and surgery, intraoperatively a bigger resection could be considered. Intraoperative histologic techniques to check the resection margins are currently being researched [24, 25]. Namin et al. [24] found a 12% of patients (6 of 51) with cancer positive findings on intraoperative bone marrow cytologic evaluation beyond the margins of the original bone resection because of occult cancellous tumor bone invasion after the mandibulectomy. This high rate of bone invasion wouldn't had been detected if only preoperative imaging without intraoperative cytologic evaluation had been performed. According to the oncological guidelines, tumor-free margins of at least 10 mm of erosive bone defects are required. Patel et al. [26] reported a difference of 45% in 5-year disease-specific survival between patients with and without positive bony margins and stressed the importance of clear bony margins in SCCa of mandible.

This condition can force to modify the size of mandibular resection during the surgery and leads the prototyped and/or prefabricated surgical devices (cutting guides and prebent reconstructive plate) to be inadequate for reconstruction with the consequent loss of money and suboptimal outcomes in functional, aesthetic, and locoregional control of tumor. Ramella et al. [27] introduced the concept of "triple-cut CAD-CAM" planning that consists in manufacturing customized osteotomies cutting guides for the mandible and the donor bone (usually fibula) that includes different cutting levels (3 per side and distances from 5 to 10 mm) to change the osteotomy dimensions planified preoperatively according to the histologic bone margins found during the surgery and adapt the reconstructive plate to different scenarios. This modification in the polyamide osteotomy guide by inserting two additional cutting levels on each side, permits two additional mandibular resections from 5 to 10 mm wide until tumor-free margins are obtained and in accordance with this, modified the size of the fibula segment for reconstruction while maintaining the prefabricated CAD-CAM reconstructive plate.

The increment of production costs with the use of preoperative CT guided planning and manufacturing prebent reconstruction plates and osteotomy guides, has been criticized. This negative point of additional expense is clearly offset by predictability of surgical outcome, decreased ischemia time and total intraoperative time that minimize the rates of flap failure, general medical complications, and patients morbidity while increasing operative efficiency [12, 28, 29]. In-house 3D printing can contribute to minimize expenses through the "low cost" production of models which can aid to study the case and to shape preoperatively standard fixation plates although patient-specific implants cannot be developed.

7.4 New Perspectives

VSP with CAD-CAM and surgical navigation have become currently a "gold standard" method applied in complex craniomaxillofacial reconstruction not only in mandibular reconstruction but in other areas as reviewed in this book, such as head and neck mid-facial oncologic resection and reconstruction, orthognathic surgery, maxillofacial trauma, TMJ reconstruction, and skull base surgery. The benefits of this new technology are well noticed in terms of improving surgical accuracy, shortening of ischemia and total surgical time, and decreasing operative costs and complications in comparison with the traditional (handmade) technique [10, 14, 30].

However, in oncologic reconstruction including soft tissues and some cases of maxillofacial trauma, especially when free composite flaps are needed, missing dots are identified in virtual and surgical phases of computer-aided mandibular reconstruction like the possibility of an accurate soft tissue resection and reconstruction planning. Software that could include the soft tissue in the 3D model should be available in order to better define the vascular pedicles, the different components of the free flap including skin, intermuscular septum, bone, muscle, location of the nutrient vessels supplying the osteoseptocutaneous skin paddle to set the right position of the osteotomies without jeopardizing the vascularization. Also the cross-section topography of bone to determine the ideal bone segment for dental implants and surgical plan flexibility should be better defined. All this points are important issues to be considered in future software programs [31].

7.5　Surgical Navigation in Mandibular Reconstruction

Intraoperative navigation has improved the accuracy of maxillofacial reconstruction as well as preventing damage from vital structures in complex reconstructions. Neurosurgery was the first discipline to adopt intraoperative navigation for the technology's ability to minimize trauma and surgical damage to the brain [32, 33]. In recent years, surgical navigation systems have been widely used in clinical practice as an outcome of medical imaging and image processing technologies in the medical field [34]. The basic principles on which intraoperative navigation is based are widely described in the surgical navigation chapter, focusing this chapter on the importance of the application of navigation in mandibular reconstruction.

Navigation has improved the reliability and results in maxillofacial reconstruction, providing real-time information to the surgeon. Recent studies reported the reliability and precision of surgical navigation applied to maxillary resection and reconstruction although navigation technology is not so frequently applied to mandibular surgery. As mentioned previously in this chapter, one of the greatest challenges in mandibular reconstruction is to accurately shape and fix vascularized bone flaps so that the symmetry and function of the face are restored optimally. The problem of the use of intraoperative navigation in the surgical treatment of the mandible is that it is a moving structure. In order to perform the navigation of lower jaw, three methods have been described according to the literature. The first is based on the use of maxillo-mandibular fixation to immobilize the jaw. The second and most used is based on the centric occlusion of the teeth by using special templates or dental splits in order to attach the lower jaw to the skull to control mobility. The jaw is placed in a reproducible position that allows its synchronization. A third method is to install a special square sensor on the jaw, thereby allowing surgeons to track the position of the mandible optically and to compensate for its continuous movement during surgery [35]. Intraoperative navigation has been proposed combined with or as an alternative method to the use of CAD/CAM 3D printed cutting guides in mandibular reconstruction with free flaps. This method provides another means to ensure operative planning success if 3D printing is not available, too time consuming, or cost prohibitive [36] (Fig. 7.4).

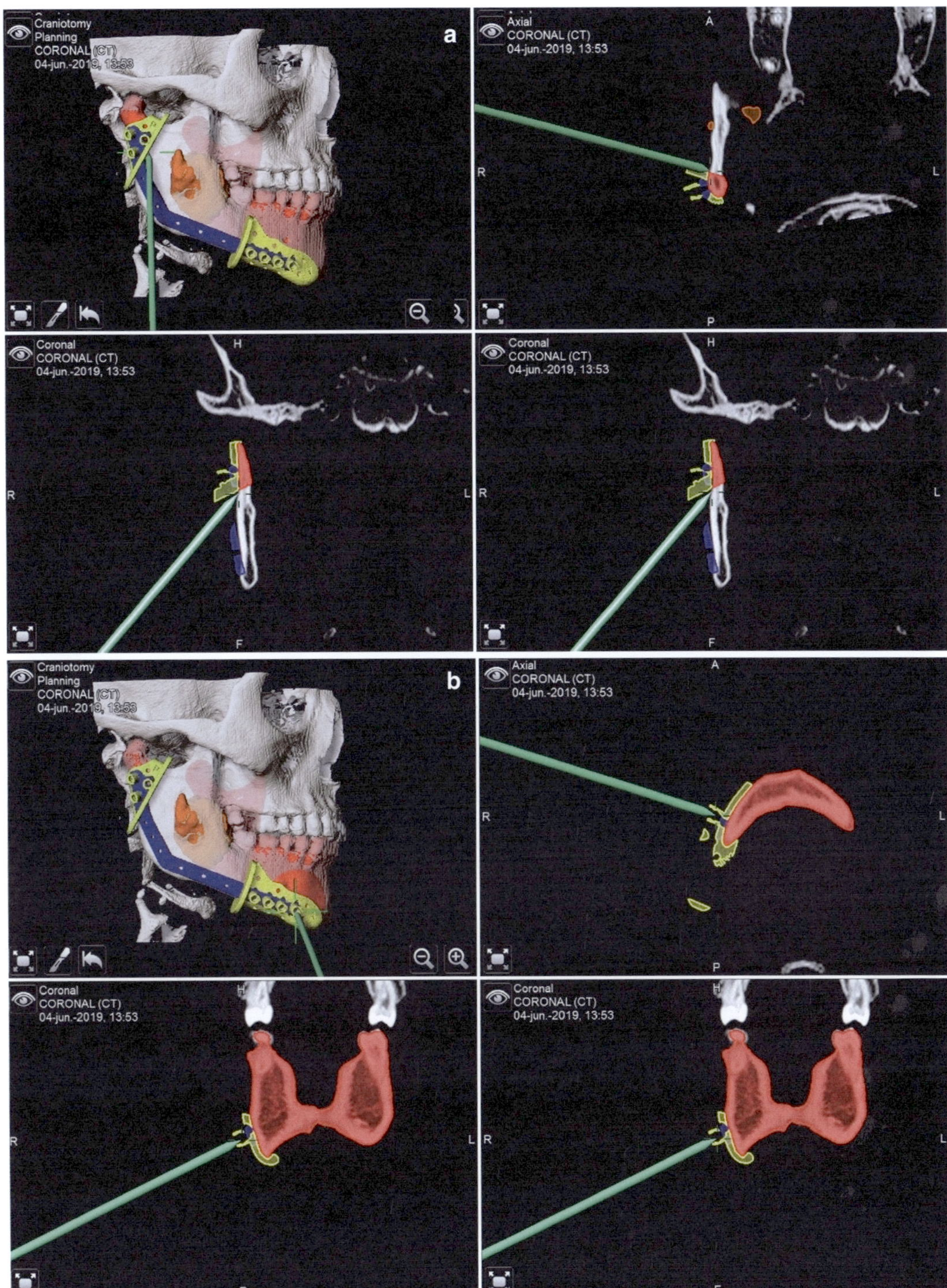

Fig. 7.4 Surgical navigation in mandibular reconstruction in a patient with mandibular ameloblastoma. (**a**) Surgical navigation. Navigating the mandibular cutting lines with overlapping STL files. (**b**) Surgical navigation. Navigating the location of osteosynthesis screws

References

1. Goh BT, Lee S, Tideman H, Stoelinga PJ. Mandibular reconstruction in adults. A review. Int J Oral Maxillofac Surg. 2008;37:597–605.
2. Hidalgo D. Fibula free flap: a new method of mandible reconstruction. Plast Reconstr Surg. 1989;84:71–9.
3. Taylor GI. Reconstruction of the mandible with free composite iliac bone grafts. Ann Plast Surg. 1982;9:361–76.
4. Gilbert A, Teot L. The free scapula flap. Plast Reconstr Surg. 1982;69:601.
5. Okay D, Al Shetawi AH, Moubayed SP, Mourad M, Buchbinder D, Urken ML. Worldwide 10-years systematic review of treatment trends in fibula free flap for mandibular reconstruction. J Oral Maxillofac Surg. 2016;74:2526–31.
6. Wang YY, Zhang HQ, Fan S, Zhang DM, Huang ZQ, Chen WL, Ye JT, Li JS. Mandibular reconstruction with the vascularized fibula flap: comparison of virtual planning surgery and conventional surgery. Int J Oral Maxillofac Surg. 2016;45:1400–5.
7. Witjes MJH, Schepers RH, Kraeima J. Impact of virtual planning on reconstruction of mandibular and maxillary surgical defects in head and neck oncology. Curr Opin Otolaryngol Head Neck Surg. 2018;26:108–14.
8. Marchetti C, Bianchi A, Mazzoni S, Cipriani R, Campobassi A. Oromandibular reconstruction using a fibula osteocutaneous free flap: four different preplating techniques. Plast Reconstr Surg. 2006;118:643–51.
9. Valentini V, Agrillo A, Battisti A, Gennaro P, Calabrese L, Iannetti G. Surgical planning in reconstruction of mandibular defect with fibula free flap: 15 patients. J Craniofac Surg. 2005;16(4):601–7.
10. Rodby KA, Turin S, Jacobs RJ, Cruz JF, Hassid VJ, Kolokythas A, Antony AK. Advances in oncologic head and neck reconstruction: systematic review and future considerations of virtual surgical planning and computer aided design/computer aided modeling. J Plast Reconstr Aesthet Surg. 2014;67(9):1171–85.
11. Ciocca L, Marchetti C, Mazzoni S, Baldissara P, Gatto MR, Cipriani R, Scotti R, Tarsitano A. Accuracy of fibular sectioning and insertion into a rapid prototyped bone plate, for mandibular reconstruction using CAD-CAM technology. J Craniomaxillofac Surg. 2015;43(1):28–33.
12. Toto JM, Chang EI, Agag R, Devarajan K, Patel SA, Topham NS. Improved operative efficiency of free fibula flap mandible reconstruction with patient specific, computer-guided preoperative planning. Head Neck. 2015;37(11):1660–4.
13. Antony AK, Chen WF, Kolokythas A, Weimer KA, Cohen MN. Use of virtual surgery and stereolithography-guided osteotomy for mandibular reconstruction with the free fibula. Plast Reconstr Surg. 2011;128(5):1080–4.
14. Sharaf B, Levine JP, Hirsch DL, Bastidas JA, Schiff BA, Garfein ES. Importance of computer-aided design and manufacturing technology in the multidisciplinary approach to head and neck reconstruction. J Craniofac Surg. 2010;21(4):1277–80.
15. Sink J, Hamlar D, Kademani D, Khariwala SS. Computer-aided stereolithography for presurgical planning in fibula free tissue reconstruction of the mandible. J Reconstr Microsurg. 2012;28(6):395–403.
16. Hirsch DL, Garfein ES, Christensen AM, Weimer KA, Saddeh PB, Levine JP. Use of computer-aided design and computer-aided manufacturing to produce orthognathically ideal surgical outcomes: a paradigm shift in head and neck reconstruction. J Oral Maxillofac Surg. 2009;67(10):2115–22.
17. Yu H, Wang X, Zhang S, Zhang L, Xin P, Shen SG. Navigation-guided en bloc resection and defect reconstruction of craniomaxillary bony tumours. Int J Oral Maxillofac Surg. 2013;42(11):1409–13.
18. Wilde F, Hanken H, Probst F, Schramm A, Heiland M, Cornelius CP. Multicenter study on the use of patient-specific CAD/CAM reconstruction plates for mandibular reconstruction. Int J Comput Assist Radiol Surg. 2015;10(12):2035–51.
19. Schepers RH, Raghoebar GM, Vissink A, Stenekes MW, Kraeima J, Roodenburg JL, Reintsema H, Witjes MJ. Accuracy of fibula reconstruction using patient-specific CAD/CAM reconstruction plates and dental implants: a new modality for functional reconstruction of mandibular defects. J Craniomaxillofac Surg. 2015;43(5):649–57.
20. Rustemeyer J, Sari-Rieger A, Melenberg A, Busch A. Comparison of intraoperative time measurements between osseous reconstructions with free fibula flaps applying computer-aided designed/computer-aided manufactured and conventional techniques. Oral Maxillofac Surg. 2015;19(3):293–300.
21. Tang NSJ, Ahmadi I, Ramakrishnan A. Virtual surgical planning in fibula free flap head and neck reconstruction: a systematic review and meta-analysis. J Plast Reconstr Aesthet Surg. 2019;72(9):1465–77.
22. Kääriäinen M, Kuuskeri M, Gremoutis G, Kuokkanen H, Miettinen A, Laranne J. Utilization of three-dimensional computer-aided preoperative virtual planning and manufacturing in maxillary and mandibular reconstruction with a microvascular fibula flap. J Reconstr Microsurg. 2016;32(2):137–41.
23. Kraeima J, Schepers RH, van Ooijen PM, Steenbakkers RJ, Roodenburg JL, Witjes MJ. Integration of oncologic margins in three-dimensional virtual planning for head and neck surgery, including a validation of the software pathway. J Craniomaxillofac Surg. 2015;43(8):1374–9.
24. Namin AW, Bruggers SD, Panuganti BA, Christopher KM, Walker RJ, Varvares MA. Efficacy of bone marrow cytologic evaluations in detecting occult cancellous invasion. Laryngoscope. 2015;125(5):E173–9.
25. Bilodeau EA, Chiosea S. Oral squamous cell carcinoma with mandibular bone invasion: intraoperative

evaluation of bone margins by routine frozen section. Head Neck Pathol. 2011;5(3):216–20.

26. Patel RS, Dirven R, Clark JR, Swinson BD, Gao K, O'Brien CJ. The prognostic impact of extent of bone invasion and extent of bone resection in oral carcinoma. Laryngoscope. 2008;118(5):780–5.

27. Ramella V, Franchi A, Bottosso S, Tirelli G, Novati FC, Arnež ZM. Triple-cut computer-aided design-computer-aided modeling: more oncologic safety added to precise mandible modeling. J Oral Maxillofac Surg. 2017;75(7):1567.e1–6.

28. Chang SY, Huang JJ, Tsao CK, Nguyen A, Mittakanti K, Lin CY, Cheng MH. Does ischemia time affect the outcome of free fibula flaps for head and neck reconstruction? A review of 116 cases. Plast Reconstr Surg. 2010;126(6):1988–95.

29. Offodile AC II, Aherrera A, Wenger J, Rajab TK, Guo L. Impact of increasing operative time on the incidence of early failure and complications following free tissue transfer? A risk factor analysis of 2,008 patients from the ACS-NSQIP database. Microsurgery. 2017;37(1):12–20.

30. Avraham T, Franco P, Brecht LE, Ceradini DJ, Saadeh PB, Hirsch DL, Levine JP. Functional outcomes of virtually planned free fibula flap reconstruction of the mandible. Plast Reconstr Surg. 2014;134(4):628e–34e.

31. Deek NF, Wei FC. Computer-assisted surgery for segmental mandibular reconstruction with the osteoseptocutaneous fibula flap: can we instigate ideological and technological reforms? Plast Reconstr Surg. 2016;137(3):963–70.

32. Shan XF, Chen HM, Liang J, Huang JW, Zhang L, Cai ZG, Guo C. Surgical navigation-assisted mandibular reconstruction with fibula flaps. Int J Oral Maxillofac Surg. 2016;45:448–53.

33. Wu J, Sun J, Shen SG, Xu B, Li J, Zhang S. Computer-assisted navigation: its role in intraoperatively accurate mandibular reconstruction. Oral Surg Oral Med Oral Pathol Oral Radiol. 2016;122(2):134–42.

34. Suchyta M, Mardini S. Innovations and future directions in head and neck microsurgical reconstruction. Clin Plast Surg. 2017;44(2):325–44.

35. Shen SY, Yu Y, Zhang WB, Liu XJ, Peng X. Angle-to-angle mandibular defect reconstruction with fibula flap by using a mandibular fixation device and surgical navigation. J Craniofac Surg. 2017;28(6):1486–91.

36. Abbate V, Orabona GDA, Solari D, Bonavolontà P, Iaconetta G, Califano L. Mandibular surgical navigation: an innovative guiding method. J Craniofac Surg. 2017;28(8):2122–6.

Advances and Innovations in Reconstruction of the Maxilla and Midface Utilizing Computer-Assisted Surgery: Technology, Principal Consideration, and Clinical Implementation

Majeed Rana and Max Wilkat

8.1 Introduction: Defects of the Maxilla

Defects of the maxilla and the midface have a spectrum of etiologies. Besides trauma and congenital deformities, neoplasia in need of resection are the most common causes [1]. These defects are accompanied by several impairments in function and aesthetics [2]. With the loss of the maxilla there is an oroantral communication which makes the normal act of swallowing impossible. With the loss of the upper teeth speaking and chewing is impaired. Without the boney support of the maxilla the midface especially the upper lip and the cheek area is hollow, patients are disfigured impairing their social life and contact behavior up to psychological illnesses. For these reasons a reconstruction "true to original" is an objective to strive for in the treatment of defects of the maxilla and the midface.

A classical approach to rehabilitation is the manufacturing of a defect prosthesis [3]. Via impression taking a model of the resection cave is produced which serves for the manufacturing process of an obturator to close the oroantral communication after resection of the maxilla. The obturator can be extended into a defect prosthesis after settlement of the wound conditions. The production process is well established, widespread available and in particular involves a containable expenditure and a comparatively small exertion for the patient. Disadvantageously, defect prosthesis might suffer from a bad retention depending on the individual anatomy of the resection cave and remaining neighboring teeth, thereby limiting oroantral seal, chewing abilities and patients' comfort. That's why this mode of rehabilitation should be limited to the elderly, severely ill, or palliative patients who could not bear elaborated reconstruction surgery [3].

The more superior restoration of maxillary defects aiming for results closer to "restitutio ad integrum" rather than "restitutio ad reparationem" is nowadays provided by reconstruction with autogenous tissue [4]. Small defects can be covered with local tissue in form of pedicled flaps such as buccinator or temporalis flap [5]. Large defects need to be treated by transplantation of autologous microvascular grafts to restore the lost hard and soft tissues [6, 7]. The introduction of computer-assisted surgery facilitates these extensive tissue transplantations and offers a precision unknown until then allowing a reconstruction

M. Rana (✉) · M. Wilkat
Department of Craniomaxillofacial Surgery,
University Hospital Düsseldorf, Heinrich Heine
University (HHU), Düsseldorf, Germany
e-mail: rana@med.uni-duesseldorf.de;
max.wilkat@med.uni-duesseldorf.de

© Springer Nature Switzerland AG 2021
J. Acero (ed.), *Innovations and New Developments in Craniomaxillofacial Reconstruction*,
https://doi.org/10.1007/978-3-030-74322-2_8

"true to original" within an even shorter surgery duration [8–11].

Surgical reconstruction can be performed primarily, which is always to favor, if the underlying disease allows it. Secondary reconstruction is applicable as well, for example in cases of defects after ablative tumor surgery of an infiltrative expanding, locally advanced malignancy and still pending of final pathohistological results regarding R0-status. However, in cases of impaired dimension of the midface after resection of the zygomatic bone or lost support of the bulbus after resection of the orbital floor one should reconstruct primarily—at least temporarily preserving the dimensions of the lost structures via application of PSIs until complete reconstruction via tissue transfer can be performed.

8.2 Virtual Planning

Three-dimensional virtual surgical planning (3DVSP) is based upon three-dimensional imaging data sets of computed tomography (CT) and magnetic resonance imaging (MRI) of the defect site as well as a CT angiography of the graft harvest site. While CT scans offer a high resolution of the hard tissue as well as the soft tissues, MRI scans can depict soft tissues even better. New software applications allow matching the data sets to combine the advantages of both imaging techniques enhancing the image quality. On the basis of these 3D data sets, virtual planning of resection and reconstruction can take place (Figs. 8.1 and 8.2). As discussed in other chapters, firstly, segmentation of the local bone and neighboring anatomical structures is performed visualizing the defect size as well as the needed bone graft as a three-dimensional object. Segmentation steps can be carried out semi-automatic saving time for the surgeon during planning procedure [12]. On the basis of this planning, the suitable kind of microvascular graft can be chosen and virtually be transplanted. During this step the intersegmental cutting of the graft to suit the defect size can already be per-

formed. The unaffected side can serve as a template during virtual reconstruction to achieve a facial symmetry and can easily be mirrored to the defect site [13, 14].

The use of virtual planning also helps to simulate an accurate dental alignment and prosthodontic rehabilitation after tumor resection and reconstruction [15]. Through prosthodontic-driven backward planning, the original intermaxillary relationships and lateral and sagittal position of the maxilla can be reproduced. In this way, the virtually reconstructed bony segments are placed in a position that later facilitate dental implant insertion and a correct occlusion for full dental rehabilitation.

In the virtual planning phase, all aspects for a reconstruction "true to original" come into consideration and all available solutions can be exercised completely non-invasive and without wasting valuable surgery time leading to the best possible result for the patient. Virtual planning can be demonstrated to the patient and with the help of virtual reality devices patient education might be even more vivid and comprehensible in future leading to full transparency of therapy plans for the patient [16, 17].

8.3 CAD/CAM of Patient-Specific Implants (PSI)

The traditional process of free-handed intraoperative plate bending and segment fixation is time consuming, unprecise and prone to errors. The use of computer-aided design/computer-aided manufacturing (CAD/CAM) techniques may aid the surgeon to efficiently and accurately perform 3D reconstructions [18, 19].

A good pre-surgical virtual planning and design of the patient-specific implants has numerous advantages over the traditional methods [20]. The PSI is designed in a way that the tumor resection boundaries are directly coded on the reconstruction plate. This eliminates the use of additional resection guides, which can be cumbersome to place and may lead to inaccuracies in

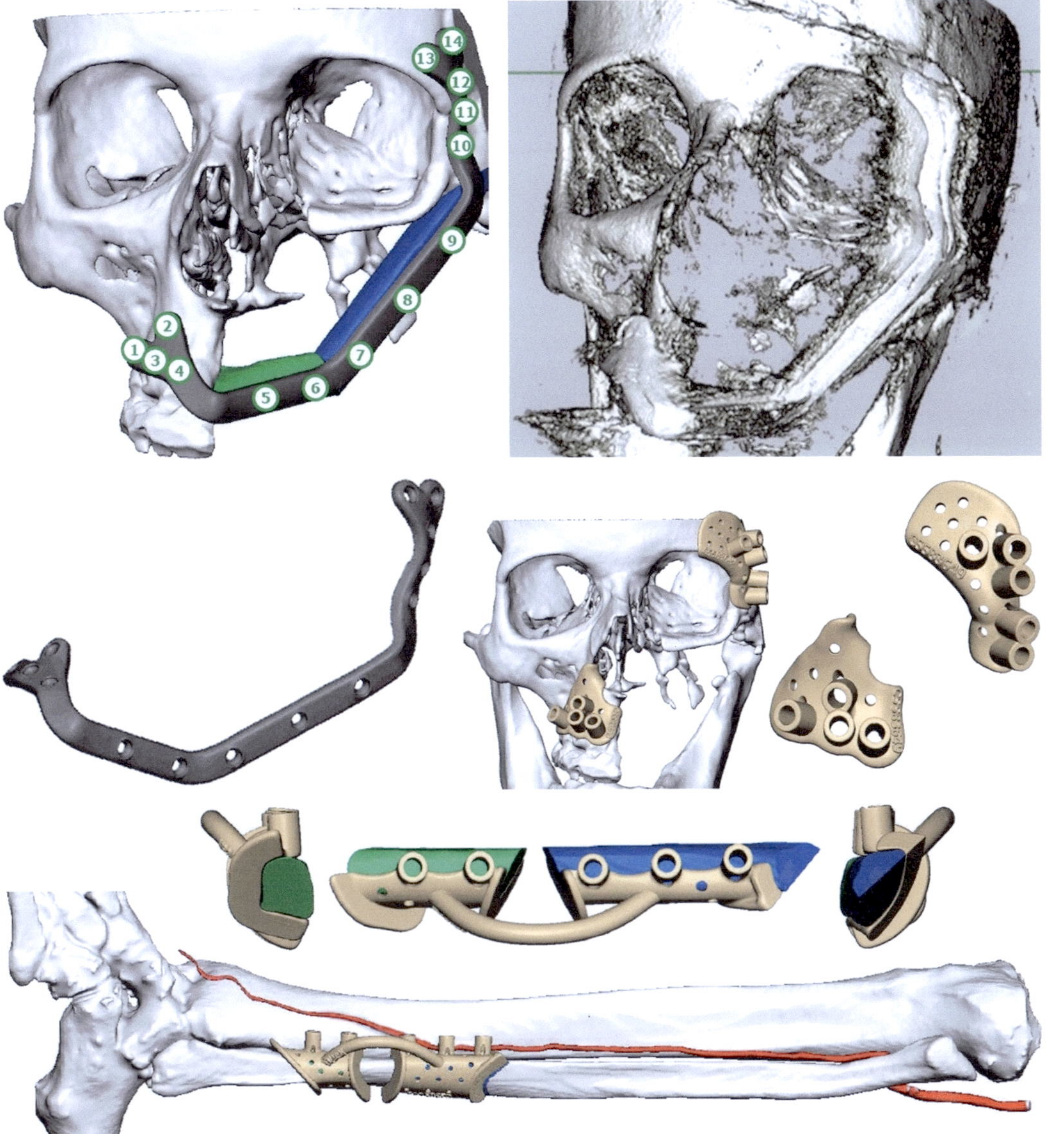

Fig. 8.1 Complete set for computer-assisted secondary reconstruction of the left maxilla with free fibula flap. During the virtual reconstruction, two segments (green and blue) of the distal fibula have been transferred to restore the maxillary arch and the crista zygomaticoalveolaris on the left side. The left orbital floor has been reconstructed before using a patient-specific implant made of titanium. For graft fixation at the recipient site, a patient-specific reconstruction plate has been designed with 14 screw holes. For each of the 14 screw holes, a suitable screw of defined length and diameter is designated for bicortical fixation at the skull and monocortical fixation at the fibula segments. Two drill guides define the positioning of the screw holes for the PSI at the anterior right maxilla and the left upper lateral orbital rim. The harvesting guide includes cutting edges indicating the osteotomy lines and drill holes for the placement of screws in the harvested fibula segments. The main vessels of the lower limb are depicted in red. In the upper right a 3D-reconstruction of the datasets of a postoperative CT scan is depicted illustrating the reconstruction true to the virtual planning illustrated on the upper left

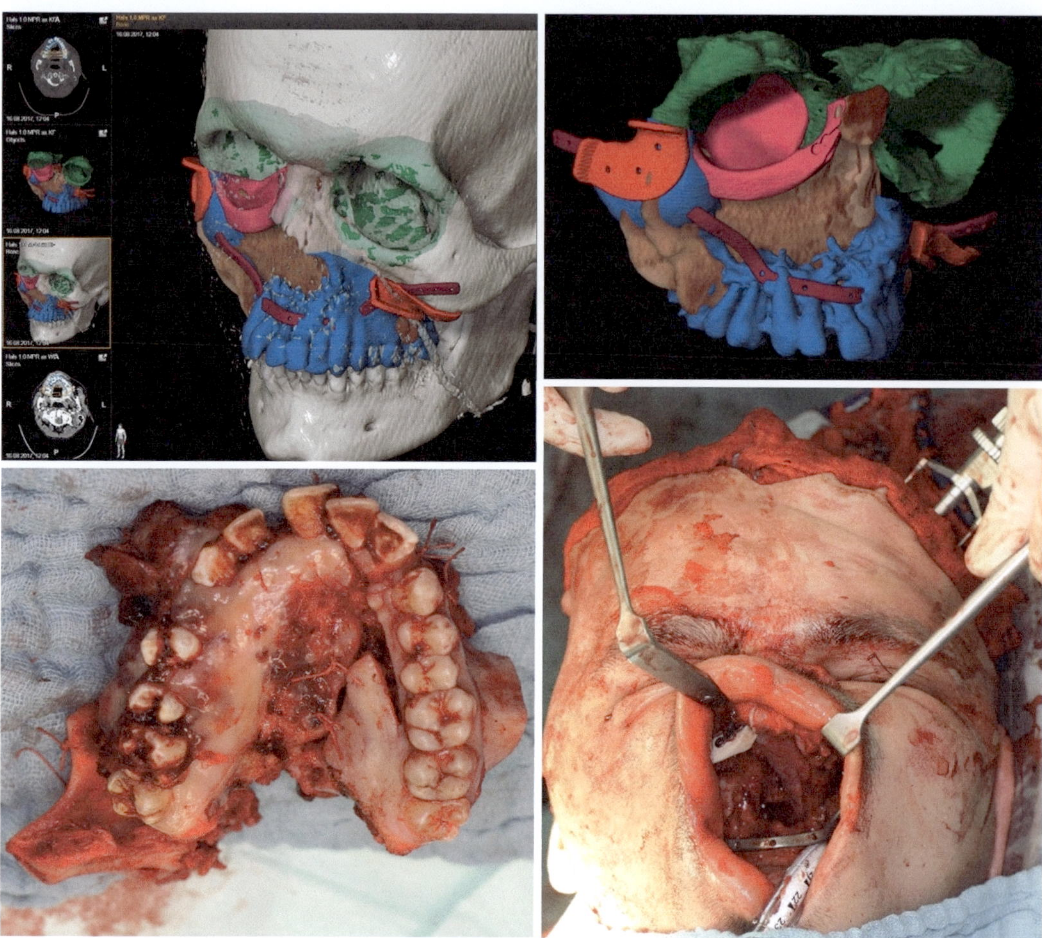

Fig. 8.2 Case of an advanced Ewing sarcoma of the right maxilla: resection virtual planning. Virtual planning allows the segmentation of volumes which define a pathophysiological, anatomical, or functional unit. The extent of the Ewing sarcoma involving the right and left maxilla, the right nasal cavity, and the right orbital floor is segmented in brown. The planned resection area is segmented in blue. The left and right orbita are segmented in green. Resection guides (red) are designed to fit at the resection borders at the right and left zygomatical bones. Along the segmented green right orbital floor a patient-specific PEEK implant (pink) is designed to reconstruct the orbital floor after resection. A reconstruction plate (purple) for preserving the sagittal dimension of the midface has been shaped to reach from the right to the left zygomatical bone for fixation after resection. The resection preparation is depicted in the lower left consisting of the complete maxilla with the right nasomaxillary and zygomaticomaxillary buttresses. The intraoperative situs after resection via transoral and bicoronal approach is illustrated in the lower right. Transorally visible, the PEEK implant and the reconstruction plate are already in place. A navigation tripod fixed to the upper left skull facilitates the matching of the virtual planning with the intraoperative situs via an infrared camera. This allows a navigated resection and an intraoperative control of the positioning of the PSIs

case that the tumor resection extends up to complex anatomical areas which is frequent in case of midfacial resections. Furthermore, the exact number, position, and angulation of the screw holes on the PSI can be determined [21, 22]. This is beneficial to obtain a good retention for the customized reconstruction plate but also to avoid interference with important anatomical structures such as the teeth. Designing the PSI-reconstructive plate in a "wrap-around"-fashion provides positioning guidance, perfect adaption and stability for the bony segments [23]. This is a crucial aspect, when comparing PSIs to traditional techniques, where intraoperative manual plate bending is an inevitable process that can be difficult and very time consuming. Frequent and extensive plate bending might be required in complex reconstructions, thus leading to mechanical weakness, decrease of strength and stability, and an increased risk of plate fracture in areas of high biomechanical loading. Finally, the use of virtual planning and PSIs eases the accurate fitting and fixation of the flap into the defect and therefore significantly reduces the ischemia time as compared to the traditional method [21, 24]. This has been shown in several comparative studies and is a powerful argument for its use, especially with less experienced microsurgeons.

The abovementioned virtual planning is exported as stereolithographic files (STL files format) and forwarded to the medical engineers to manufacture the individual cutting guides and the customized reconstruction plate/patient-specific implants (PSI) via selective laser melting (SLM). An example of a patient-specific reconstruction plate with drill guides is depicted in Fig. 8.1.

8.4 Microvascular Grafts Suitable for Computer-Assisted Reconstruction of the Maxilla

Surgical resections for conditions such as malignant and benign tumors, osteomyelitis, osteoradionecrosis, or medication-related osteonecrosis of the jaw (MRONJ) may result in complex maxillary defects. Adequate functional and aesthetic reconstruction of the maxilla usually requires microvascular free tissue transfer via fibula, iliac crest or scapula flaps [25, 26]. All of these three microvascular bone grafts are compatible with the workflow of computer-assisted surgery as presented above.

The primary goal is to restore the maxillary arch, facial support and masticatory function. This is achieved by reshaping and positioning of the osteotomized bone tissue of the flap in a way that the original position and outer contour of the maxilla can be re-established. The contour of the bony segments is maintained by fixation with mini-plates or a reconstruction plate which can be designed as a patient-specific implant according to the principles mentioned above. Based on angiography of the donor site, the ideal section of the donating bone is identified and virtually adjusted until it fits the defect and the original dental profile. Harvesting guides are designed and superimposed on the donor site to incorporate a maximum amount of cutaneous perforators on the skin island. Cutting edges in these guides are designed to indicate the planned osteotomy lines, drilling holes are added to facilitate the correct positioning of the reconstruction plate at the harvested bone segments even before the nutrifying vessels are cut, thereby shortening the ischemia time and overall surgery duration. Examples of harvesting guides are depicted in Fig. 8.3.

8.4.1 Free Fibula Flap

The free fibula flap (FFF) that can be harvested as osseous, myo-osseous, or osteo-cutaneous is considered a suitable graft for the reconstruction of segmental and composite maxillectomy defects [27–29]. Its versatility, predictability, shape, and good cortical bone quality favor its use for later dental implant placement and full oral rehabilitation [30]. Advantages of the fibula transplant over the iliac crest and the scapula lie in the longer segments available for harvesting allowing the reconstruction of a hole maxilla. Moreover, the long vessel pedicle eases the anastomosis at cervical vessels. Donor site morbidity is normally low and there are no serious impairments of the lower limb after surgery. Because of the distance between donor and recipient site, there is enough space for a two-team approach reducing surgery duration. A complete reconstruction plan with the needed PSI, drill and harvesting guides is illustrated in Fig. 8.1. A case of a 42-year-old male patient with a keratocyst of the right maxilla and computer-assisted secondary reconstruction with a fibula transplantation is depicted in Fig. 8.4a–c.

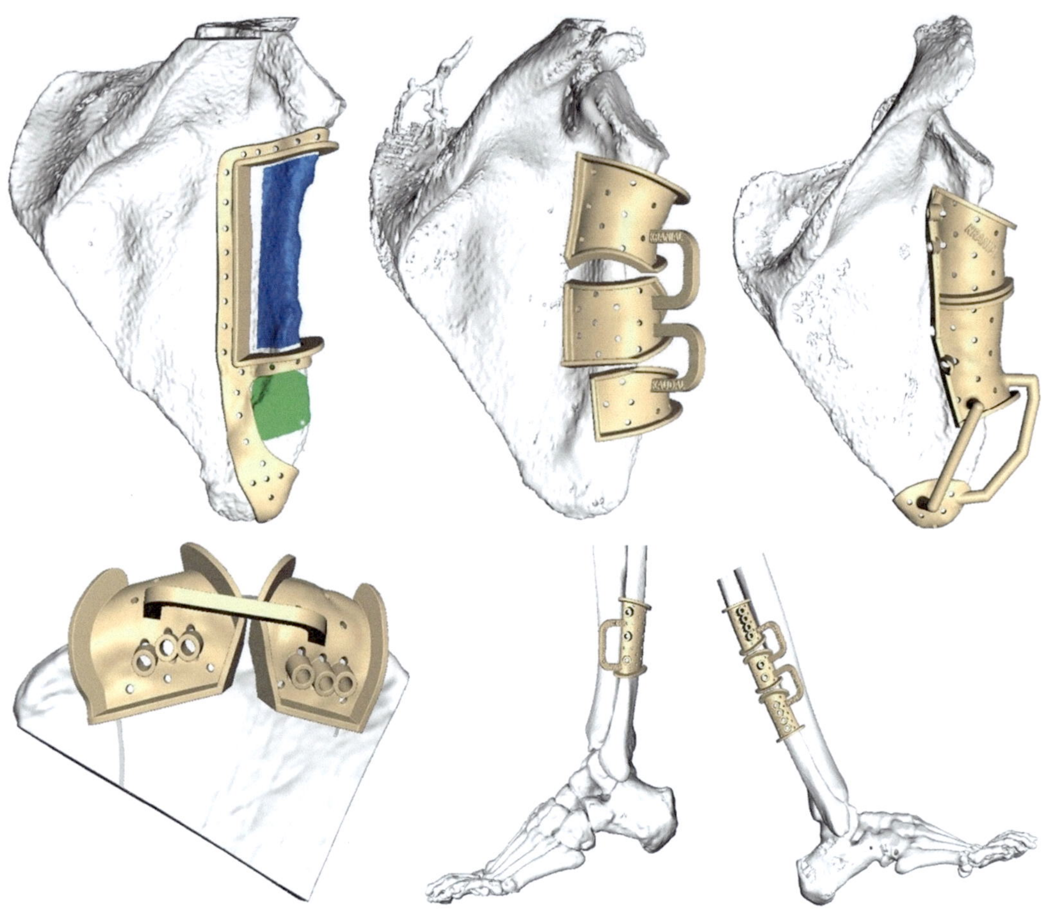

Fig. 8.3 Examples of different harvesting guides virtually designed for scapula (upper line), iliac crest (lower left), and fibula (lower right). After identifying the needed bone segments (single- or multi-segmental) at the donor site (colored in green and blue at a right scapula depicted in the upper left as an example), harvesting guides can be designed virtually. There are different shapes of harvesting guides individually fitted for the specific patient. Design of harvesting guides should include surfaces, landmarks and small drilling holes that ensure a secured and reproducible positioning, cutting edges along the desired osteotomy lines and guided drilling holes for later screw application that automatically fit the screw holes of the PSI

8.4.2　Microvascular Iliac Crest

The assets of a microvascular iliac crest transplantation are found in the good bone quality and geometrical height of the bone level which facilitates later implantation for dental rehabilitation [31–33]. On the downside of this graft, there is a limitation to the length, which does not offer the reconstruction of the full dental arch. Moreover, the anastomosis of the pedicle vessels is more intricate. First, pedicle vessels are shorter limiting the possibilities of anastomosis localizations. Second, the transplant can be harvested as a myo-osseous or myo-osteo-cutaneous transplant: The more tissue one harvests the more one is advised to prepare two pedicle vessels for anastomosis as just one nitrifying vessel might not be sufficient within this transplant. However, iliac crest bone can be harvested as free bone graft without a microvascular pedicle. This should be limited to smaller defects and to cases of recipient sites without previous contamination, inflammation, or radiation.

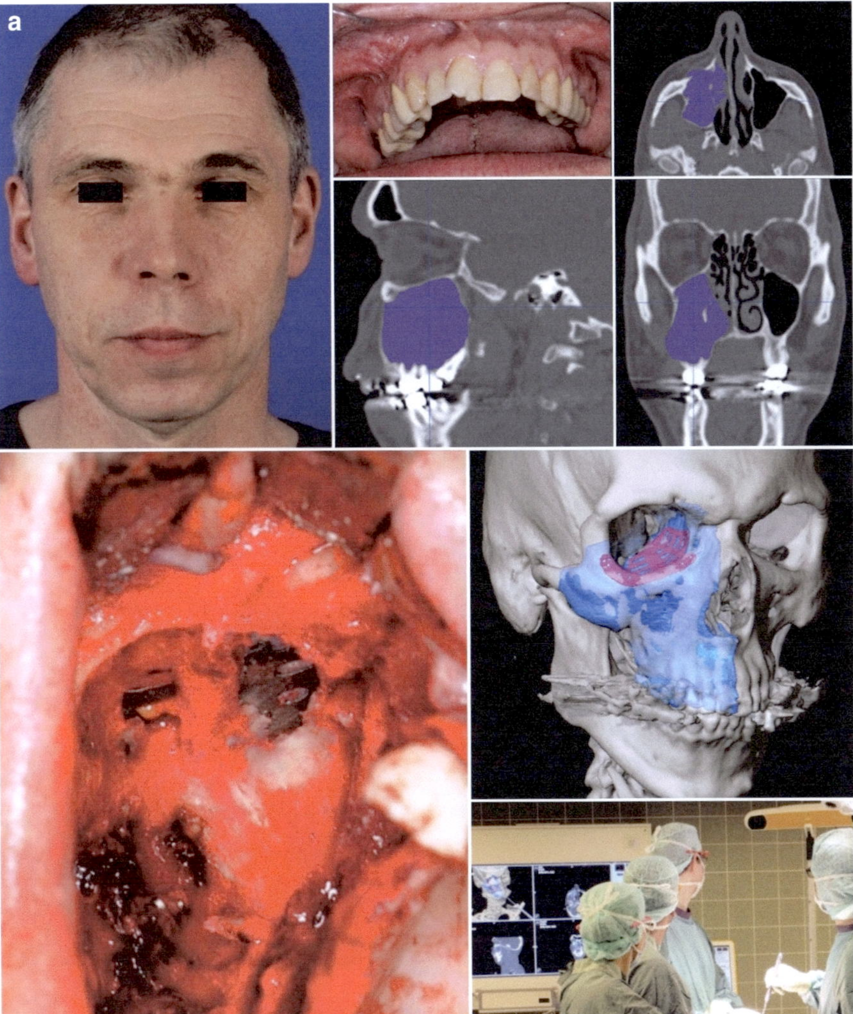

Fig. 8.4 (**a**) Case of a 42-year-old male patient with a keratocyst of the right maxilla. Extra- and intraoral clinical pictures show no sign of the displacing growth of the keratocyst, which has completely suspended the right maxillary sinus. CT images show that the cyst reaches out to the nasal cavity and to the right orbital floor having started to resorb its thin bone layer, which supports the right bulbus. A 3D-reconstruction of the skull shows the parts of the facial skeleton segmented and displayed in blue, which are involved in the keratocyst's extent; a PSI has been designed (displayed in pink color), which serves for the reconstruction of the orbital floor after the planned resection of the keratocyst. The intraoperative image shows the view from intraorally through the resected keratocyst/right maxillary sinus area onto the partially removed right orbital floor which has been reconstructed by the implanted PSI. Via navigation probe and infrared camera, the surgeon can control the positioning of the PSI intraoperatively. (With permissions of Brainlab AG). (**b**) Case of a 42-year-old male patient with a defect of the right maxilla after resection of a keratocyst: early secondary reconstruction with PSI and microvascular fibula flap. Matching 3D-reconstruction of the facial skull after (beige) and before (blue) resection of the keratocyst allows virtual designing of an PSI mesh (purple) re-establishing the outer contour of the original right maxilla. Left fibula can be virtually transplanted with the vessel pedicle (red) and cut into segments to fit the original shape of the right maxilla. Intraoperatively after skin marking and surgical exposure of the left fibula, cutting the fibula segments and their fixation to the PSI are facilitated by the combined cutting/drilling guides, which are manufactured to translate the virtual planning into reality during surgery. (**c**) Case of a 42-year-old male patient after early secondary reconstruction with PSI and microvascular fibula flap of a defect of the right maxilla after resection of a keratocyst. Clinical photographs of the patient from different angles show the facial symmetry especially in the region of the facial wall of the maxillary sinus which could be restored except for a slightly sunken right upper lip due to the still missing support of the lateral teeth. Intraoral photographs show a viable and adequately healed transplant ready for dental rehabilitation as the final step to concluding reconstruction

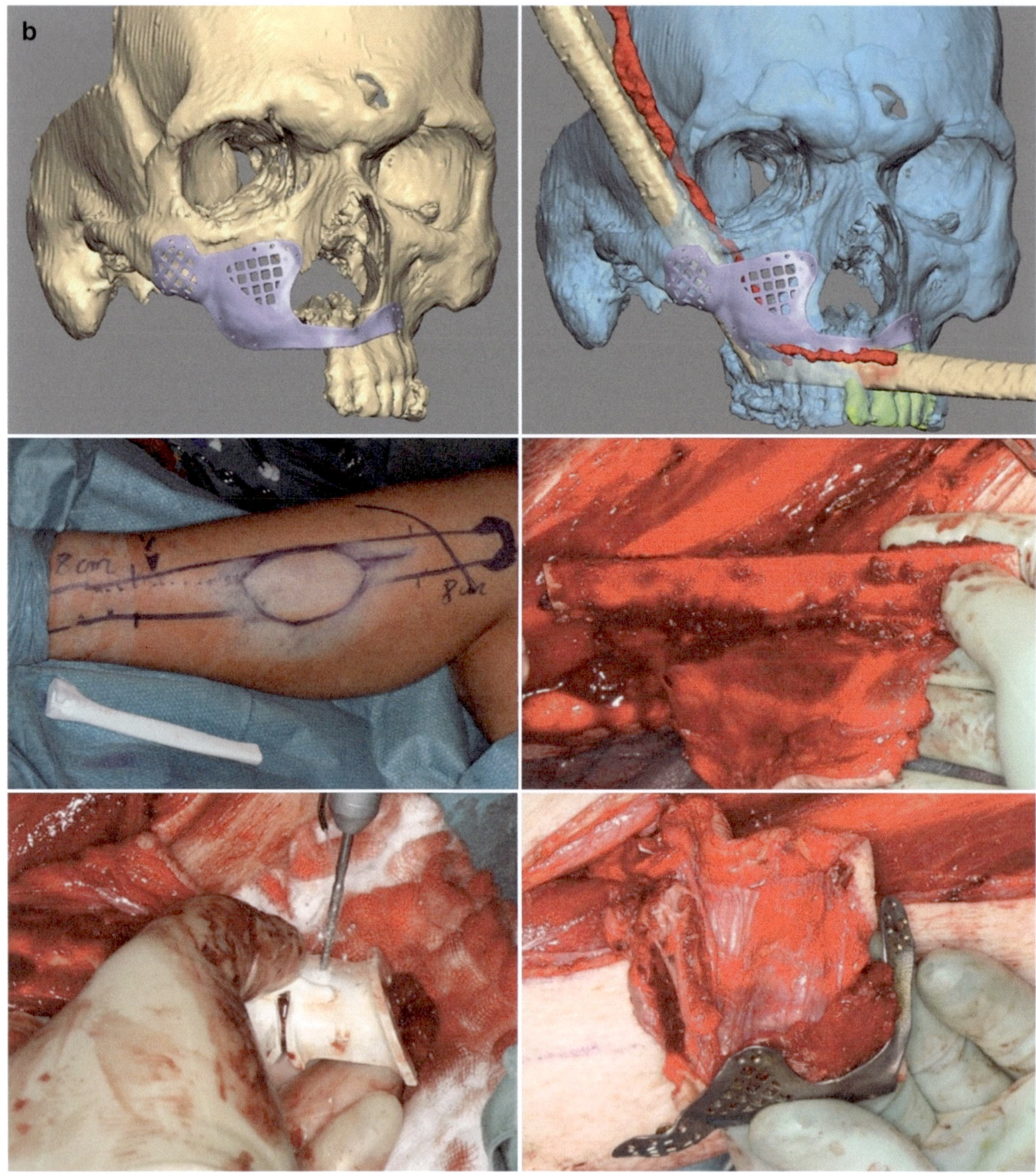

Fig. 8.4 (continued)

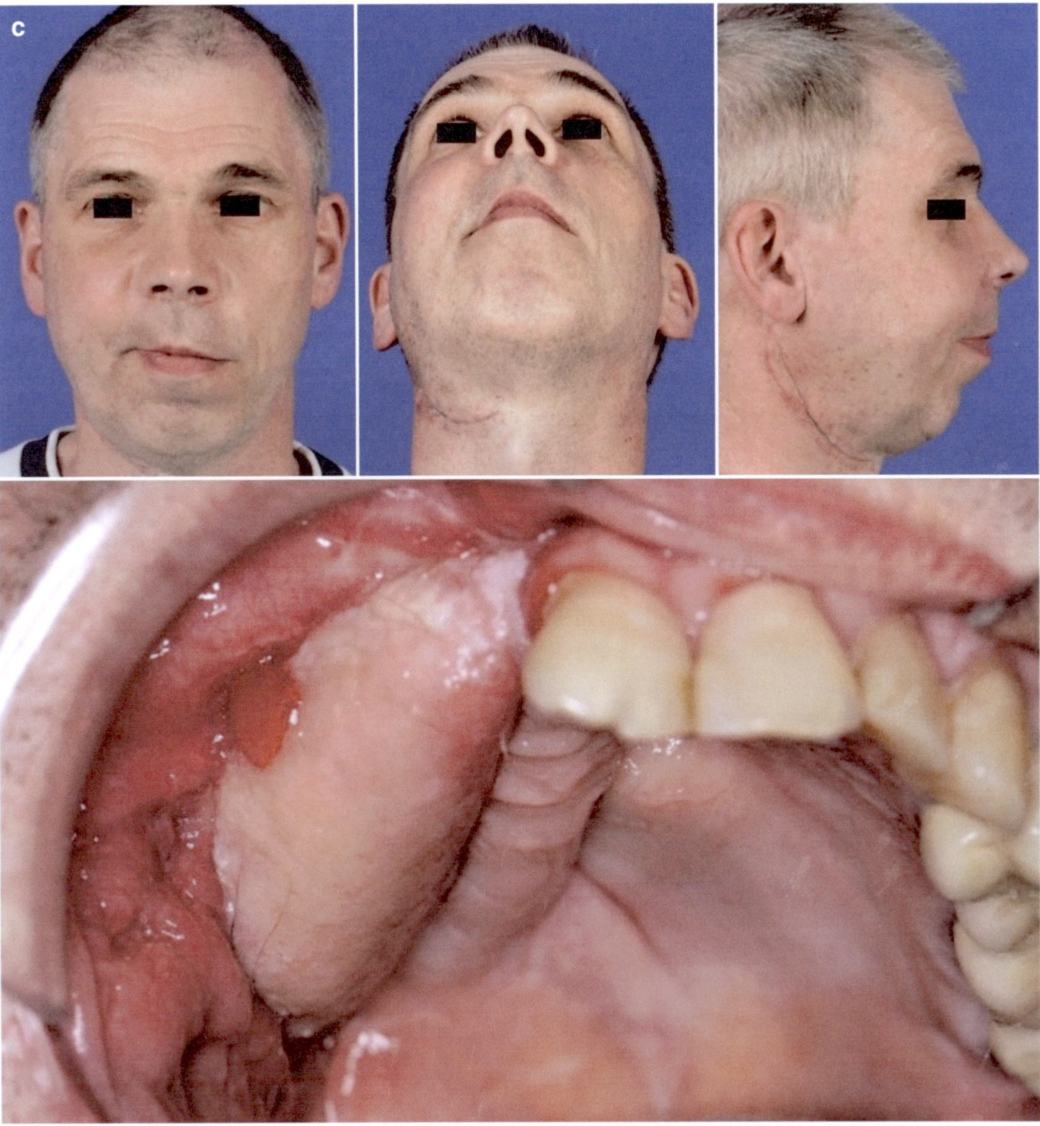

Fig. 8.4 (continued)

8.4.3 Free Scapula Flap

The free scapula flap is a suitable graft for reconstruction of maxillary and midface defects [34, 35]. Although the bone of the lateral margin can be small in dimension compared to the other flaps presented above, the soft tissue coat can be harvested with a variable quantity adapted to the present defect. Moreover, the harvested soft tissue offers a flexibility in terms of positioning facilitating replacement of extra-oral skin as well as intraoral mucosal surface defects. As such, it can be for example used for covering the defects in case of a required exenteration of the orbital cavity accompanying the maxillary resection. The donor site can be closed primarily due to mobilization of surrounding tissue. A disadvantage in usage of the scapula flap is the requirement of an intraoperative change of positioning. This makes a two-team approach impossible lengthening the surgery duration. A guided harvesting of a scapula flap is illustrated in Fig. 8.5.

8.5 Evaluation of Reconstruction Result

Due to swelling of the soft tissue and an operation situs partially not accessible to direct vision, a correct translation of the virtual planning into the surgical reality can be hard to be evaluated clinically [36, 37]. Therefore, intraoperative navigation can be applied [38]. Insertion of navigation markers in form of screws or dental splints previously to taking the pre-operative 3D imaging data sets allows the intraoperative matching of virtual planning environment to the real clinical situation via infrared camera system and a navigation tripod temporarily fixed to the skull (see Fig. 8.2). Thus the virtual plan can be evaluated for its correct surgical realization in real time ensuring high precision reconstruction "true to planning." Postoperative CT scans compared to the virtual planning via matching can enhance the evaluation of the reconstruction result even further [39].

8.6 Virtual Reality

In the context of virtual planning and computer-assisted surgery, new advances concerning the use of virtual reality and augmented or rather mixed reality are being made in the field of oral and maxillofacial surgery [16].

Virtual reality describes a computer-generated three-dimensional environment presented to the viewer. Concerning the way of possible interactions with multi-sensual feedback of the virtual environment, it can be described as non-immersive to fully immersive [40]. The above presented procedures of virtual planning and computer-assisted designing (CAD) of PSIs are in a way a version of a non-immersive virtual reality being displayed on a computer monitor and allowing the interactions via the computer mouse.

A step further to immersiveness is achieved by VR headsets, which present two slightly different video signals to each eye for a three-dimensional impression and integrates head movements into these signals. This immersive display of a virtual reality without sophisticated methods of interacting with it is used for presenting intricate head and neck anatomy during medical education [41, 42]. Moreover by scanning not only the hard tissues via CBCT but also the soft tissues with the facial surface via stereophotogrammetry and the use of sophisticated planning software, pre- and postoperative simulations of the patient's face for orthognathic and reconstructive surgery can be presented to the patient via VR headsets [43–45]. This offers a more immersive impression of a simulated surgery result to the patient which may lead to an improved patient education followed by a better compliance and adherence to postoperative behavior instructions [17].

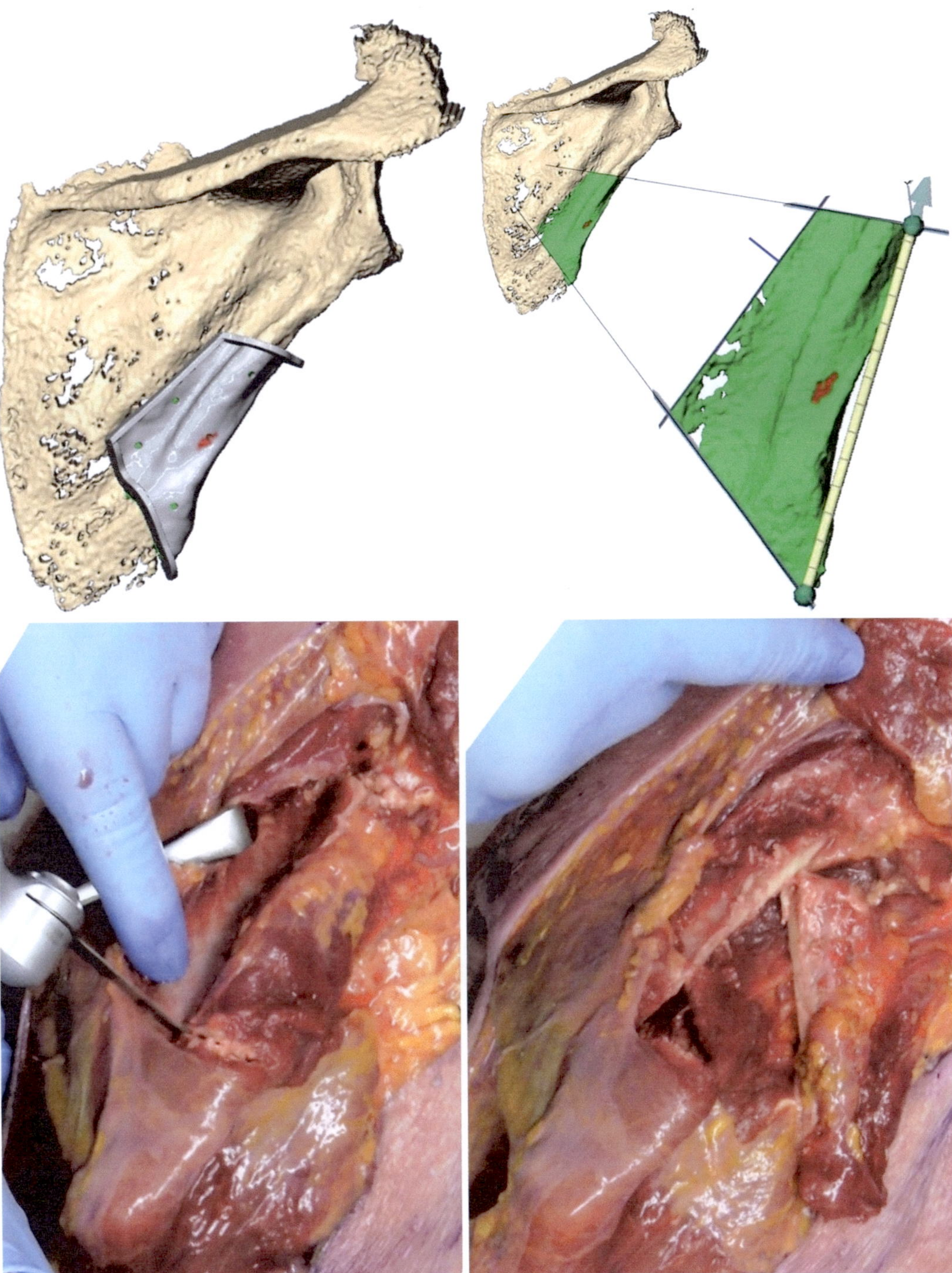

Fig. 8.5 Harvesting of a free scapula flap with the help of a harvesting guide. Virtual model of a scapula with the bone segment desired for transplantation in green and the accordingly designed harvesting guide in grey. Surgical flap harvesting is demonstrated at a body donor as depicted in the lower pictures. Once the lateral margin of the scapula is prepared, fitting of the virtually designed harvesting guide can take place to define the osteotomy lines. Osteotomy is performed along the cutting edges. The lateral margin of the scapula can be harvested along with a variable amount of soft tissue. Transplantation takes place after the bone transplant has been fixed to the patient-specific reconstruction plate and the recipient site has been prepared

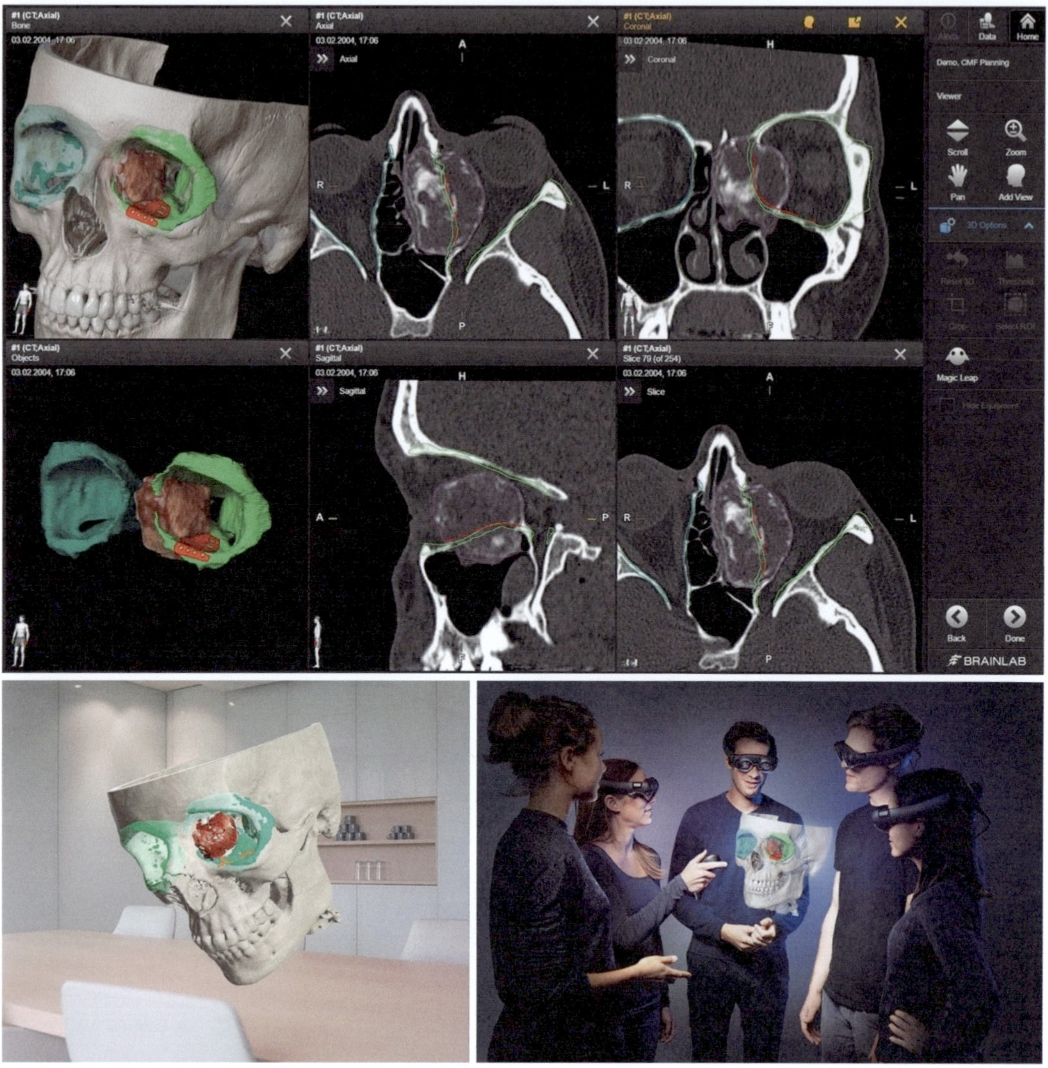

Fig. 8.6 The virtual planning of a PSI for reconstruction of the orbital floor can be visualized three-dimensionally by augmented reality. (With permission by Brainlab AG, Munich, Germany). The segmented left (light green) and right (dark green) orbital cavities are designed to reconstruct the left orbital floor with a PSI (red) after the resection of the segmented tumor (brown) has taken place. This virtual planning can be demonstrated three-dimensionally for medical educating purposes or during the education of the patient leading to a more immersive and comprehensible experience facilitated by augmented reality devices

An even more immersive virtual reality is offered by integration of possibilities of interaction via tracking of hand or eye movements and giving haptic feedback to the performed interactions. Those technologies are currently used in different scenarios for surgical training [46–49].

Augmented reality or mixed reality takes place when you superimpose the display of a virtual reality or aspects of a virtual reality on to the real environment using semitransparent VR headsets [50] (see Fig. 8.6). In oromaxillofacial surgery, systems are in development that allow the projection of critical anatomical structures within the hard tissues such as the greater palatine foramen with its emerging vessels and nerves or the mandibular canal containing the inferior alveolar nerve into the surgeon's view of the operation situs [51]. This technique may help the surgeon to preserve these structures during surgery. While there are some studies about phantom operations, few first clinical studies in the field of orthognathic surgery and dental implantation yield promising results so far [52–54].

References

1. Futran ND, Mendez E. Developments in reconstruction of midface and maxilla. Lancet Oncol. 2006;7(3):249–58.
2. Brown JS, Shaw RJ. Reconstruction of the maxilla and midface: introducing a new classification. Lancet Oncol. 2010;11(10):1001–8.
3. Phasuk K, Haug SP. Maxillofacial prosthetics. Oral Maxillofac Surg Clin North Am. 2018;30(4):487–97.
4. O'Connell DA, Futran ND. Reconstruction of the midface and maxilla. Curr Opin Otolaryngol Head Neck Surg. 2010;18(4):304–10.
5. Dalgorf D, Higgins K. Reconstruction of the midface and maxilla. Curr Opin Otolaryngol Head Neck Surg. 2008;16(4):303–11.
6. Costa H, Zenha H, Sequeira H, et al. Microsurgical reconstruction of the maxilla: algorithm and concepts. J Plast Reconstr Aesthet Surg. 2015;68(5):e89–e104.
7. McCarthy CM, Cordeiro PG. Microvascular reconstruction of oncologic defects of the midface. Plast Reconstr Surg. 2010;126(6):1947–59.
8. Rana M, Essig H, Eckardt AM, et al. Advances and innovations in computer-assisted head and neck oncologic surgery. J Craniofac Surg. 2012;23(1):272–8.
9. Wang Y, Fan S, Zhang H, Lin Z, Ye J, Li J. Virtual surgical planning in precise maxillary reconstruction with vascularized fibular graft after tumor ablation. J Oral Maxillofac Surg. 2016;74(6):1255–64.
10. Zhang WB, Yu Y, Wang Y, et al. [Surgical reconstruction of maxillary defects using a computer-assisted techniques]. Beijing Da Xue Xue Bao. 2017;49(1):1–5.
11. Numajiri T, Morita D, Nakamura H, et al. Using an in-house approach to computer-assisted design and computer-aided manufacturing reconstruction of the maxilla. J Oral Maxillofac Surg. 2018;76(6):1361–9.
12. Rana M, Modrow D, Keuchel J, et al. Development and evaluation of an automatic tumor segmentation tool: a comparison between automatic, semi-automatic and manual segmentation of mandibular odontogenic cysts and tumors. J Cranio Maxillofacial Surg. 2015;43(3):355–9.
13. Essig H, Dressel L, Rana M, et al. Precision of posttraumatic primary orbital reconstruction using individually bent titanium mesh with and without navigation: a retrospective study. Head Face Med. 2013;9(1):1–7.
14. Yu H, Zhang S, Wang X, Lin Y, Wang C, Shen G. [Application of computer-assisted navigation in oral and maxillofacial surgery: retrospective analysis of 104 consecutive cases]. Shanghai Kou Qiang Yi Xue. 2012;21(4):416–21.
15. Essig H, Rana M, Kokemueller H, et al. Pre-operative planning for mandibular reconstruction—a full digital planning workflow resulting in a patient specific reconstruction. Head Neck Oncol. 2011;3:45.
16. Ayoub A, Pulijala Y. The application of virtual reality and augmented reality in oral & maxillofacial surgery. BMC Oral Health. 2019;19(1):238.
17. Pandrangi VC, Gaston B, Appelbaum NP, Albuquerque FC, Levy MM, Larson RA. The application of virtual reality in patient education. Ann Vasc Surg. 2019;59:184–9.
18. Sonmez N, Gultekin P, Turp V, Akgungor G, Sen D, Mijiritsky E. Evaluation of five CAD/CAM materials by microstructural characterization and mechanical tests: a comparative in vitro study. BMC Oral Health. 2018;18(1):5.
19. Wagner M, Gander T, Blumer M, et al. [CAD/CAM revolution in craniofacial reconstruction]. Praxis (Bern 1994). 2019;108(5):321–8.
20. Bell RB, Markiewicz MR. Computer-assisted planning, stereolithographic modeling, and intraoperative navigation for complex orbital reconstruction: a descriptive study in a preliminary cohort. J Oral Maxillofac Surg. 2009;67(12):2559–70.
21. Wilde F, Hanken H, Probst F, Schramm A, Heiland M, Cornelius C-P. Multicenter study on the use of patient-specific CAD/CAM reconstruction plates for mandibular reconstruction. Int J Comput Assist Radiol Surg. 2015;10(12):2035–51.
22. Cornelius C-P, Giessler GA, Wilde F, Metzger MC, Mast G, Probst FA. Iterations of computer- and template assisted mandibular or maxillary reconstruction with free flaps containing the lateral scapular border—evolution of a biplanar plug-on cutting guide. J Cranio Maxillofacial Surg. 2016;44(3):229–41.
23. Mascha F, Winter K, Pietzka S, Heufelder M, Schramm A, Wilde F. Accuracy of computer-assisted mandibular reconstructions using patient-specific implants in combination with CAD/CAM

fabricated transfer keys. J Cranio Maxillofacial Surg. 2017;45(11):1884–97.

24. Wilde F, Cornelius C-P, Schramm A. Computer-assisted mandibular reconstruction using a patient-specific reconstruction plate fabricated with computer-aided design and manufacturing techniques. Craniomaxillofac Trauma Reconstr. 2014;7(2):158–66.

25. Lenox ND, Kim DD. Maxillary reconstruction. Oral Maxillofac Surg Clin North Am. 2013;25(2):215–22.

26. Wilkman T, Husso A, Lassus P. Clinical comparison of scapular, fibular, and iliac crest osseal free flaps in maxillofacial reconstructions. Scand J Surg. 2019;108(1):76–82.

27. Chen C, Zhang L-M, Ren W-H, et al. [Optimal design by customized plate on reconstruction of maxillary unilateral defect via free fibula flap]. Shanghai Kou Qiang Yi Xue. 2018;27(5):455–460.

28. Fu K, Liu Y, Gao N, Cai J, He W, Qiu W. Reconstruction of maxillary and orbital floor defect with free fibula flap and whole individualized titanium mesh assisted by computer techniques. J Oral Maxillofac Surg. 2017;75(8):1791.e1–9.

29. Zhang WB, Wang Y, Liu XJ, et al. Reconstruction of maxillary defects with free fibula flap assisted by computer techniques. J Craniomaxillofac Surg. 2015;43(5):630–6.

30. Patel A, Harrison P, Cheng A, Bray B, Bell RB. Fibular reconstruction of the maxilla and mandible with immediate implant-supported prosthetic rehabilitation: jaw in a day. Oral Maxillofac Surg Clin North Am. 2019;31(3):369–86.

31. Osborn TM, Helal D, Mehra P. Iliac crest bone grafting for mandibular reconstruction: 10-year experience outcomes. J Oral Biol Craniofacial Res. 2018;8(1):25–9.

32. Bianchi B, Ferri A, Ferrari S, Copelli C, Boni P, Sesenna E. Iliac crest free flap for maxillary reconstruction. J Oral Maxillofac Surg. 2010;68(11):2706–13.

33. Kelly CP, Moreira-Gonzalez A, Ali MA, et al. Vascular iliac crest with inner table of the ilium as an option in maxillary reconstruction. J Craniofac Surg. 2004;15(1):23–8.

34. Wu Y, Li D, Wang X, Xu Z. [Application of scapula osteomyocutaneous flap in the repair of maxillary defect]. Zhonghua Er Bi Yan Hou Tou Jing Wai Ke Za Zhi. 2015;50(10):814–7.

35. Tang AL, Bearelly S, Mannion K. The expanding role of scapular free-flaps. Curr Opin Otolaryngol Head Neck Surg. 2017;25(5):411–5.

36. Heiland M, Habermann CR, Schmelzle R. Indications and limitations of intraoperative navigation in maxillofacial surgery. J Oral Maxillofac Surg. 2004;62(9):1059–63.

37. Mischkowski RA, Zinser MJ, Ritter L, Neugebauer J, Keeve E, Zöller JE. Intraoperative navigation in the maxillofacial area based on 3D imaging obtained by a cone-beam device. Int J Oral Maxillofac Surg. 2007;36(8):687–94.

38. Schramm A, Suarez-Cunqueiro MM, Barth EL, et al. Computer-assisted navigation in craniomaxillofacial tumors. J Craniofac Surg. 2008;19(4):1067–74.

39. Scolozzi P, Schouman T. [Interventional multidimodal hybrid unit: from pre-operative planning to immediate post-operative control]. Rev Stomatol Chir Maxillofac. 2012;113(2):115–23.

40. Bartella AK, Kamal M, Scholl I, et al. Virtual reality in preoperative imaging in maxillofacial surgery: implementation of "the next level"? Br J Oral Maxillofac Surg. 2019;57(7):644–8.

41. Towers A, Field J, Stokes C, Maddock S, Martin N. A scoping review of the use and application of virtual reality in pre-clinical dental education. Br Dent J. 2019;226(5):358–66.

42. Weiner CK, Skålén M, Harju-Jeanty D, et al. implementation of a web-based patient simulation program to teach dental students in oral surgery. J Dent Educ. 2016;80(2):133–40.

43. Ayoub AF, Xiao Y, Khambay B, Siebert JP, Hadley D. Towards building a photo-realistic virtual human face for craniomaxillofacial diagnosis and treatment planning. Int J Oral Maxillofac Surg. 2007;36(5):423–8.

44. Naudi KB, Benramadan R, Brocklebank L, Ju X, Khambay B, Ayoub A. The virtual human face: superimposing the simultaneously captured 3D photorealistic skin surface of the face on the untextured skin image of the CBCT scan. Int J Oral Maxillofac Surg. 2013;42(3):393–400.

45. de Waard O, Baan F, Verhamme L, Breuning H, Kuijpers-Jagtman AM, Maal T. A novel method for fusion of intra-oral scans and cone-beam computed tomography scans for orthognathic surgery planning. J Craniomaxillofac Surg. 2016;44(2):160–6.

46. Wu F, Chen X, Lin Y, et al. A virtual training system for maxillofacial surgery using advanced haptic feedback and immersive workbench. Int J Med Robot. 2014;10(1):78–87.

47. Khelemsky R, Hill B, Buchbinder D. Validation of a novel cognitive simulator for orbital floor reconstruction. J Oral Maxillofac Surg. 2017;75(4):775–85.

48. Pohlenz P, Gröbe A, Petersik A, et al. Virtual dental surgery as a new educational tool in dental school. J Craniomaxillofac Surg. 2010;38(8):560–4.

49. Pulijala Y, Ma M, Pears M, Peebles D, Ayoub A. Effectiveness of immersive virtual reality in surgical training—a randomized control trial. J Oral Maxillofac Surg. 2018;76(5):1065–72.

50. Kim Y, Kim H, Kim YO. Virtual reality and augmented reality in plastic surgery: a review. Arch Plast Surg. 2017;44(3):179–87.
51. Zhu M, Liu F, Chai G, et al. A novel augmented reality system for displaying inferior alveolar nerve bundles in maxillofacial surgery. Sci Rep. 2017;7:42365.
52. Kwon H-B, Park Y-S, Han J-S. Augmented reality in dentistry: a current perspective. Acta Odontol Scand. 2018;76(7):497–503.
53. Holzinger D, Juergens P, Shahim K, et al. Accuracy of soft tissue prediction in surgery-first treatment concept in orthognathic surgery: a prospective study. J Craniomaxillofac Surg. 2018;46(9):1455–60.
54. Pellegrino G, Mangano C, Mangano R, Ferri A, Taraschi V, Marchetti C. Augmented reality for dental implantology: a pilot clinical report of two cases. BMC Oral Health. 2019;19(1):158.

Computer Assisted Surgery and Navigation in Cranio-orbital Resection and Reconstruction

Julio Acero and Patricia de Leyva

9.1 Introduction

The cranio-orbital region is a complex anatomical area delimited by the frontal bone, the orbits, and the anterior skull base as well as the anterior and lateral aspects of the middle cranial fossa. This area includes structures of great importance such as the brain, vascular structures like the internal carotid artery and the cavernous sinus, the cranial nerves including the olfactory nerves, the optic nerves and chiasm, and the orbital contents with the eye globes, extraocular muscles, fat and the lacrimal gland. A wide variety of primary or secondary benign and malignant tumors of epithelial or mesenchymal origin can affect this area and spread through the anatomical spaces to affect the different structures of the region. The most frequent type of tumors affecting this region are squamous cell carcinoma (SCC), adenocarcinoma, different types of sarcoma, meningioma, and osteoma [1]. Fibro-osseous lesions, inflammatory processes, and traumatic injuries can also cause defects in this area. Major cosmetic and functional impairment can result after surgical treatment of lesions affecting this region, thus requiring reconstruction.

Treatment of tumors of the cranio-orbital region is a challenge for the surgeon. The complex anatomy of this region offers a limited access and reduced visualization. Moreover, a complete exposure of the surgical site is often difficult to achieve, thus endoscopic accesses to the skull base have been introduced although open approaches are still necessary in many situations. Appropriate presurgical evaluation and planning of the surgical resection and the reconstructive approach must be carefully designed in order to obtain a favorable oncologic result with a good aesthetic and functional outcome. A peculiarity of skull base surgery is the need of providing a hermetic sealing in order to isolate the intracranial structures from the upper aerodigestive tract. Reconstruction of the resulting defects must be carefully planned in order to avoid severe complications such as cerebrospinal fluid (CSF) leak and meningitis.

Traditionally, surgical planning was based on two-dimensional (2D) imaging for treatment planning of a three-dimensional (3D) patient with less predictable results, mostly based on the surgeon's experience since Cushing in 1938 and Dandy in 1941 firstly described a combined transcranial-facial access to approach orbital tumors and Smith referred in 1954 the first combined craniofacial resection in a patient affected by a malignant tumor arising in the frontal sinus [2]. Computer assisted 3D planning techniques, computer-aided design of the reconstruction and manufacturing of patient-specific implants (CAD/CAM procedures) as well as surgical navigation

J. Acero (✉) · P. de Leyva
Department of Oral and Maxillofacial Surgery,
University Hospital Ramón y Cajal, University of
Alcala, Madrid, Spain

© Springer Nature Switzerland AG 2021
J. Acero (ed.), *Innovations and New Developments in Craniomaxillofacial Reconstruction*,
https://doi.org/10.1007/978-3-030-74322-2_9

constitute a major advance in the treatment of tumors affecting the craniofacial region providing the possibility of an accurate planning of the tumor resection as well as performing complex three-dimensional reconstructions with highly predictable postoperative results. Navigation allows the surgeon to visualize in real time the actual position in the surgical field in relation with essential anatomical structures such as the optic nerve or the cavernous sinus, thus increasing safety of the procedure which is a critical concept in cranio-orbital surgery [3].

The conceptual basis for these techniques has been previously described in other chapters of this book. It is necessary to remark that although an accurate 3D planning and computer assisted surgery improve predictability and precision of the procedure, the technical complexity and additional cost could be a major drawback [4].

9.2 Surgical Anatomy

Knowledge of the craniofacial anatomy is essential when planning the surgical treatment of tumors affecting this area and the reconstruction of the defect. The cranio-orbital region includes the upper third of the face and the upper portion of the middle third of the face. It is a protective structure for the brain and the eye and its bony framework also provides the support for the overlying soft tissue. The anterior skull base forms the floor of the anterior cranial fossa and roof of the orbits. It extends from the posterior wall of the frontal sinus anteriorly to the posterior border formed by the lesser wing of the sphenoid bone posteriorly. Medially, the floor of the anterior cranial fossa is formed by the roof of the nasal cavity and ethmoid sinus. Laterally, the roof of the orbit, formed by the orbital plate of the frontal bone, constitutes the largest surface of the anterior cranial fossa [5]. The middle cranial fossa is a butterfly-shaped depression of the skull base, narrow medially and wider and deeper laterally. The medial portion presents the chiasmatic groove, the tuberculum sellae and sella turcica, the carotid grooves and the clinoid processes. The chiasmatic groove ends bilaterally at the optic foramen, with the optic

nerve and ophthalmic artery passing into the orbital cavity (Fig. 9.1).

The orbits are conical structures with an irregular pyramidal shape, perforated by foramina and fissures. They contain the eyeball and optic nerves, extraocular muscles, the lacrimal gland, vessels, nerves, fat, and fasciae. The four walls of the orbit are curvilinear in shape in order to maintain the projection of the ocular globe and to cushion it when affected by blunt forces. The apex and margins or base of the pyramid of the orbits are composed of thick bone, whereas the walls are thinner. The orbit is a well-designed and protective structure, which shields the eye. It is composed of seven bones. The lateral wall is formed by the greater wing of the sphenoid, the frontal bone, and the zygomatic bone. The floor is formed from the sphenoid, the orbital process of the palatine bone, and the orbital process of the maxillary bone. The medial wall is formed from the lesser wing of the sphenoid, the ethmoid bone, the lacrimal bone, and the frontal process of the maxilla. Finally, the roof of the orbit is formed from the sphenoid and the frontal bones [1].

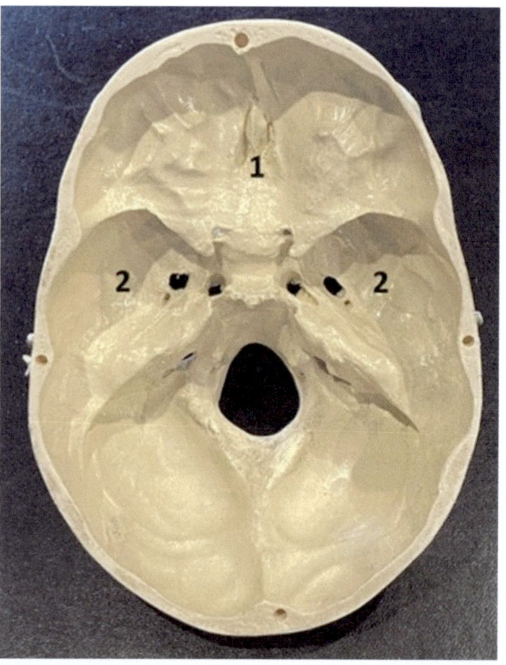

Fig. 9.1 Skull base: intracranial view. (1) Anterior skull base, (2) middle cranial fossa

Important vascular structures of this region include the carotid arteries and the vertebrobasilar system. The cavernous sinus is a dural venous sinus located bilaterally on either side of the sella turcica in the middle cranial fossa. The cavernous sinus houses the cavernous portion of the internal carotid artery and is crossed by important nerve structures on their way to the orbit: the abducens nerve or cranial nerve VI (CN VI) and the carotid plexus (post-ganglionic sympathetic nerve fibers) course through the cavernous sinus while through the lateral wall of the sinus travel the oculomotor nerve (CN III), the trochlear nerve (CN IV), and the ophthalmic and maxillary branches of the trigeminal nerve (V1 and V2). The superior orbital fissure is the communication between the cavernous sinus and the apex of the orbit. It is straddled by the tendinous ring of Zinn which is the common origin of the four rectus muscles (extraocular muscles). The abducens nerve (CN VI), the inferior ramus of the oculomotor nerve (CN III), and the inferior ophthalmic vein enter the orbits through the medial portion of the superior orbital fissure; the superior ramus of the oculomotor nerve (CN III), the trochlear nerve (CN IV), the ophthalmic branch of the trigeminal nerve (V1), and the superior ophthalmic vein enter through the lateral portion of the fissure. The inferior orbital fissure lies in the floor of the orbit and it is bounded superiorly by the greater wing of sphenoid, inferiorly by the maxilla and orbital process of the palatine bone, and laterally by the zygomatic bone. It opens into the posterolateral aspect of the orbital floor and it is crossed by the zygomatic and infraorbital branches of the trigeminal nerve, the infraorbital artery and vein as well as ganglionic branches from the pterygopalatine ganglion to the maxillary nerve.

The pterygopalatine fossa is a small space of the cranial base located between the maxillary bone anteriorly, the pterygoid process posteriorly, and the orbital apex superiorly. It is of great importance in cranial base surgery as it is a neurovascular crossroad of the nasal cavity, masticatory space, orbit, oral cavity, and middle cranial fossa and therefore constitutes a pathway for the spread of neoplastic processes. The pterygopalatine fossa communicates laterally with the infratemporal fossa via the pterygomaxillary fissure and anteriorly with the orbit via the inferior orbital fissure. It also communicates medially with the nasal cavity via the sphenopalatine foramen (crossed by the sphenopalatine artery, the nasopalatine nerve, and the posterior superior nasal nerves); posteriorly and superiorly with the Meckel cave and cavernous sinus via the foramen rotundum (crossed by the maxillary nerve -V2-); posteriorly and inferiorly with the middle cranial fossa via the vidian canal (crossed by the vidian nerve); posteriorly and medially with the nasopharynx, via the palatovaginal canal (crossed by the pharyngeal nerve and the pharyngeal branch of the maxillary artery); and inferiorly with the palate via the greater and lesser palatine canals.

The infratemporal fossa lies posterolateral to the maxillary sinus below the skull base, between the pharyngeal sidewall and the ramus of the mandible. It communicates with the temporal fossa via the space deep to the zygomatic arch, with the pterygopalatine fossa via the pterygomaxillary fissure, and with the middle cranial fossa via the foramina ovale and spinosum. It contains the medial and lateral pterygoid muscles, the temporalis muscle, the maxillary artery and its branches, the pterygoid venous plexus, the mandibular nerve and its branches (including the lingual nerve), the chorda tympani nerve and the posterior superior alveolar nerve of maxillary nerve [6].

9.3 Tumors of the Cranio-orbital Region: Principles of Treatment

Management of tumors involving the fronto-orbital and temporal region depends on histology, location, staging, resectability, reconstructive options, and patients' compliance. Surgical excision of tumors in this region is challenging because of the complex anatomy and limited access of this area as well as the lack of visibility of the surgical field that may lead to difficulty in identifying anatomical landmarks during the surgical procedure. A multidisciplinary approach is necessary requiring a careful presurgical planning with clinical examination, imaging techniques including computed tomography (CT) scan and magnetic resonance imaging (MRI) as well as angiography if indicated. Radiological evaluation of the craniofacial skeleton should be performed with a submillimeter data set, reconstructed in the axial, coronal, and sagittal planes [7].

Treatment of benign tumors is based on conservative resection or enucleation while in malignant tumors a complete surgical en bloc resection, usually followed by adjuvant radiotherapy or chemoradiation, has proven to show the best outcomes [1]. Neoplasms arising in this area are frequently originated in deep anatomical spaces such as the sinonasal tract, the posterior orbit or intra-cranially and can grow to a considerable size before any symptoms are noticed, leading to a delayed diagnosis. Surgical resection can therefore be extensive and carry a high risk due to the involvement of critical structures at the orbit or cranial base. Complete en bloc resections can be difficult to achieve in these situations, with a rate of positive margins in SCC of the sinonasal tract between 10 and 63% [8–10].

Assessment of resectability or technical ability to obtain clear margins according to the NCCN Guidelines [11] includes the preoperative evaluation of potential gross extension of the tumor to the skull base especially with involvement of the cavernous sinus, involvement of the pterygopalatine fossa, encasement of the internal carotid artery defined as tumor surrounding the artery by 270° or greater and/or direct extension to prevertebral fascia or cervical vertebrae. In selected cases, depending on the type of tumor, some of these sites of involvement could be considered as non-absolute contraindications and the widest possible resection should be performed combined with postoperative radiation/chemoradiation therapy.

Surgical approaches to the craniofacial region are summarized in Table 9.1. Endoscopic approaches can provide a safe trans-nasal approach to anterior skull base tumors especially located in the midline [12]. In extended tumors, especially malignancies affecting the orbit, facial skin, and skull base, an open approach is still frequently required. In order to avoid facial skin incisions in case of

Table 9.1 Surgical approaches to the craniofacial region

• Endoscopic approach
• Coronal approach, frontal craniotomy
• Lateral approach (temporal-orbito-zygomatic approach)
• Anterolateral approach (fronto-temporal + orbito-zygomatic)
• Combined approaches: transoral/transfacial: mandibulotomy, midfacial translocation

orbital exenterations associated with skull base or midfacial resections, we have introduced a combined coronal-transconjunctival approach, which allows to expose the whole frontal-orbital and midfacial skeleton by associating a coronal approach with a perilimbic-transconjunctival incision, preserving the conjunctival sac [13].

## 9.4	Principles of Craniofacial Reconstruction

Reconstruction of the cranio-orbital region is challenging. Reconstructive goals in this area should include:

– Repair of dural defects and interposition of a barrier of viable tissue between the intracranial contents and the sinonasal tract in order to avoid complications like CSF fistula or meningitis.
– Restoration of facial harmony. To restore the three-dimensional appearance of the face, reconstruction of the craniofacial bony architecture will be required in case of anatomic or functional deformity. Restoration of soft tissue bulk in order to achieve an acceptable aesthetic contour is also required.
– Repair of facial skin defects after resections of cutaneous tissue. Extensive craniofacial resections of tumors including the eyelids or nose can require the reconstruction of these anatomical structures. Total amputation of the eyelids is frequently associated with exenteration.
– Orbital repair: Filling of the orbital cavity and coverage of the defect is necessary after exenteration while an accurate orbital wall reconstruction providing support to the eye globe must be provided in case of eye preservation.

As discussed in other chapters, the ultimate goal in orbital reconstruction is to restore form and function through correctly re-establishing the 3D architecture of the orbital frame and orbital volume [14]. Achieving these objectives, in case of preservation of the ocular globe, helps to prevent complications such as enophthalmos and dystopia, extraocular muscle restriction, and diplopia. Postsurgical enophthalmos and diplopia as a result of inaccurate restoration of orbital anatomy are relatively frequent after complex reconstruction. These complications are most commonly due to enlargement of the bony orbit volume especially in patients with complex orbital injuries involving the deep orbit posterior to the equator of the globe. When the orbit anatomy is disrupted, loss of anatomical references can make difficult the accurate positioning of bone grafts or mesh plates to repair the defect. In these scenarios, an adequate preoperative planning and intraoperative computer assisted surgery with navigation adds accuracy, safety, and predictability to implant positioning [14].

The different reconstructive options which can be used to repair craniofacial defects in order to achieve the mentioned goals are summarized in Table 9.2. Dural tears have to be sutured in order to prevent CSF leaks. Adhesive sealants can also be used. In large dura tears or when a portion of dura is missing and cannot be sutured, an onlay or suturable dural graft using biological or synthetic dural substitutes may be preferable to the use of pericranium or fascia lata (Fig. 9.2). Local and regional flaps like the galeal-pericranial flap or the temporalis muscle flap can be used to cover moderate bone defects in order to seal the skull base or to fill the orbital cavity after exen-

teration. Pericranial flaps and the nasoseptal flap vascularized by the sphenopalatine artery (Hadad flap) can also be used in endoscopic endonasal skull base procedures [15].

Repair of bone defects at the skull base and craniofacial region requires a careful evaluation of the cosmetic and functional impact. Defects without aesthetic or functional significance do not need any bone reconstruction once a satisfactory stability for the intracranial content after dura repair and sealing with a galeal-pericranial flap has been achieved (Fig. 9.2). Bone remodeling to improve the facial contour can be an option in some cases of fibrous dysplasia. Significant craniofacial defects with anatomic deformity in the cranio-orbito-facial region or functional consequences, require an accurate repair of bone defects in order to restore the facial contour and to protect vital structures like the brain or the eye globe. Bone reconstruction in this area can be accomplished by using bone grafts or alloplastic materials. Split calvarial bone grafts have been used for bone reconstruction in the cranio-orbital región but show disadvantages like the limited source of bone, the unpredictable resorption of the bone graft, and potential infection leading to graft loss. Reconstruction with alloplastic implants avoids morbidity at the donor site and its use has become the standard for the repair of bone defects in this area. Although controversy remains and a variety of materials such as titanium, polyethylene, hydroxyapatite, poly-DL-lactic acid (PDLLA), calcium phosphate, and polyether-ether-ketone (PEEK) have been proposed to reconstruct defects of the craniofacial region, titanium meshes seem to be particularly adequate for reconstructing the orbital walls after tumor resection or large orbital fractures [16]. Polymers like PEEK show a combination of strength and excellent biocompatibility and can be tailored to fit to the exact shape and size of the defects affecting the cranial vault and orbital rims. Outcomes of craniofacial reconstruction with PEEK implants are satisfactory although complications like infection or wound related problems have been reported [17, 18]. Coverage with a galeal-pericranial flap could contribute to avoid implant-related complications such as exposure of the material.

Table 9.2 Skull base reconstruction techniques

• Dural repair
• Local flaps (galeal-pericranial flaps)
• Skull base endoscopic reconstruction
Different options: pericranial scalp flap, synthetic dural substitute, fat grafting, nasoseptal flap (Hadad flap)
• Regional pedicled flaps (temporalis muscle flap)
• Osseous reconstruction
• Massive resections: free microvascular flaps

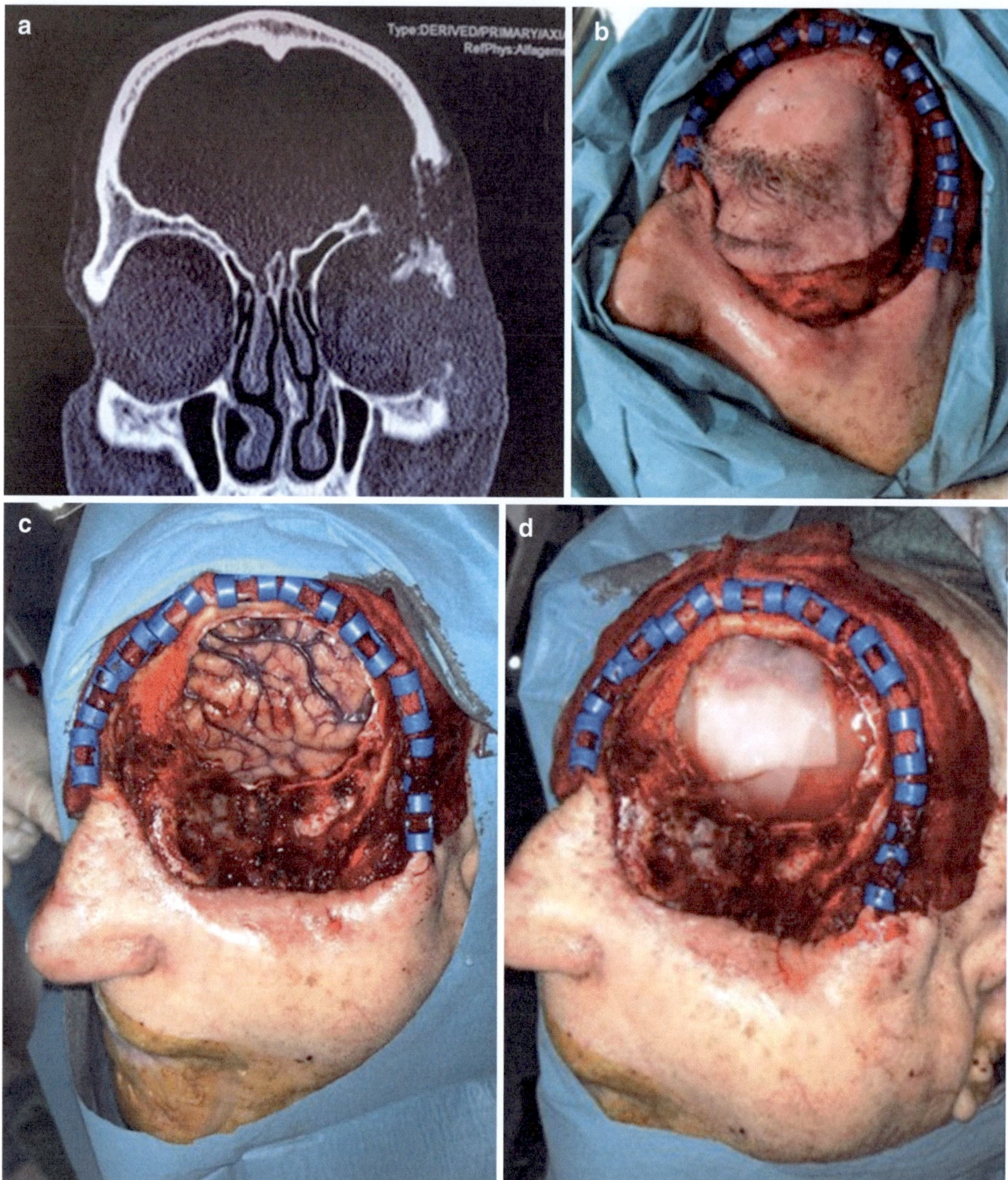

Fig. 9.2 Adenocarcinoma of the lacrimal gland with intracranial and cutaneous involvement. (**a**) CT imaging showing extensive orbito-cranial bone destruction. (**b**, **c**) Composite cranio-orbital resection including facial skin, orbital exenteration, skull and dural resection. (**d**) Dural reconstruction. (**e**) Rectus abdominis free flap. (**f**) Postoperative image of the patient. No bone reconstruction has been performed

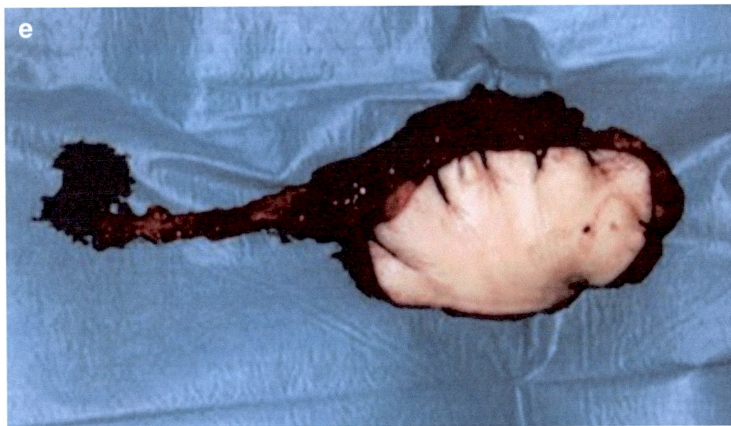
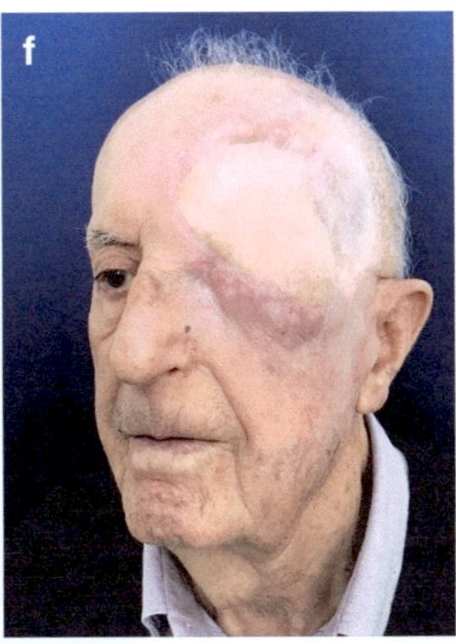

Fig. 9.2 (continued)

Finally, in case of massive resections in the craniofacial region, microvascular flaps will be required to repair wide defects affecting the skull base, facial contour, and large skin areas. Microvascular free flaps can provide a reliable, well-vascularized barrier to separate the intracranial and the extracranial spaces, sufficient bulk to obliterate the dead space after resections of large tumors as well as cutaneous coverage for the skin or mucosal lining, thus helping to prevent complications like CSF fistula or infection [19]. Selection of flap depends on the anatomical structures, the size and type of tissues to be restored, and the surgeon's experience. The rectus abdominis, the anterolateral thigh (ALT), and the osteocutaneous fibula free flaps are frequently used in skull base reconstruction since all have a long vascular pedicle in order to perform the microvascular anastomosis at the cervical level if the superficial temporal vessels are not available. Subscapular system flaps including the scapula or the latissimus dorsi can be raised as chimeric flaps to repair complex composite defects [20] (Figs. 9.2 and 9.3).

9.5 Virtual Planning: Computer-Assisted Surgery

Introduction of computer-based technology led to a major change in craniofacial surgery. Computer-assisted 3D planning techniques, computer-aided design of the reconstruction and manufacturing of 3D models, surgical guides and patient-specific implants as well as surgical navigation have contributed to make oncologic cranio-orbital surgery more accurate and reliable. Furthermore, these innovative technologies have enabled an optimal reconstructive surgery in the craniofacial region [21].

9.5.1 Computer-Aided Presurgical Planning

Preoperative planning of the ideal reconstruction should be performed together with the resection planning in the craniofacial region. As mentioned before, the incorporation of digital imaging modalities such as 3D CT and MRI, angiography, etc. facilitates the full comprehension of the complex 3D anatomy of this region and the relation of the tumor with vital structures such as the internal carotid artery [3, 4]. In skull base surgery, preoperative planning allows to determine tumor resection margins and to outline anatomical structures and operative landmarks before surgery. Preoperative virtual surgery can be performed in the computer including the design of computer-generated cutting guides (Fig. 9.4). The surgical guides can be printed to be placed in the surgical field in order to transfer the virtual design of the craniofacial osteotomies to the patient. 3D printed surgical cutting guides must fit in a precise position in order to achieve intraoperative accuracy although intraoperative fitting

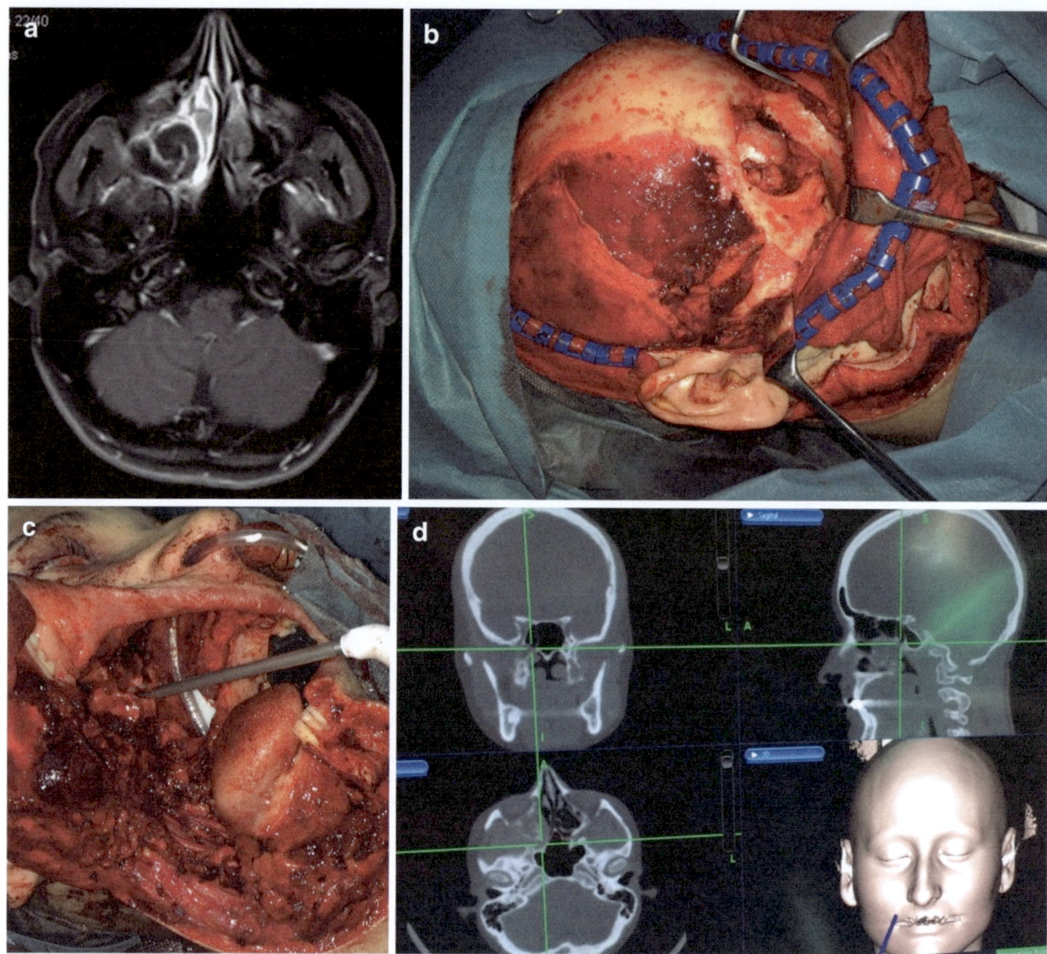

Fig. 9.3 Young patient affected by chondrosarcoma involving the upper maxilla, orbit, infratemporal fossa, and skull base with foramen rotundum and vidian canal infiltration. (**a**) MRI imaging, axial view. (**b**) Avoiding midfacial incisions: coronal approach combined with perilimbic-transconjunctival and lip split-mandibulotomy approach. (**c**, **d**) Subcranial navigation assisted skull base resection. (**e**) Surgical specimen: en bloc extended maxillectomy with orbital exenteration. (**f**) Reconstruction with a chimeric dorso-scapular flap including the tip of the scapula and a latissimus dorsi free flap. (**g**) Facial postoperative aspect with temporary eye prosthesis

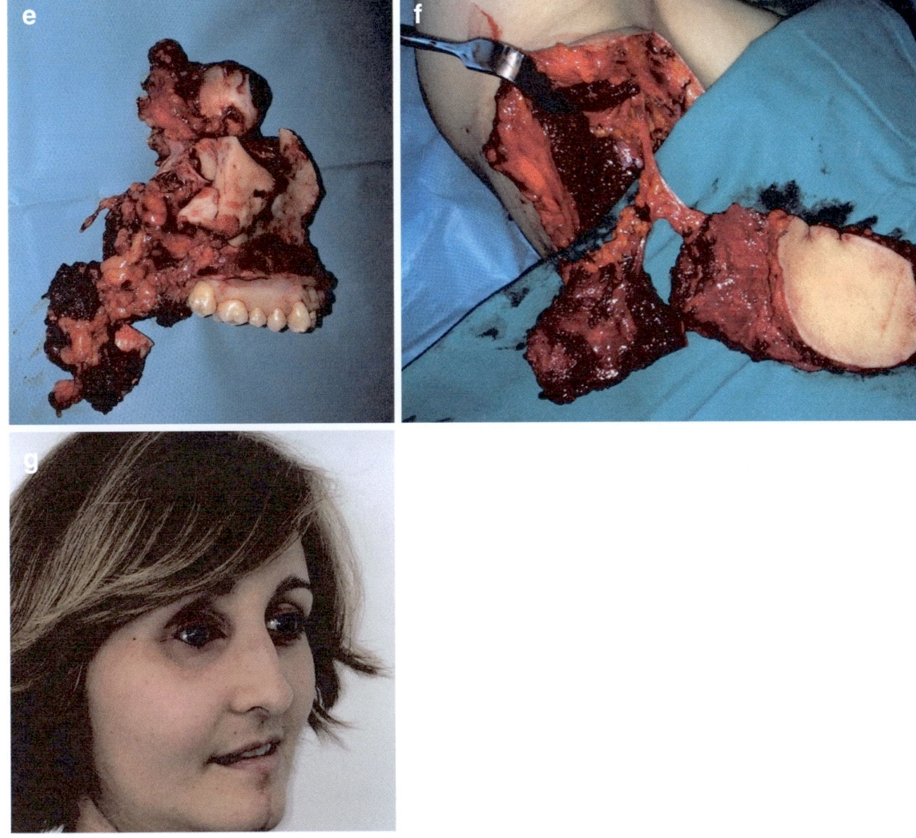

Fig. 9.3 (continued)

of the guides could be difficult in some regions such as the infratemporal fossa. Non-printed virtual guides combined with navigation to transfer the virtual planning to the patient during surgery can also be used.

Planning of the resection should be followed by the virtual design of the reconstruction including planning of bone flaps or alloplastic implants geometry. Virtual presurgical reconstruction enables to obtain symmetry of the cranio-orbital region by segmentation and virtual mirroring of the contralateral side. A 3D model of the skull including the planned bone reconstruction can be printed in order to perform the preoperative bending of the fixation plates or titanium meshes although patient-specific implants (PSI) such as customized titanium meshes, fixation plates, or PEEK implants designed for orbital and skull base reconstruction can be manufactured directly based on the ideal virtual reconstruction. Customized implants can be designed to repair a pre-existing surgical defect in case of secondary reconstruction or a virtual defect in cases of virtual planning of primary resection and immediate reconstruction. Presurgical fabrication of the implants according to the size and shape of the defect allows shorter operating time with quick and easy positioning and good cosmetic results [22] also avoiding donor site morbidity [23]. Patient-specific PEEK implants in the cranio-orbital region are accurate in complex orbito-fronto-temporal reconstruction [24], although they are not an option in the growing patient. PEEK implants offer excellent biocompatibility and good mechanical strength as mentioned before. Since this material is radiologically translucent, it does not produce artifacts and permits a good imaging follow-up in either CT scan or

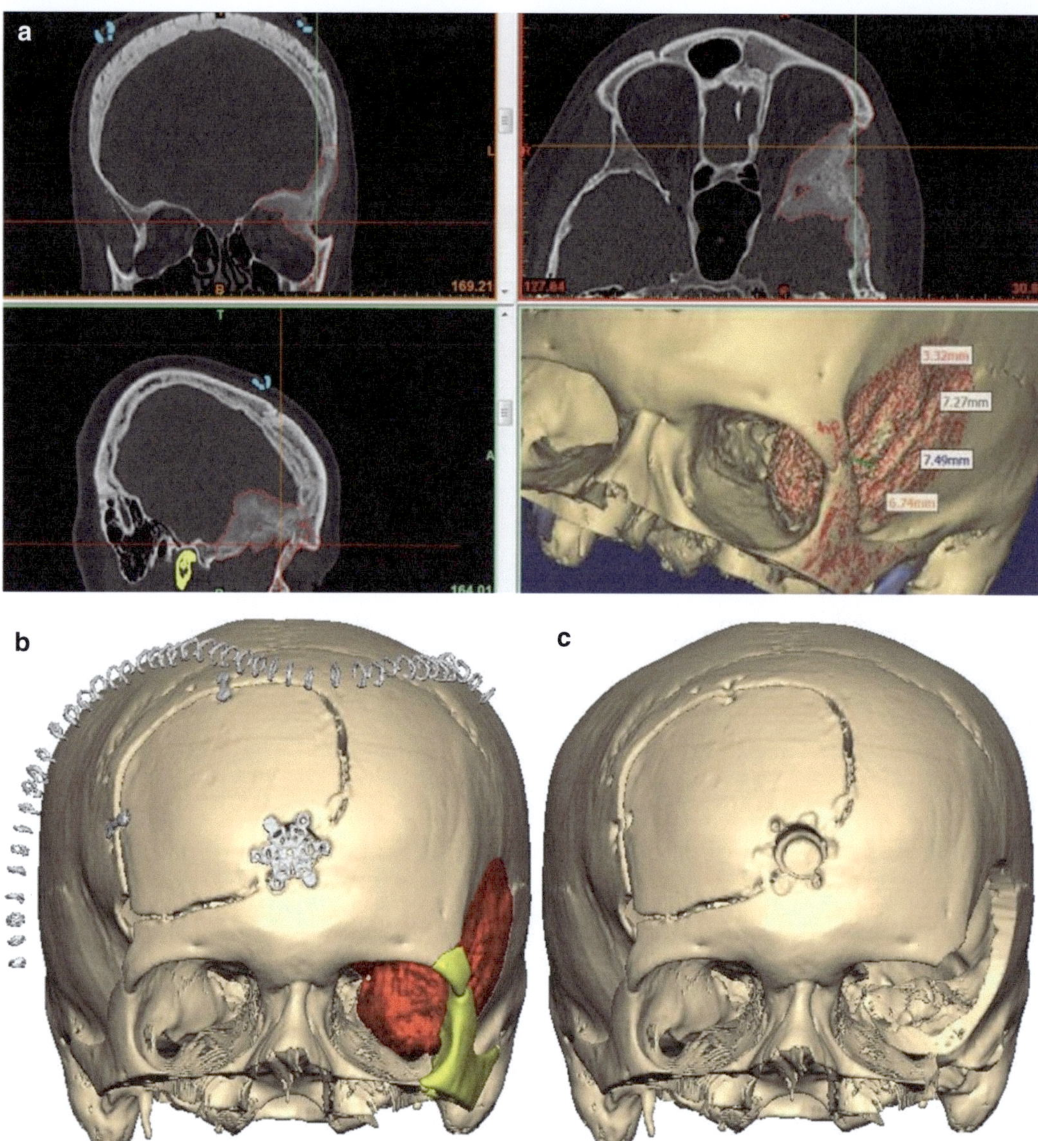

Fig. 9.4 Intraosseous meningioma of the left sphenoid bone affecting the lateral wall of the orbit and extended to the temporal bone. (**a**) CT views with 3D reconstruction. (**b–d**) Virtual resection and design of a PEEK specific implant to repair the defect. A zygomatic osteotomy is planned to approach the tumor. (**e**, **f**) Virtual and 3D printed cutting guides. (**g**) Orbito-cranial resection. (**h**) PEEK implant placed to cover the defect. (**i**) Postoperative view of the patient showing excellent aesthetic result

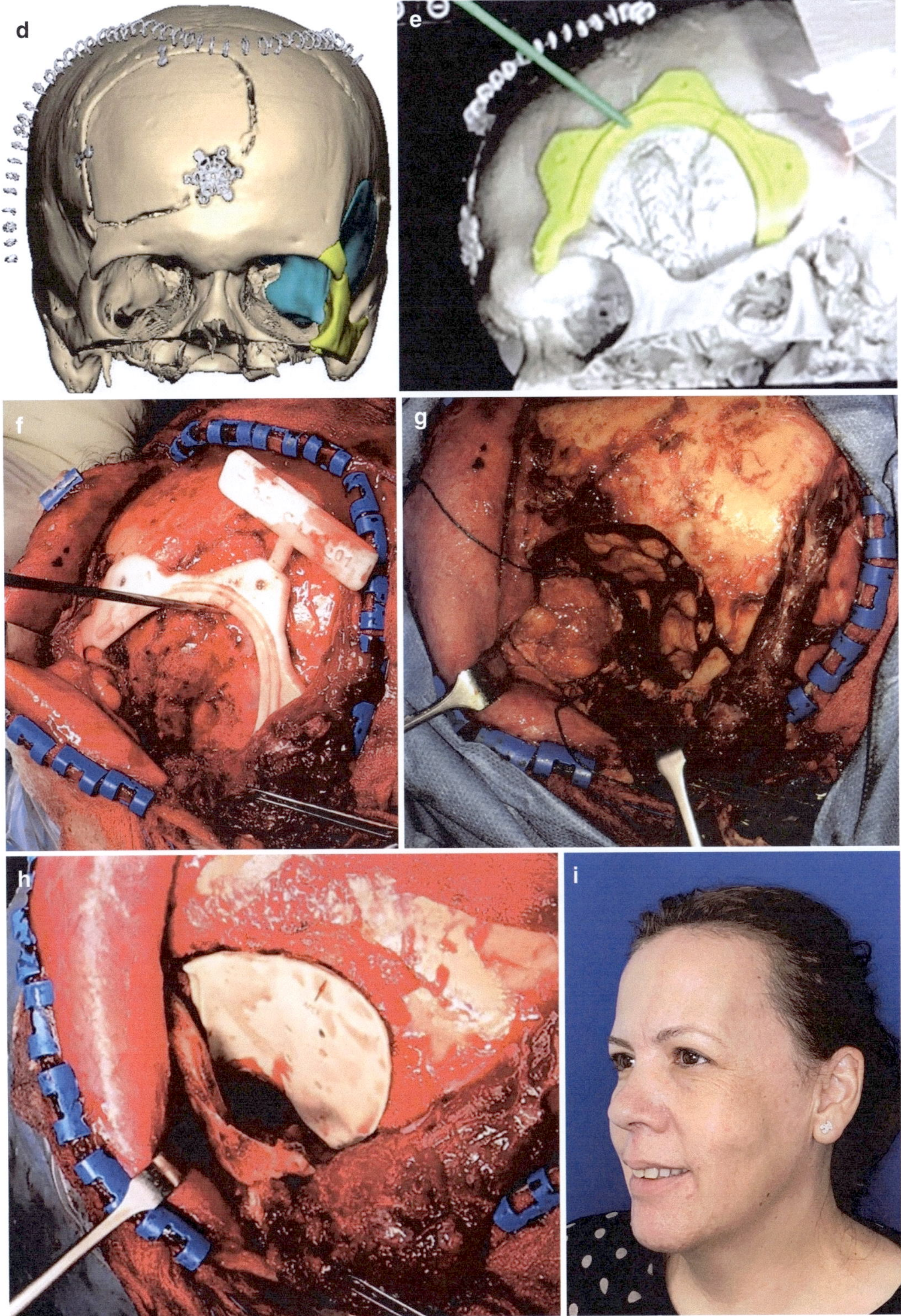

Fig. 9.4 (continued)

MRI [23]. Another advantage of PEEK implant is that they can be drilled to precisely fit in the surgical defect if necessary (Figs. 9.4, 9.5 and 9.6).

9.5.2 Value of Navigation in Craniofacial Oncologic Surgery

Image-guided navigation has many potential applications in surgery, especially in areas of complex anatomy where precision is required such as the craniofacial region [25]. Intraoperative navigation in head and neck oncologic surgery can help to provide safer margins of resections and a more precise intraoperative orientation in order to respect vital structures. Navigation can also assist to perform an accurate reconstruction.

Concerning tumor resection, navigation assisted surgery can precisely locate tumors and vital structures [26], helping the surgeon to assess the resection margins during tumor excision which is critical in complex anatomical areas. Safety of the resection is improved due to the intraoperative control of the anatomical relations of the tumor with vital structures such as the internal carotid artery, the optic chiasm, or the cavernous sinus. Current computer-based technology also allows for a preoperative volumetric virtual planning of the resection margins using the anatomical landmarks on CT scan. The volumetric tumor resection planning combined with a navigation guided resection taking in account the planned margins instead of the lesion appear to contribute to an improvement in the control of surgical margins in extended tumors involving the deep anatomical spaces related to the midface [27] (Fig. 9.7).

Navigation has also a value in craniofacial reconstructive surgery. Intraoperative navigation is a very useful tool to check the osteotomy design or the situation after placement of implants/grafts in relation with the preoperative planning, thus being a valuable tool in the intraoperative assessment of the accuracy of the reconstruction and the correct restoration of anatomy, volume, and contour [28] (Fig. 9.5). Navigation also helps the surgeon in an inverse way to transfer the 2D virtual planned surgery of the screen to the 3D reality in the operating room: after the preoperative planning of the resection in the craniofacial region and manufacturing of a patient-specific implant according to the planned resection, the digital data including the virtual planning of the resection and implant placement can be downloaded into the navigation system, thus allowing for an accurate intraoperative navigation assisted design of the resection in the patient during the surgical procedure according to the previous planning and a quick and precise implant placement [23] (Figs. 9.4 and 9.6).

9.5.3 Intraoperative Imaging

Although there are limited data available, advances in intraoperative imaging technology have contributed to a better evaluation of complex craniomaxillofacial trauma providing immediate information about the positioning of the bony fragments allowing the surgeon to check intraoperatively the results of the treatment, as it has been pointed out in other chapters of this book. Currently available intraoperative imaging, including CT and MRI, can be considered in oncologic and reconstructive craniofacial surgery not only as a tool to check the accuracy of the reconstruction but also to confirm whether the extent of the resection performed includes the previously planned margins especially concerning the bone structures [29] (Fig. 9.8).

Fig. 9.5 Giant fronto-ethmoidal osteoma with right orbital extension. (**a**) Facial preoperative aspect of the patient. Proptosis and inferior displacement of the globe. (**b**, **c**) CT Axial projection and 3D CT imaging. (**d–g**) CAD/CAM surgical planning. Virtual resection of the tumor. Mirroring of the contralateral side and design of customized titanium mesh to repair the defect. (**h**, **i**) Anterior approach: Frontal craniotomy and supraorbital bar osteotomy to access the anterior skull base. (**j–l**) Navigation assisted tumor excision and placement of the titanium implant to repair the orbital walls defect. (**m**) Repositioning of the bone fragments. Miniplate fixation and coverage with a pericranial flap. (**n**) Aspect of the patient 9 months after operation showing good postoperative evolution. (**o**) Control CT. No tumor relapse. Correct implant positioning

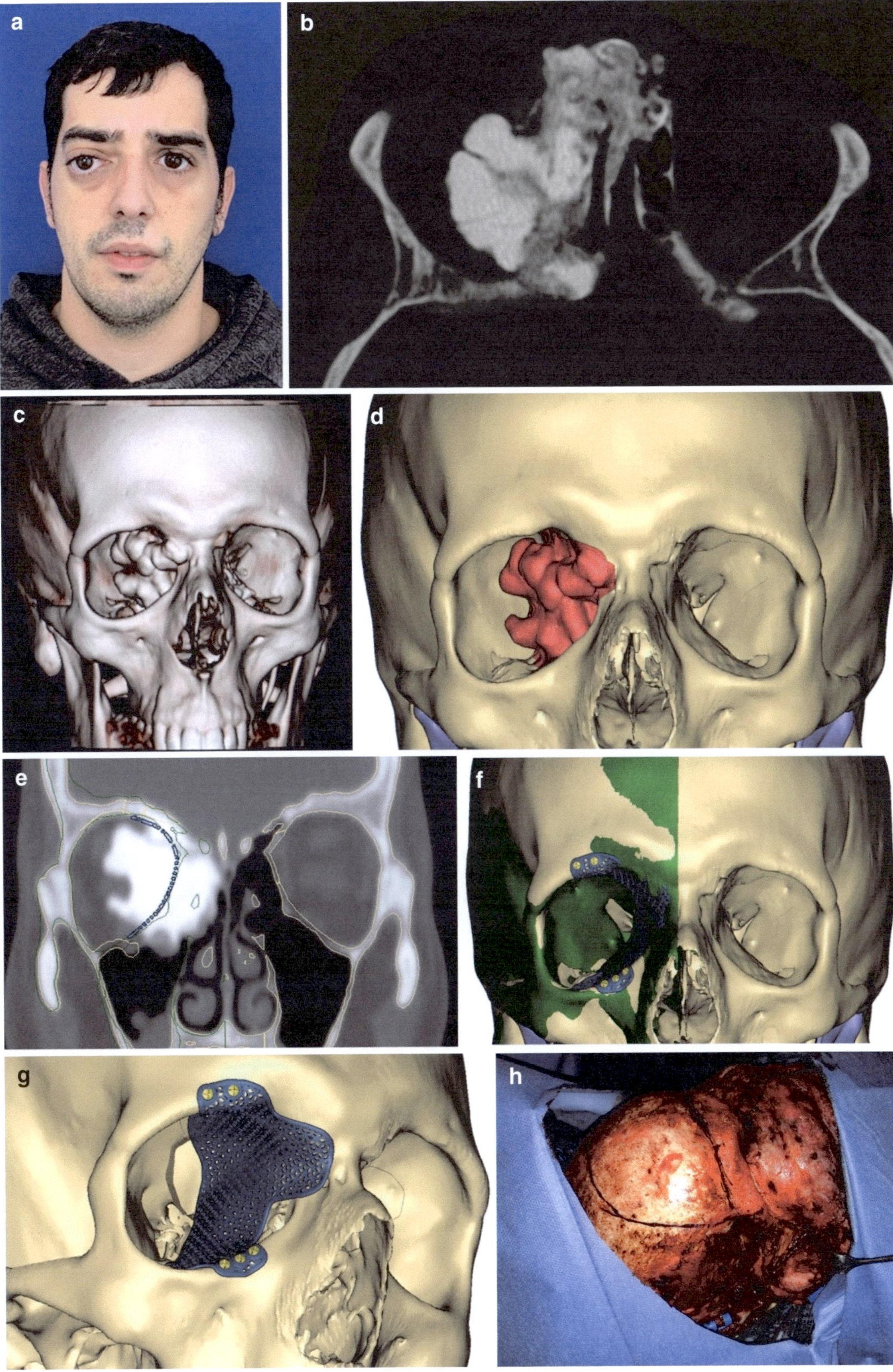

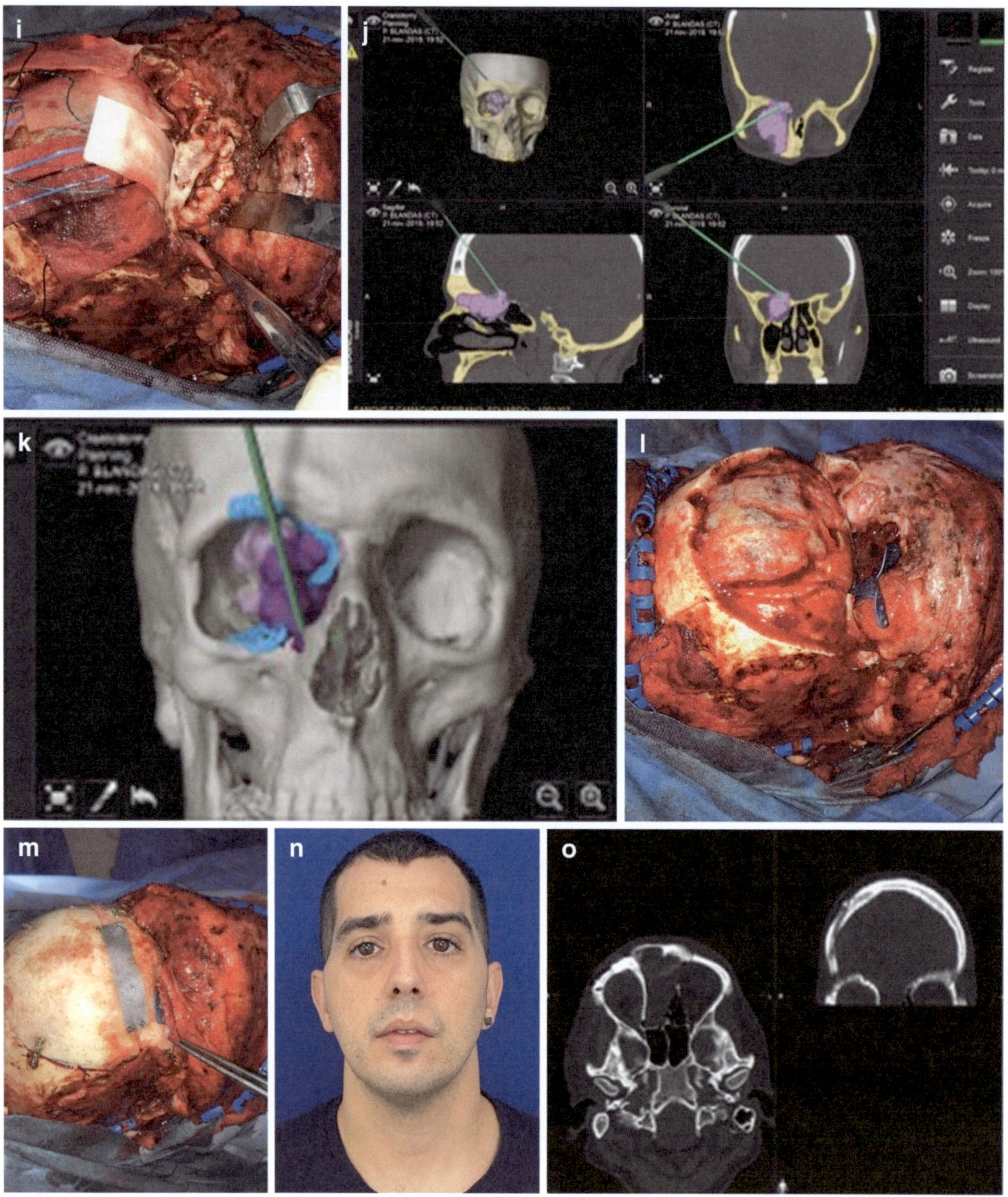

Fig. 9.5 (continued)

Fig. 9.6 Relapsing fronto-orbito-zygomatic intraosseous meningioma with extensión to the infratemporal fossa. (**a**) CT imaging: coronal view. (**b**) Surgical planning. 3D reconstruction showing the extraosseous component of the tumor with intraorbital and infratemporal extension. (**c–f**) CAD/CAM virtual planning of extended craniofacial resection and design of a patient-specific PEEK implant. (**g, h**) Navigation assisted transfer of the surgical planning into the surgical field. Design of the cranial osteotomies according to the preoperative planning. (**i, j**) PEEK implant placed in the surgical defect. Covering the implant with a galeal/pericranial flap while the temporalis muscle is filling the infratemporal and retro-orbital spaces

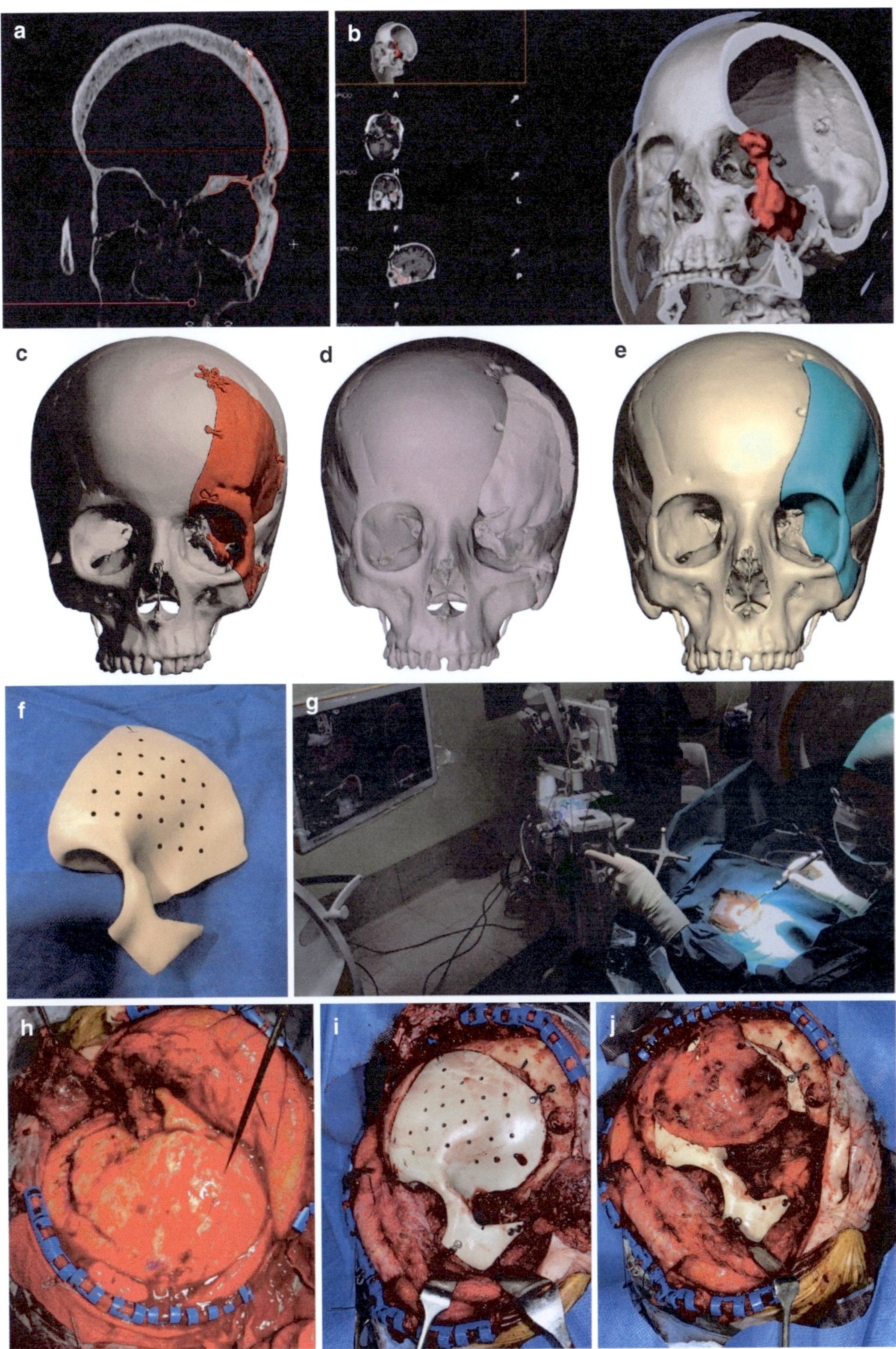

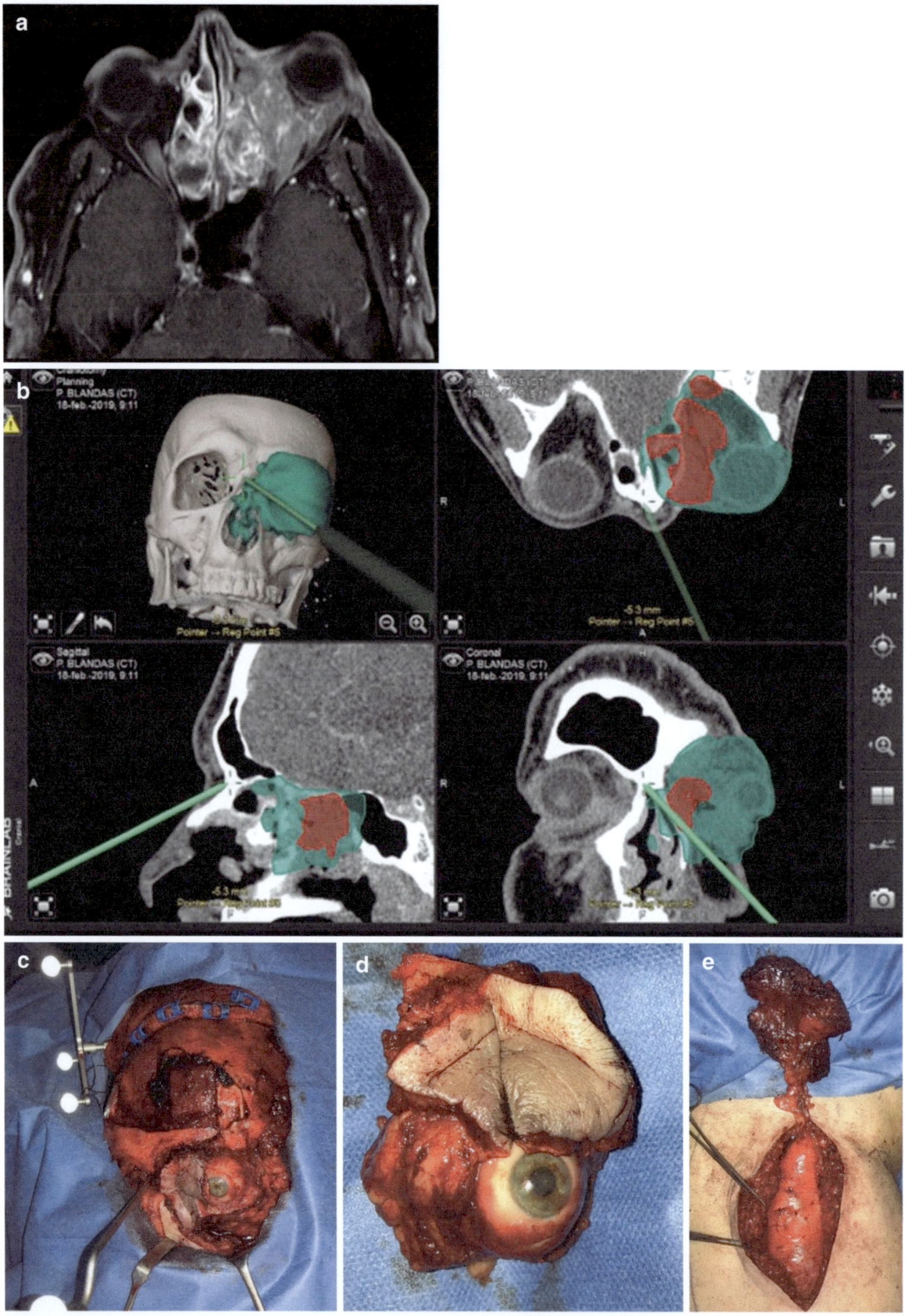

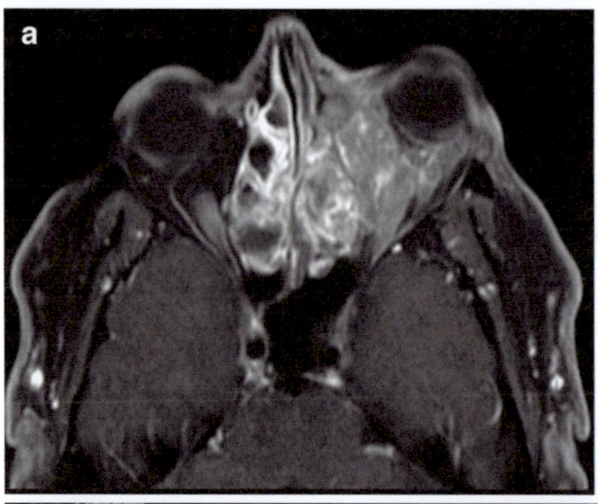

Fig. 9.7 Clear cell carcinoma of the orbit. (**a**) Axial CT showing extensive orbital involvement. (**b**) Volumetric tumor resection planning. The tumor is marked in red and the planned surgical margins in green. (**c, d**) Navigation assisted orbito-cranial resection including exenteration. Accurate sur-gical margins can be checked intraoperatively according with the previous planning. (**e, f**) Microvascular rectus abdominis muscle free flap raised to cover the defect. A barrier of well-vascularized tissue is established between the upper airway and the cranial cavity. (**g**) Final aspect of the patient

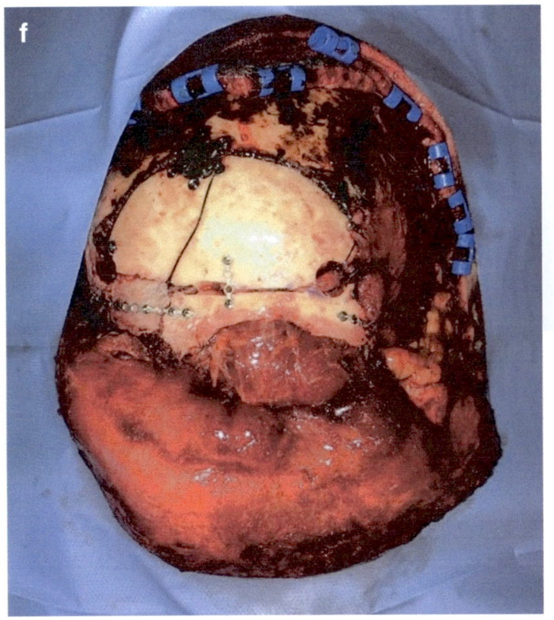

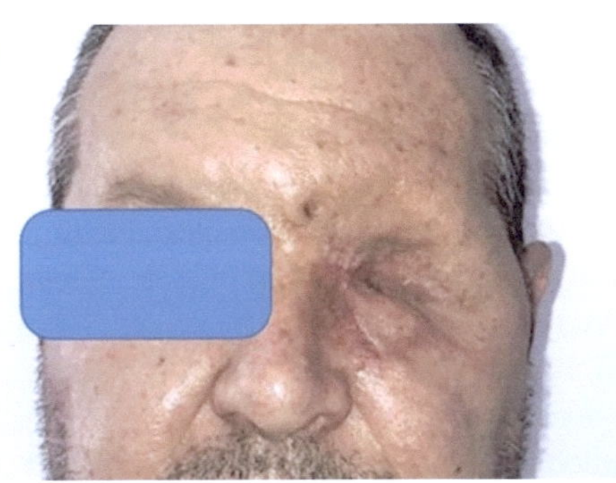

Fig. 9.7 (continued)

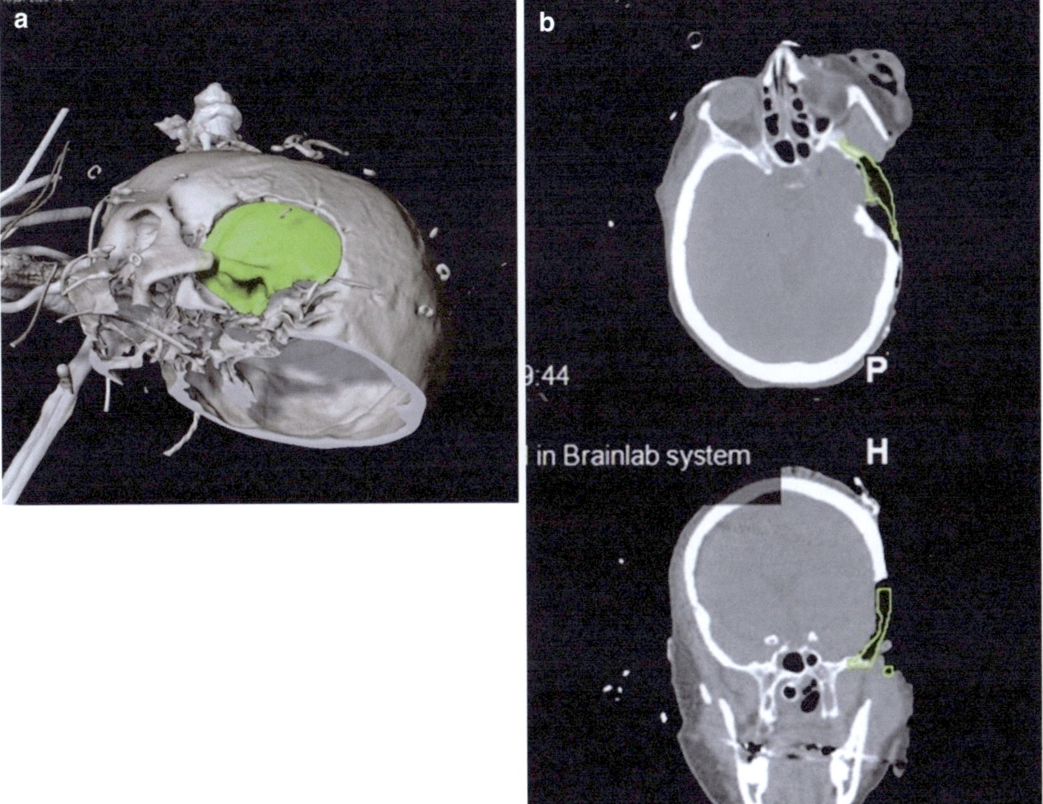

Fig. 9.8 Intraoperative CT control of meningioma resection in the temporal región of the skull base. (**a**, **b**) Resection planning identified as the green object. Intraoperative CT after resection shows remnant affected areas pending of excision. Once identified, resection can be completed under navigation

9.6 Conclusion

As a complex anatomical area, the cranio-orbital region has the singularity that structures of vital importance are comprised in close proximity: the skull base and anterior and middle cranial fossa with the optic chiasm, internal carotid artery and cavernous sinus on the inside. Moreover, this region of the face is an area of mayor aesthetic importance, responsible of a great part of a human's social function. So not only life is at risk when this region is surgically violated, but also the individual's visual and social functions. Computer assisted surgery including preoperative planning of tumor excision and reconstruction, design and manufacturing of 3D models or patient specific implants, navigation and digital intraoperative imaging open a new world helping the surgeon to enhance safety of tumor resection as well as to obtain an optimal aesthetic and functional result.

References

1. Acero J, Maza C, Salmerón J, Ochandiano S. Reconstruction of the cranio-orbital region. In: Navarro-Vila C, editor. Reconstructive oral and maxillofacial surgery. New York: Springer; 2015. p. 77–102.
2. Smith R, Klopp C, Williams J. Surgical treatment of cancer of the frontal sinus and adjacent areas. Cancer. 1954;7(5):991–4.
3. Sukegawa S, Kanno T, Furuki Y. Application of computer-assisted navigation systems in oral and maxillofacial surgery. Jpn Dent Sci Rev. 2018;54(3):139–49.
4. Lübbers H-T, Jacobsen C, Matthews F, Grätz KW, Kruse A, Obwegeser JA. Surgical navigation in craniomaxillofacial surgery: expensive toy or useful tool? A classification of different indications. J Oral Maxillofac Surg. 2011;69(1):300–8.
5. Parmar H, Gujar S, Shah G, Mukherji SK. Imaging of the anterior skull base. Neuroimaging Clin N Am. 2009;19(3):427–39.
6. Rouviere H. Human anatomy. 2013th ed. Paris: Masson; 2007. 2696p.
7. Schmitt PJ, Barrett DM, Christophel JJ, Leiva-Salinas C, Mukherjee S, Shaffrey ME. Surgical perspectives in craniofacial trauma. Neuroimaging Clin N Am. 2014;24(3):531–52.
8. Bobinskas AM, Wiesenfeld D, Chandu A. Influence of the site of origin on the outcome of squamous cell carcinoma of the maxilla—oral versus sinus. Int J Oral Maxillofac Surg. 2014;43(2):137–41.
9. Patel SG, Singh B, Polluri A, Bridger PG, Cantu G, Cheesman AD, et al. Craniofacial surgery for malignant skull base tumors. Cancer. 2003;98(6):1179–87.
10. Vidhyadharan S, Augustine I, Kudpaje AS, Iyer S, Thankappan K. Site-wise differences in adequacy of the surgical resection margins in head and neck cancers. Indian J Surg Oncol. 2014;5(3):227–31.
11. Adelstein D, Gillison ML, Pfister DG, Spencer S, Adkins D, Brizel DM, et al. NCCN guidelines insights: head and neck cancers, version 2. J Natl Compr Cancer Netw. 2017;15(6):761–70.
12. Carrau RL, Kassam AB, Snyderman CH, Duvvuri U, Mintz A, Gardner P. Endoscopic transnasal anterior skull base resection for the treatment of sinonasal malignancies. Oper Tech Otolayngol Head Neck Surg. 2006;17(2):102–10.
13. de Leyva P, Pezzi M, Picón M, Núñez J, Almeida F, Baranda E, Acero J, et al. Craniofacial resections with orbital exenteration. Avoiding cutaneous midfacial incisions. The transconjunctival technique. Int J Oral Maxillofac Surg. 2019;48:269.
14. Bell RB, Markiewicz MR. Computer-assisted planning, stereolithographic modeling, and intraoperative navigation for complex orbital reconstruction: a descriptive study in a preliminary cohort. J Oral Maxillofac Surg. 2009;67(12):2559–70.
15. Hadad G, Bassagasteguy L, Carrau RL, Mataza JC, Kassam A, Snyderman CH, et al. A novel reconstructive technique after endoscopic expanded endonasal approaches: vascular pedicle nasoseptal flap. Laryngoscope. 2006;116(10):1882–6.
16. Dubois L, Steenen SA, Gooris PJJ, Bos RRM, Becking AG. Controversies in orbital reconstruction—III. Biomaterials for orbital reconstruction: a review with clinical recommendations. Int J Oral Maxillofac Surg. 2016;45(1):41–50.
17. Rammos CK, Cayci C, Castro-Garcia JA, Feiz-Erfan I, Lettieri SC. Patient-specific polyetheretherketone implants for repair of craniofacial defects. J Craniofac Surg. 2015;26(3):631–3.
18. Oh J. Recent advances in the reconstruction of craniomaxillofacial defects using computer-aided design/computer-aided manufacturing. Maxillofac Plast Reconstr Surg. 2018;40:2.
19. Nouraei S, Ismail Y, Gerber C, Crawford P, McLean N, Hodgkinson P. Long-term outcome of skull base surgery with microvascular reconstruction for malignant disease. Plast Reconstr Surg. 2006;118(5):1151–8.
20. Macía G, Picón M, Nuñez J, Almeida F, Alvarez I, Acero J. The use of free flaps in skull base reconstruction. Int J Oral Maxillofac Surg. 2016;45(2):158–62.
21. Azarmehr I, Stokbro K, Bell RB, Thygesen T. Surgical navigation: a systematic review of indications, treatments, and outcomes in oral and maxillofacial surgery. J Oral Maxillofac Surg. 2017;75(9):1987–2005.
22. Gerbino G, Bianchi FA, Zavattero E, Tartara F, Garbossa D, Ducati A. Single-step resection and reconstruction using patient-specific implants in the treatment of benign cranio-orbital tumors. J Oral Maxillofac Surg. 2013;71(11):1969–82.

23. Jalbert F, Boetto S, Nadon F, Lauwers F, Schmidt E, Lopez R. One-step primary reconstruction for complex craniofacial resection with PEEK custom-made implants. J Craniomaxillofac Surg. 2014;42(2): 141–8.
24. Scolozzi P, Martinez A, Jaques B. Complex orbito-fronto-temporal reconstruction using computer-designed PEEK implant. J Craniofac Surg. 2007;18(1):224–8.
25. Yu H, Shen SG, Wang X, Zhang L, Zhang S. The indication and application of computer-assisted navigation in oral and maxillofacial surgery-Shanghai's experience based on 104 cases. J Craniomaxillofac Surg. 2013;41(8):770–4.
26. Gao D, Fei Z, Jiang X, Zhang X, Liu W, Fu L, et al. The microsurgical treatment of cranio-orbital tumors assisted by intraoperative electrophysiologic monitoring and neuronavigation. Clin Neurol Neurosurg. 2012;114(7):891–6.
27. Ricotta F, Cercenelli L, Battaglia S, Bortolani B, Savastio G, Marcelli E, et al. Navigation-guided resection of maxillary tumors: can a new volumetric virtual planning method improve outcomes in terms of control of resection margins? J Craniomaxillofac Surg. 2018;46(12):2240–7.
28. Luebbers H-T, Messmer P, Obwegeser JA, Zwahlen RA, Kikinis R, Graetz KW, et al. Comparison of different registration methods for surgical navigation in cranio-maxillofacial surgery. J Craniomaxillofac Surg. 2008;36(2):109–16.
29. Cuddy K, Khatib B, Bell RB, Cheng A, Patel A, Amundson M, et al. Use of intraoperative computed tomography in craniomaxillofacial trauma surgery. J Oral Maxillofac Surg. 2018;76(5):1016–25.

E. Belli, A. Kapitonov, and M. Zappalà

10.1 Introduction

The application of endoscopic surgery was first theorized by Bozzini in the early years of the nineteenth century, and the endoscope became a valuable instrument in the surgeon's hands only after the modification performed by Hopkins in the 1950s [1] and subsequently made popular by Carl Storz.

In the second half of twentieth century thanks to Messerkingler's monumental work, endoscopy was finally applied to managing sinonasal inflammatory pathologies. The real revolution was to try to restore normal ventilation in the diseased sinuses, so the type of surgery changed dramatically from a non-functional to a functional technique.

With the development of endoscopic techniques in 1981, Wigand first performed an endonasal endoscopic closure of an iatrogenic fistula after a sphenoethmoidectomy [2].

This crucial event was a turning point in the development and the application of endoscopic techniques for skull base reconstruction and for the treatment of endocranial lesions.

Endoscopic techniques have undergone significant advancement in the last three decades.

With the development of angled endoscopes, high-definition monitors, frameless navigation systems, high-resolution imaging and the improvement of anatomic knowledge, it is now possible not only to treat inflammatory sinonasal disease but also to manage sinus and skull base tumours [3–5], to perform orbital decompression [6, 7], to approach the orbital apex, clivus [8, 9] and pituitary gland [10] and to repair CSF leaks and meningoencephaloceles [11, 12] (Figs. 10.1 and 10.2).

These approaches allow good visualization of difficult-to-access locations with decreased morbidity and shorter recovery periods when compared with standard open approaches [13].

10.2 Skull Base Reconstruction

The standard endoscopic surgical treatment of skull base lesions can be described by three fundamental steps: approach, resection and reconstruction.

One of the most challenging steps of skull base defects reconstruction after tumour resection is effective watertight repair. This provides a barrier between the contaminated extracranial spaces and the sterile intradural compartment that assure an adequate dural seal. An unsuccessful reconstruction may lead to significant complications: meningitis, cerebrospinal fluid

E. Belli · A. Kapitonov (✉) · M. Zappalà
Maxillo-Facial Unit, MESMOS Department,
Ospedale S. Andrea "Università La Sapienza",
Rome, Italy

© Springer Nature Switzerland AG 2021
J. Acero (ed.), *Innovations and New Developments in Craniomaxillofacial Reconstruction*,
https://doi.org/10.1007/978-3-030-74322-2_10

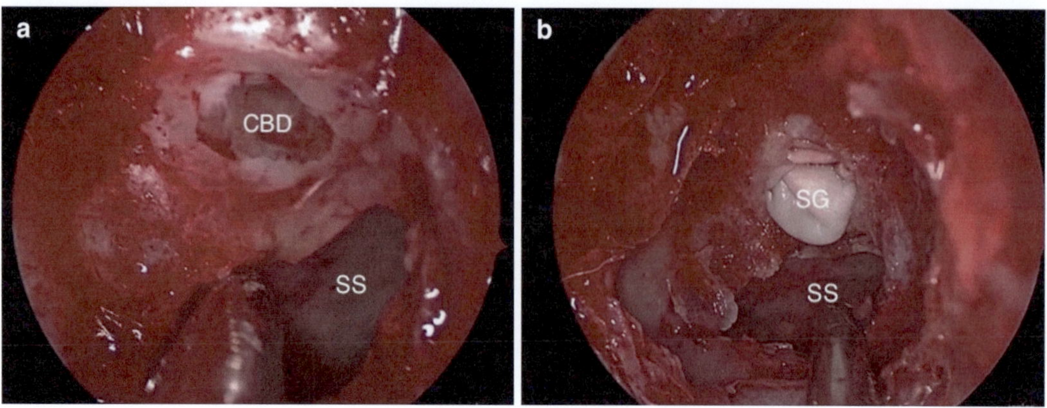

Fig. 10.1 Meningoencephalocele. *CBD* cranial base defect, *SS* sphenoidal sinus, *SG* synthetic graft

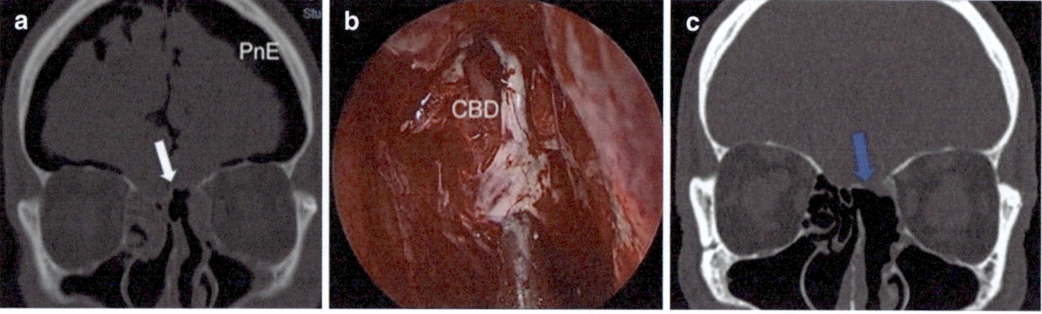

Fig. 10.2 Iatrogenic skull base fracture. (**a**) Preoperative CT scan WHITE ARROW Iatrogenic cranial base fracture. *PnE* pneumocephalus, (**b**) CBD cranial base defect, endoscopic view, (**c**) control CT scan 2 years after the fracture repair *blue arrow* repaired fracture

(CSF) leak, brain herniation and tension pneumocephalus [14].

Nowadays, endoscopic endonasal approach (EEA) has become the standard for the care of the majority of anterior cranial fossa CSF leaks [12, 15].

Current and frequent repair techniques include:

- Purely endoscopic approach:
  - Free autografts
  - Synthetic dural replacement grafts
  - Vascularized intranasal flaps
    Random flaps
    Pedicle flaps
- Transcranial endoscopically assisted approach:
  - Pericranial flap

10.2.1 Free Autografts

Autologous tissues represent the first options for skull base reconstruction, and these include free mucosal graft, fat/dermal fat graft, fascia lata and bone graft.

Free mucosal grafts may be taken from the septum, inferior or middle turbinate, but the last site is the most preferred considering that the middle turbinate is typically removed during standard endoscopic approaches to the skull base.

These types of graft are used as an onlay graft to seal small site defects, and it is of primary importance to ensure that the graft is applied with the mucosal side out to prevent mucocele.

The fat grafts typically harvested from abdominal adipose tissue provide a suitable subdural inlay to fill cavities after tumour removal [16]. Dermal fat grafts represent a valid alternative because of its characteristics. Dermis permit better manipulation of the operating site and the laminal surface makes it more suitable for consequent multi-layered reconstruction.

Fascia lata represent a durable onlay material, easy to harvest but characterized by major drawbacks due to possible wound-related issues especially in physically active patients.

Bone grafts can be used when is needed for rigid repair mainly in obese patients who have a higher risk to develop brain or meningeal herniation over time [17, 18].

Platelet-rich fibrin is a concentrated suspension of growth factors found in platelets, which act as bioactive surgical additives that are applied locally to induce wound healing [19] (Fig. 10.3).

10.2.2 Synthetic Dural Replacement Grafts

This kind of grafts may be used in inlay or onlay technique. In the inlay technique, it can be placed in the epidural plane (between dura and skull bone) or in the subdural plane (between brain and dura), and in both techniques, it should be placed up to 10 mm beyond the dural margin to prevent CSF leakage, and it could be surrounded by another onlay graft or flap.

When it is used as onlay graft, complete removal of underlying mucosa should be done to prevent any mucocele formation.

The selection of the type and brand is to surgeon's discretion. The main advantage of this grafts is the absence of the associated morbidity of the donor site [16].

10.2.3 Vascularized Flaps

The most frequently used flaps are here described.

10.2.3.1 Intranasal Vascularized Flaps

Since 2006 the **Hadad-Bassagasteguy flap** [20] (nasoseptal flap) has become the contemporary strong point of endoscopic repair of large skull base defects, drastically improving postoperative CSF leak rates (Figs. 10.4 and 10.5).

The NSF is composed of mucoperiosteum and mucopericondrium and characterized by consistent vascularity (superior septal artery, terminal branch of internal maxillary artery), long and robust pedicle, ease to harvest and good adaptability [21].

Careful elevation of this flap permits to obtain up to 25 cm^2 of vascularized tissue that is superior to any other local flap.

To tailor this flap, the inferior turbinates are outfractured bilaterally, and the ipsilateral middle turbinectomy can be performed. To harvest this flap, three cuts in the nasalseptal mucosa should be made. The first superior cut begins along the

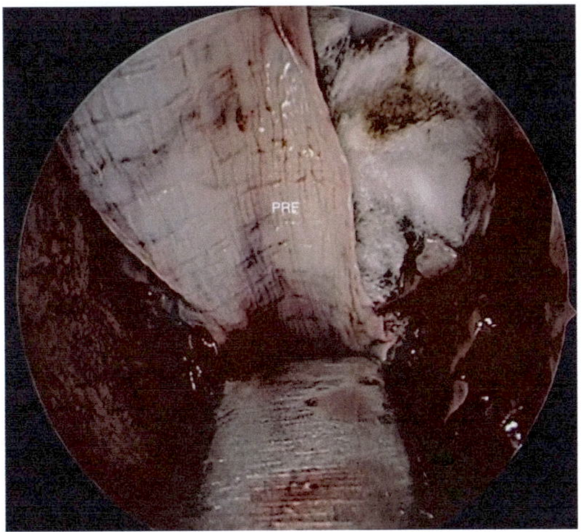

Fig. 10.3 The last step of multilayer reconstruction with PRF membrane

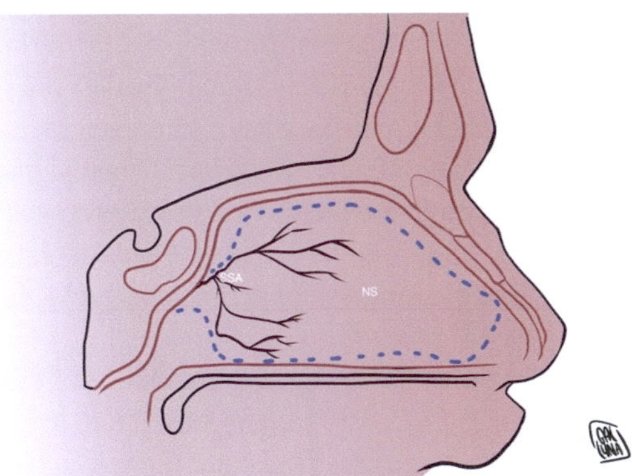

Fig. 10.4 Scheme of nasoseptal flap. *NS* nasal septum, *SSA* superior septal artery

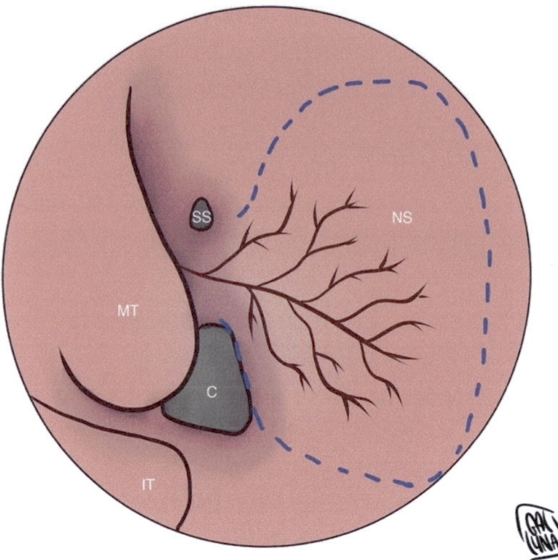

Fig. 10.5 Nasoseptal flap, schematic endoscopic view. *IT* inferior turbinate, *MT* middle turbinate, *SS* sphenoid sinus, *C* choana, *NS* nasal septum

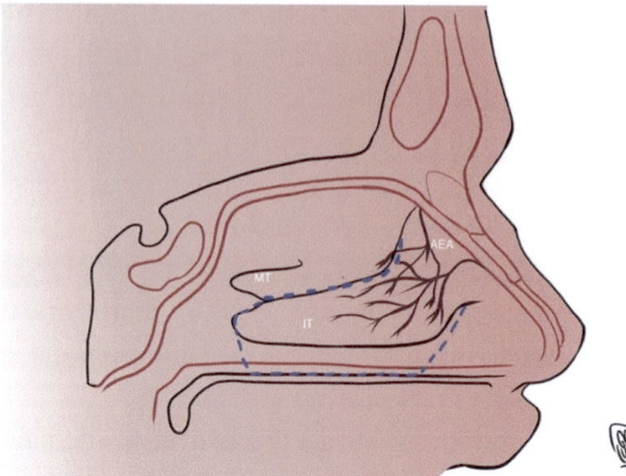

Fig. 10.6 Scheme of anterior pedicled lateral nasal wall flap. *AEA* anterior ethmoid artery, *NS* nasal septum, *IT* inferior turbinate, *MT* middle turbinate

sphenoid bone and continues along the septum anteriorly, below the cribriform plate to preserve the olfactory epithelium [20, 21].

The second inferior incision is performed from the superior margin of the choana, then it goes across to the posterior margin of the vomer and along the junction of the septum and the nasal floor, and it could be modified by extending the cut laterally to include the nasal floor to obtain a larger flap. Careful attention must be paid to not damage the soft palate.

The two previous incisions are connected anteriorly by a vertical incision. It can be extended anteriorly up to the mucocutaneus junction.

The flap is carefully dissected from the underlying bone or cartilage preserving the posterior vascular pedicle, and it is placed in the nasopharynx or ipsilateral maxillary sinus to prevent damage during the surgical procedure. Finally, the flap is gently applied directly on the dura or over a fat graft. To fix the flap, biologic glue is used and a nasal packing is applied to compress the flap against the defect.

Contraindication to the surgical choice of this flap includes previously surgery of septum, sphenoid or pterygopalatine fossa and tumour herein located.

Thanks to the introduction of nasoseptal flap the postoperative CSF leak rate has been reduced to less than 5% [22].

When the use of nasoseptal flap is inappropriate for insufficient blood supply (previous septoplasty, skull base surgery or functional sinus surgery), other local pedicle flaps should be addressed.

One of such options can be **anterior pedicled lateral nasal wall flap** (Fig. 10.6). A mucoperiosteum flap of lateral nasal wall vascularized by the anterior ethmoid artery. Anterior incision extents from the caudal part of nasal bones towards the head of the inferior turbinate, the posterior incision follows the superior aspect of the inferior turbinate up to its posterior extent and continues medially the floor of the nose [23].

This flap is suited to cover anterior skull base defects and frontal sinus posterior table defects [21, 24].

Posterior pedicled middle turbinate flap is supplied by a branch of the sphenopalatine artery (Fig. 10.7). The use of this flap is limited by its small dimension, arc of rotation and its technical difficulty in harvesting. In the author's experience, after removing osteo-cartilaginous structures, the whole turbinate can be rotated laterally basing on sphenopalatine artery and middle turbinate's mucosa.

It has to be considered as an alternative for small fovea ethmoidalis, planum and sella defects

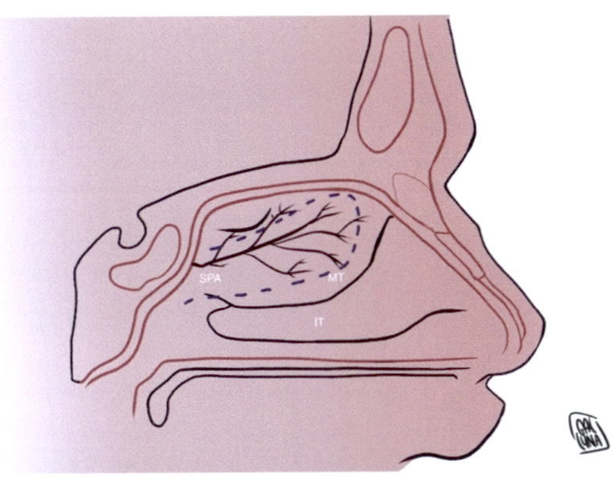

Fig. 10.7 Scheme of posterior pedicled middle turbinate flap. *SpA* branch of sphenopalatine artery, *IT* inferior turbinate, *MT* middle turbinate

especially when nasoseptal flap cannot be performed [24].

10.2.3.2 Extranasal Vascularized Flaps

Before the endoscopic era, different regional myocutaneous flaps were used to repair CFS leaks, dural and skull base defects. Some of these techniques have been modified for endoscopic surgery.

Zanation introduced the use of the **pericranial flap** for endoscopic anterior skull base reconstruction [25]. The blood supply is based on supraorbital and supratroclear artery. This flap is an excellent alternative in case of tumour invasion of nasal septum or if the nasoseptal flap is impossible to use. This flap is harvested by performing 2-cm midline incision and 1-cm lateral port incision along the coronal plane. Supraorbital and supratroclear arteries should be identified using a Doppler scan. Once performed a subgaleal careful dissection, periostium is separated from the calvarium. A 1-cm transverse glabellar incision is performed to dissect down to the periosteum of the nasion. The flap is transposed in the nasal cavity through a bony opening in drilled nasion. Nevertheless, according to the authors, traditional coronal incision and frontal osteotomy are more frequently indicated when wide skull base defects must be addressed by transcranial nasoendoscopic approach (Fig. 10.8).

The use of pericranial flap is convenient in case of defects anterior to the sella turcica [26].

10.2.4 Synthetic Absorbable Sealants and Glues

Despite the adopted surgical option absorbable glues and sealants assure the firmness of the multilayer sandwich. The general rule of the use of this resorbable materials is that none of them must be placed underneath the graft.

10.3 Selection of Reconstruction Options

The selection of specific endoscopic reconstructive techniques is tailored upon many factors such as [27]: the site, the size and the shape of the skull base defect, the quality of the surrounding bone and remaining dura, the amount of CSF leak (high-flow, low-flow, no flow), the individual anatomy of the nasal septum and lateral nasal wall, previous history of surgery, trauma or radiation therapy, and the expected need for adjuvant radio- or chemotherapy.

Concerning the practical choice of the specific reconstructive option probably the most important guiding factor is the CSF leak type. CSF leak can be classified into three main types: no leak, low flow, high flow (the defect communicates with the ventricle or cistern) [16]. In cases in which no intraoperative CSF flow was noted, the outcomes were excellent regardless of whether the cranial base defect was repaired or not [28].

According to the author, it is of great help the use of simple synthetic graft placed epidural or subdural that can be strengthened with the addiction of an autograft.

According to literature in case of low-flow CSF leak, there is no difference whether multilayer non-vascularized or vascularized grafts are used [16].

Higher flow leaks were repaired with greater success rates when vascularized tissue and multilayer repair were used as reported by Patel et al. [29] and Soudry et al. [28].

There are several independent factors that help the surgeon to choose the suitable technique.

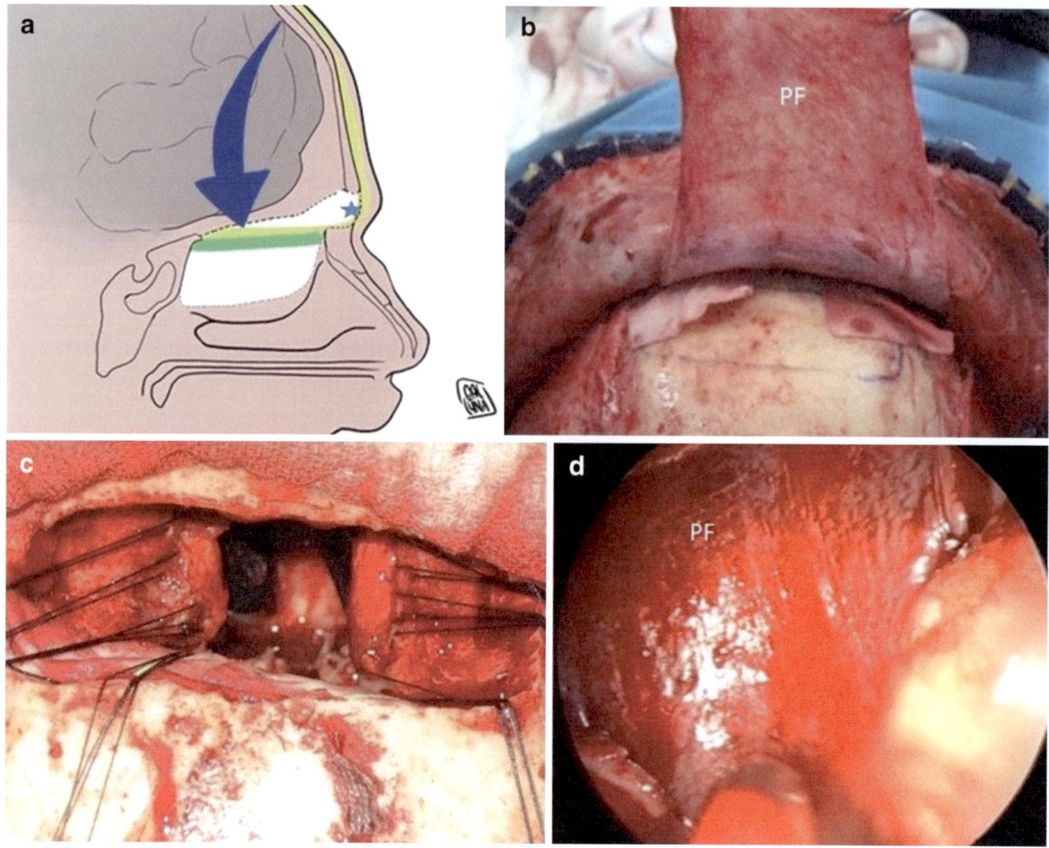

Fig. 10.8 Transcranial endoscopically assisted pericranial flap harvesting. *PF* pericranial flap. (**a**) *yellow line* pericranial flap *green line* multilayer *blue arrow* flap rota-tion *blue star* bone opening, (**b**, **c**) pericranial flap harvesting, intraoperative view, (**d**) endoscopic view of the pericranial flap

As claimed by Harvery et al. [30], vascularized flaps were associated with a lower rate of postoperative CSF leaks when compared with free tissue grafts in the reconstruction of large dural defects.

Regarding the site of the skull base defect, there is no clear differences between vascularized and non-vascularized reconstruction techniques except the tuberculum sella and the clivus. Resection of lesion in these areas leads to a higher risk of high-flow CSF leak; therefore, the defect may benefit more from vascularized flap reconstruction.

Specific disorders such as meningiomas, craniopharyngiomas, Cushing disease and obesity increase the risk for postoperative CFS leaks, and the use of vascularized flap for skull base reconstruction should be strongly considered.

Another key point is the need for future or the history of radiation therapy. In these cases, the use of vascularized flap is indicated because it seems that vascularized tissues are more likely to resist the long-term effects of radiation [16].

10.4 Lumbar Drain

Nowadays, the indication for perioperative placement of a lumbar drain (LD) is not clear because it has not been shown to reduce postoperative CSF leak rate. However, it has been evidenced that LD may be advocated as a first line treatment in postoperative persistent CSF leak. In the case of failure of LD management, surgery is required [28].

10.5 Clinical Consideration on Radiotherapy in Skull Base Surgery

Neo-adjuvant and adjuvant radiotherapy is an important step in the management of malignant skull base tumours. Radiation is usually performed postoperatively, and it may be combined with chemotherapy.

In general, skull base could receive 70–76 Gy in fractions of 1.8–2 Gy with low risk of osteonecrosis.

In case of malignancies, the timing of RT application is crucial for survival improvement. As soon as surgical field is adequately healed, the RT should be started.

Since vascularized flap techniques assure an adequate and fast healing, the earlier delivery of radiation is possible.

Frequent endoscopic postoperative examination is fundamental for detecting satisfactory healing of the wound in order to schedule the early start of RT [31, 32].

References

1. Doglietto F, Prevedello DM, Jane JA Jr, Han J, Laws ER Jr. Brief history of endoscopic transsphenoidal surgery–from Philipp Bozzini to the first world congress of endoscopic skull base surgery. Neurosurg Focus. 2005;19(6):E3. Review.
2. Wigand ME. Transnasal ethmoidectomy under endoscopical control. Rhinology. 1981;19(1):7–15.
3. Thaler ER, Kotapka M, Lanza DC, Kennedy DW. Endoscopically assisted anterior cranial skull base resection of sinonasal tumors. Am J Rhinol. 1999;13(4):303–10.
4. Tufano RP, Thaler ER, Lanza DC, Goldberg AN, Kennedy DW. Endoscopic management of sinonasal inverted papilloma. Am J Rhinol. 1999;13(6):423–6.
5. Schlosser RJ, Mason JC, Gross CW. Aggressive endoscopic resection of inverted papilloma: an update. Otolaryngol Head Neck Surg. 2001;125(1):49–53.
6. Kennedy DW, Goodstein ML, Miller NR, Zinreich SJ. Endoscopic transnasal orbital decompression. Arch Otolaryngol Head Neck Surg. 1990;116(3):275–82.
7. Metson R, Dallow RL, Shore JW. Endoscopic orbital decompression. Laryngoscope. 1994;104(8 Pt 1):950–7.
8. Kelley TF, Stankiewicz JA, Chow JM, Origitano TC. Endoscopic transsphenoidal biopsy of the sphenoid and clival mass. Am J Rhinol. 1999;13(1):17–21.
9. Kingdom TT, Delgaudio JM. Endoscopic approach to lesions of the sphenoid sinus, orbital apex, and clivus. Am J Otolaryngol. 2003;24(5):317–22.
10. Sethi DS, Pillay PK. Endoscopic management of lesions of the Sella turcica. J Laryngol Otol. 1995;109(10):956–62.
11. Mattox DE, Kennedy DW. Endoscopic management of cerebrospinal fluid leaks and cephaloceles. Laryngoscope. 1990;100(8):857–62.
12. Lanza DC, O'Brien DA, Kennedy DW. Endoscopic repair of cerebrospinal fluid fistulae and encephaloceles. Laryngoscope. 1996;106(9 Pt 1):1119–25.
13. DelGaudio JM. Endoscopic transnasal approach to the pterygopalatine fossa. Arch Otolaryngol Head Neck Surg. 2003;129(4):441–6.
14. Gil Z, Abergel A, Leider-Trejo L, Khafif A, Margalit N, Amir A, Gur E, Fliss DM. A comprehensive algorithm for anterior skull base reconstruction after oncological resections. Skull Base. 2007;17(1):25–37.
15. Martin TJ, Loehrl TA. Endoscopic CSF leak repair. Curr Opin Otolaryngol Head Neck Surg. 2007;15(1):35–9. Review.
16. Zanation AM, Thorp BD, Parmar P, Harvey RJ. Reconstructive options for endoscopic skull base surgery. Otolaryngol Clin N Am. 2011;44(5):1201–22. https://doi.org/10.1016/j.otc.2011.06.016. Review.
17. Kim GG, Hang AX, Mitchell CA, Zanation AM. Pedicled extranasal flaps in skull base reconstruction. Adv Otorhinolaryngol. 2013;74:71–80. https://doi.org/10.1159/000342282. Epub 2012 Dec 18. Review.
18. Zuniga MG, Turner JH, Chandra RK. Updates in anterior skull base reconstruction. Curr Opin Otolaryngol Head Neck Surg. 2016;24(1):75–82. https://doi.org/10.1097/MOO.0000000000000223. Review.
19. Kiran NK, Mukunda KS, Tilak Raj TN. Platelet concentrates: a promising innovation in dentistry. J Dent Sci Res. 2011;2:50–61.
20. Hadad G, Bassagasteguy L, Carrau RL, Mataza JC, Kassam A, Snyderman CH, Mintz A. A novel reconstructive technique after endoscopic expanded endonasal approaches: vascular pedicle nasoseptal flap. Laryngoscope. 2006;116(10):1882–6.
21. Clavenna MJ, Turner JH, Chandra RK. Pedicled flaps in endoscopic skull base reconstruction: review of current techniques. Curr Opin Otolaryngol Head Neck Surg. 2015;23(1):71–7. https://doi.org/10.1097/MOO.0000000000000115. Review.
22. Van Zele T, Bachert C. Endoscopic skull base reconstruction after endoscopic endonasal approach. B-ENT. 2011;7(Suppl 17):41–6.
23. Hadad G, Rivera-Serrano CM, Bassagaisteguy LH, Carrau RL, Fernandez-Miranda J, Prevedello DM, Kassam AB. Anterior pedicle lateral nasal wall flap: a novel technique for the reconstruction of anterior skull base defects. Laryngoscope. 2011;121(8):1606–10. https://doi.org/10.1002/lary.21889.
24. Meier JC, Bleier BS. Anteriorly based pedicled flaps for skull base reconstruction. Adv Otorhinolaryngol.

2013;74:64–70. https://doi.org/10.1159/000342281. Epub 2012 Dec 18. Review.

25. Zanation AM, Snyderman CH, Carrau RL, Kassam AB, Gardner PA, Prevedello DM. Minimally invasive endoscopic pericranial flap: a new method for endonasal skull base reconstruction. Laryngoscope. 2009;119(1):13–8. https://doi.org/10.1002/lary.20022.

26. Sigler AC, D'Anza B, Lobo BC, Woodard TD, Recinos PF, Sindwani R. Endoscopic skull base reconstruction: an evolution of materials and methods. Otolaryngol Clin N Am. 2017;50(3):643–53. https://doi.org/10.1016/j.otc.2017.01.015. Epub 2017 Mar 31. Review.

27. Cavallo LM, Messina A, Esposito F, de Divitiis O, Dal Fabbro M, de Divitiis E, Cappabianca P. Skull base reconstruction in the extended endoscopic transsphenoidal approach for suprasellar lesions. J Neurosurg. 2007;107(4):713–20.

28. Soudry E, Turner JH, Nayak JV, Hwang PH. Endoscopic reconstruction of surgically created skull base defects: a systematic review. Otolaryngol Head Neck Surg. 2014;150(5):730–8. https://doi.org/10.1177/0194599814520685. Epub 2014 Feb 3. Review.

29. Patel MR, Stadler ME, Snyderman CH, Carrau RL, Kassam AB, Germanwala AV, Gardner P, Zanation AM. How to choose? Endoscopic skull base reconstructive options and limitations. Skull Base. 2010;20(6):397–404. https://doi.org/10.1055/s-0030-1253573.

30. Harvey RJ, Parmar P, Sacks R, Zanation AM. Endoscopic skull base reconstruction of large dural defects: a systematic review of published evidence. Laryngoscope. 2012;122(2):452–9. https://doi.org/10.1002/lary.22475. Epub 2012 Jan 17.Review.

31. Thorp BD, Sreenath SB, Ebert CS, Zanation AM. Endoscopic skull base reconstruction: a review and clinical case series of 152 vascularized flaps used for surgical skull base defects in the setting of intraoperative cerebrospinal fluid leak. Neurosurg Focus. 2014;37(4):E4. https://doi.org/10.3171/2014.7.FOCUS14350. Review.

32. Jang JW, Chan AW. Prevention and management of complications after radiotherapy for skull base tumors: a multidisciplinary approach. Adv Otorhinolaryngol. 2013;74:163–73. https://doi.org/10.1159/000342293. Epub 2012 Dec 18. Review.

Preoperative Assessment and Monitoring of Free Flaps

11

J. Collin and R. Fernandes

11.1 Preoperative Assessment

11.1.1 Clinical

Preoperative assessment for any type of surgery will, of course, include a thorough clinical evaluation of the patients and their suitability to undergo the proposed procedure with an acceptable level of risk relative to the expected benefit. Free-tissue transfer increases the operative time in almost all cases, and in patients with significant comorbidity, it may be prudent to consider more expedient reconstructive options utilizing local or regional pedicled flaps. In terms of factors directly affecting the risk of free-flap failure, those commonly acknowledged include operative time, increasing age, female gender, obesity, malnutrition, nicotine use, anaemia, previous irradiation, diabetes mellitus and systemic vascular disease [2, 3]. Atherosclerosis affecting the donor or recipient vessels is more likely with many of these risk factors, which increases the technical difficulty of free-flap reconstruction and the associated complication rate.

Previous surgery, injury or neurovascular deficit determined from the clinical history and examination may preclude the harvest of certain flaps. The patient's employment and recreational interests can also affect the choice of donor site. There are now myriad reliable options for free tissue transfer, and the reconstructive surgeon should consider carefully which donor site(s) will provide the best balance of functional and cosmetic reconstruction with lowest risk of flap failure.

11.1.2 Radial Flap Assessment

The modified Allen's test, originally devised by Edgar Van Nuys Allen [4] to examine for poor vascular supply distal to the wrist, has been adapted to determine if collateral ulnar artery supply is adequate for harvest of the radial artery without causing ischaemia of the hand:

1. The hand is elevated, and the patient is asked to clench their fist.
2. The ulnar and the radial arteries are occluded with three digits of each of the examiners hands (this will also occlude any significant palmar carpal branch of the radial artery with an abnormally proximal origin [5]).
3. The patient fully opens and clenches again to exsanguinate the hand.

J. Collin (✉)
Department of Oral and Maxillofacial Surgery,
Bristol Royal Infirmary, Bristol, UK
e-mail: John.Collin@nhs.net

R. Fernandes
Division of Head and Neck Surgery, Department of
Oral and Maxillofacial Surgery, University of Florida,
Jacksonville, FL, USA
e-mail: Rui.Fernandes@jax.ufl.edu

© Springer Nature Switzerland AG 2021
J. Acero (ed.), *Innovations and New Developments in Craniomaxillofacial Reconstruction*,
https://doi.org/10.1007/978-3-030-74322-2_11

4. Still elevated, the patient's hand is then partially opened (hyperextension of the hand and wide separation of the fingers can lead to a false-positive result by occlusion of the transpalmar arch [6]) and pallor should be observed.
5. Ulnar pressure is released while radial pressure is maintained, and the colour should return within 6 s, particularly to the thenar eminence. If this is not observed, the test is considered positive or abnormal.

The predictive value of a normal (negative) Allen's test is 0.8%, and therefore, no further preoperative investigations are necessary with this finding. The predictive value of an abnormal (positive) test is only 53%, however so does not necessarily preclude radial artery harvest. In such cases, photoplethysmography of the thumb can be assessed with and without occlusion of the radial artery. Alternatively, or in addition, duplex ultrasonography studies of the upper limb vasculature can be obtained.

11.1.3 Fibular Flap Assessment

Palpation of pulses at the ankle can determine suitable vasculature for harvest of a fibular flap. This can be supplemented with Doppler pulse assessment, which can also be used to identify perforating arteries that would support a cutaneous paddle. More recently, thermal imaging (Fig. 11.1) has been used to identify

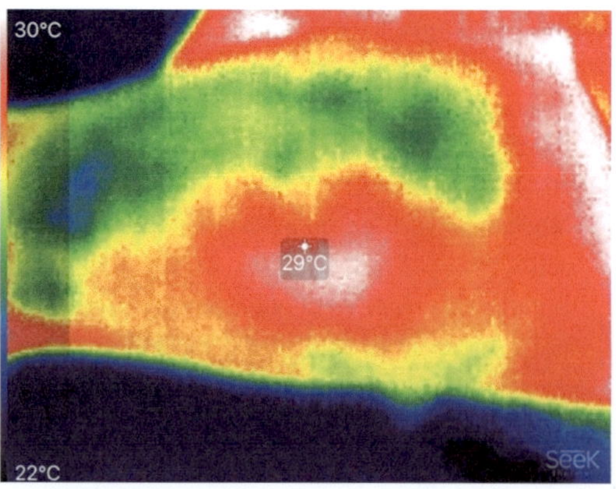

Fig. 11.1 Thermal image demonstrating perforating vessels supplying skin over the lateral aspect of the thigh after application of an ice pack

perforating arteries to guide free-flap skin paddle design [7]. Some surgeons may be happy to rely on clinical examination alone if distal pulses are palpable [8], requesting contrast studies only in cases of abnormal pulses or previous serious lower leg trauma. The majority of clinicians, however, prefer some form of vascular imaging to reduce the potential risk of lower limb ischaemia particularly as the peroneal pulse can mimic posterior tibial and dorsalis pedis pulses.

11.1.4 Radiological Assessment

For many years, conventional digital subtraction angiography (DSA) was considered the gold standard in preoperative assessment of the fibular flap, largely to exclude significant atherosclerosis and peronea magna. Conventional angiography is invasive, with risks of renal ischaemia, groin or retroperitoneal heamatoma, pseudoaneurysm, thromboembolism and intimal damage. For these reasons, the first-line imaging modality of choice is either computerized tomography angiography (CTA) or magnetic resonance angiography (MRA). The former also provides bone data for use in virtual surgical planning (VSP) of osseous flaps, while the latter avoids radiation exposure. There is still a role for conventional angiography, however, where detailed delineation of vessels is required due to equivocation over potential flow limiting lesions. CTA often requires substantially more contrast than an equivalent conventional DSA, and in densely calcified vessels, can struggle to distinguish opacified lumen from calcified atheromatous plaque. MRA has neither of those problems, but is prone to exaggerate vessel narrowing, and is therefore less accurate in quantifying the degree of stenosis.

CTA of the head and neck can also be used to help identify the presence of suitable recipient vessels when considering free-flap reconstruction in a previously operated and/or radiotherapized patient [9, 10]. Magnetic resonance angiography (MRA) can be used to assess the leg vasculature in place of CTA prior to fibular flap harvest. As with CTA, it is less invasive than digital subtraction angiography (DSA), but also has the benefit of avoiding radiation exposure. Patients with ferrous implants or foreign bodies may be precluded from MRI, and those with claustrophobia may not tolerate traditional narrow scanners, however. MRA is able to provide imaging equivalent in quality to tibioperoneal trunk DSA for the purpose of excluding vascular variations or peripheral vascular disease [11] and has been validated in fibular flap assessment [12]. Furthermore, MRA has been shown to be capable of evaluating septocutaneous perforators for composite fibular flap planning [13, 14]. With increasing resolution of newer scanners, MRA has the potential for evaluating vasculature for perforator harvest sites throughout the body.

Colour duplex ultrasound examination can be used as an alternative to contrast angiography for fibular flap assessment; however, it has no standard of reference, and is therefore rather subjective, while it does not generate data of use to the surgeon to guide dissection intraoperatively. Furthermore, additional imaging is still necessary to assess bony volume, provide data for VSP and exclude unidentified previous trauma.

11.2 Intraoperative Assessment

11.2.1 Clinical

Most surgeons will rely on their clinical assessment of intraoperative flap perfusion by evaluating colour, capillary refill time, turgor and bleeding of the flap margins. Obviously, this is highly subjective, dependent on the surgeon's experience and limited to the period between completion of the anastomosis and the end of surgery. A double-forceps 'strip test' is usually performed to confirm venous outflow from the flap downstream of the anastomosis using two pairs of micro-forceps, although this manoeuvre will only differentiate 'some flow' from 'no flow'. One animal study showed that even with up to 95% thrombotic reduction of the lumen, almost 50% of the anastomoses were classified as fully patent using this method [15].

11.2.2 Fluorescent Angiography

In view of the indistinct threshold between clinically adequate but decreased perfusion, and that which will lead to postoperative flap necrosis, a method that quantifies perfusion and also differentiates between arterial and venous compromise is of great benefit. Intraoperative angiography can help provide this information, affording visualization of arterial and venous flow, and soft tissue perfusion (Fig. 11.2). The drawbacks of traditional contrast angiography include the requirement for radiographers, bulky equipment and the additional radiation exposure to staff and patients. Fluorescein arteriography has been used mainly experimentally in free-flap surgery, but is extravasated quickly and can only delineate very superficial vasculature [16]. Indocyanine green near-infrared fluorescent angiography provides an attractive alternative to radiopaque contrast and fluorescein.

The technique involves peripheral intravenous administration of indocyanine green (ICG), a water soluble tricarbocyanine dye that has a long established role in measuring cardiac output, liver function and ocular choroidal angiography. ICG absorbs near-infrared light maximally at 805 nm and has peak fluorescence at 835 nm in vivo. Absorption of these wavelengths by dermal chromophores like haemoglobin and water is low; therefore, intravascular ICG can be visualized with a near-infrared light and suitable cam-

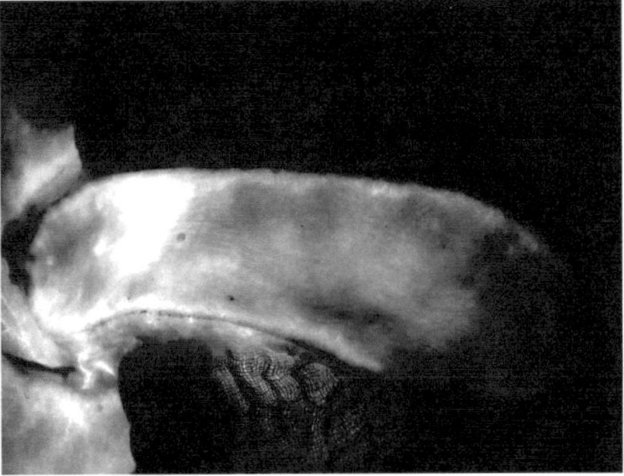

Fig. 11.2 Indocyanine green angiography demonstrating good perfusion of a supraclavicular island flap after raising and prior to inset

era up to 2 cm from the surface. This makes the deep dermal plexus readily apparent, compared with fluorescein imaging that is limited to the superficial dermis. Furthermore, ICG binds large plasma proteins (B-lipoprotein) that keep the dye in the intravascular compartment by preventing capillary exudate, while its short half-life of 3–4 min permits sequential perfusion monitoring, as previous boluses will not obscure subsequent imaging. ICG undergoes biliary excretion via the liver, and adverse reactions are extremely rare [17]. Pregnancy, hepatic impairment, uraemia and previous history of anaphylaxis with intravenous contrast are contraindications. The usual dose for perfusion imaging is within the range of 0.1–1 mg/kg, and toxicity is not seen below 5 mg/kg [18]. As well as a lower risk of contrast-related side effects, there is no radiation exposure to the patient and staff as with traditional angiography.

Near-infrared video cameras for ICG angiography include the SPY Elite (LifeCell Corporation), IC View and PDE systems (Pulsion Medical Systems and Hamamatsu Photonics). This technology can also be integrated into the optical path of surgical microscopes to permit micro-angiography of vessels less than 1 mm in diameter. During harvest, ICG angiography can provide information about the distribution of blood flow to a flap and the extent of tissue supplied by the vascular pedicle. This information is especially important when raising extended flaps for large, complex reconstructions. ICG angiography has also been shown in experimental and clinical studies to have a high sensitivity in identifying perforators and their supplied territory for use in perforator flaps. Although perforator flaps have many advantages, the high variability in perforator vessel anatomy and territories they supply means that verification of these prior to flap harvest with ICGA potentially increases the reliability and success rate while decreasing harvest time.

ICG angiography allows objective assessment of anastomotic patency—the primary determinant for initial microvascular free-flap survival, at the earliest stage before the patient leaves the operating theatre. Confirmation and quantification of both arterial and venous flow can be obtained. Furthermore, adequacy of blood supply to all regions of the flap can be assessed after insetting when parts may have become kinked or compressed. This final assessment of perfusion can be helpful in avoiding partial flap necrosis [19]. ICGA is also useful when undertaking flap salvage surgery to identify the cause and location of the vascular compromise, be it due to thrombosis, arterial spasm, kinking or external compression of the vascular pedicle, hematoma and vasospasm. Early or small microvascular thrombotic occlusions are hard to confirm with subjective clinical assessment; therefore, surgical exploration is almost always undertaken and often re-anastomosis performed. In large flap salvage series, microvascular thrombosis is only found in approximately half of cases [20]. This means that potentially around 50% of cases are subjected to unnecessary surgical exploration. The use of ICGA to determine first if re-exploration is required, and then intraoperatively to identify if re-anastomosis is needed, may prevent potentially harmful surgery and unnecessary manipulation of the microvascular anastomosis when vascular flow is actually present. In summary ICGA requires minimal equipment and peripheral administration of safe contrast agent without radiation exposure to provide extremely helpful quantitative information pre, intra and post-operatively to help reduce partial flap necrosis and need for re-exploration in microvascular and also pedicle flap reconstruction. Presently the cost of the imaging equipment is the only significant drawback, and hopefully, this will continue to decrease with time [21].

11.3 Postoperative Monitoring

Rates of free flap failure due to postoperative vascular compromise are around 2–5% [22, 23] with over 95% of failures occurring within the first 72 h following surgery. In these cases, the chance of successful salvage is highly time dependent [24, 25]. The gold standard for monitoring of flaps is still clinical assessment, and this incurs minimal expense with negligible discomfort and risk to the patient. Most institutions will have a protocol for assessment of flap colour, capillary refill, turgor and sometimes surface temperature 1–4 hourly within the first 24–48 h, when the risk of vascular complications is greatest and the chance of salvage best. Pin-prick bleeding and scratch bleeding time can also be tested; however, some clinicians would prefer not to injure the flap in any way. The emphasis on appearance and in particular the hue of the flap as a guide to perfusion means that high colour rendering index LED light sources have been advocated when examining flaps postoperatively [26]. If clinical assessment is to be relied upon alone, then admission to a high or medium dependency unit is helpful to ensure adequate staffing to carry out the checks at the required frequency. Clinical monitoring is therefore labour intensive, largely subjective, dependent on the experience of the observer and intermittent in nature.

Obviously clinical assessments are only possible where there is a visible skin paddle. If this is not the case, then a strong argument can be made for using internal monitoring devices. While there is evidence to show that they work and some indications that flap salvage rates improve compared with other series, there have been no randomized controlled trials to date [27]. Noninvasive techniques include hand-held acoustic Doppler ultrasound, infrared thermography, polarized spectral imaging and laser Doppler perfusion imaging. Invasive techniques include implantable Doppler probes, micro-dialysis and venous pressure measurements. No one system has been universally adopted.

11.3.1 Thermal Assessment

Some clinicians have used thermistor or thermocouple probes to provide continuous monitoring of flap surface temperature [28, 29]. A drop of around 3 degrees relative to adjacent native skin is suggestive of arterial occlusion, whereas smaller drops of 1–2 degrees can be due to venous compromise [30]; however, there is a delay in temperature change following vascular obstruction, and the technique is not suitable for intra-oral or buried flaps. Thermal imaging has been employed for monitoring of flaps with an external cutaneous component, noting the position of perforators identified preoperatively [31]. This technique is intermittent and relatively subjective in nature though.

11.3.2 Doppler Assessment

11.3.2.1 Acoustic Doppler Probes

Acoustic Doppler probe assessment can be used as an adjunct to clinical examination of a skin paddle. It can also be a reliable means of assessing perfusion of buried flaps with a superficially lying pedicle. Obviously, some care is needed to ensure the probe is not detecting a native vessel and therefore providing false reassurance. Often the surgical team will denote the correct position for Doppler examination of the pedicle with an ink or suture marking the overlying skin. In these cases flow can be confirmed through the pedicle, however this does not necessarily mean that there is perfusion of the entirety of the flap.

11.3.2.2 Colour Duplex Ultrasonography

A refinement of the Doppler principle is colour duplex ultrasonography. This adds visual representation of flow velocity to the acoustic Doppler signal, with different velocities assigned different colours displayed on a viewing monitor. Again, this is noninvasive and can be useful in the assessment of buried flaps. There is much greater expense compared with hand held probes due to the equipment and personnel required. Each examination may require the involvement of an ultrasonographer, radiologist, and the microvascular surgeon, which currently makes frequent observations in the postoperative period unfeasible. Instead it has mainly been used an adjunct to other monitoring techniques, particularly for buried flaps when there is suspicion of vascular compromise [32–35].

11.3.2.3 Implantable Doppler Probes

The implantable Doppler probe was first described in 1988 by Swartz for monitoring of buried free flaps [36]. It became commonly known as the Cook-Swartz probe and is now in widespread use. The device consists of a piezoelectric crystal mounted to a silicone cuff that can be attached to the pedicle artery and/or vein to convert small changes in pressure into electrical current. Wires extend transcutaneously to connect with a device that converts the electrical current to an audible tone, comparable with a standard acoustic Doppler. This arrangement provides continuous information about intravascular flow through the pedicle. An instant alert to vascular compromise in theory allows a quicker return to theatre and increased chance of flap salvage. A systematic review and meta-analysis of flaps for head and neck, breast and extremity reconstruction in 2016 provided evidence to support this, with significantly greater flap salvage rates and overall flap success rates when an implanted Doppler was employed compared with clinical monitoring alone [37]. Furthermore, the majority of the positive benefit is observed in head and neck reconstruction [38]. However, this meta-analysis also identified an 8–17% false-positive rate, and therefore, a significant number of patients were subjected to the risks of surgical exploration unnecessarily [37]. These false positives are due to either malfunction or malposition of the probe [39, 40], so the former may improve with further refinement, and the latter with operator technique and experience. Eventually, wireless probes could help reduce dislodgement in the future too [41]. Obviously, the use of implantable Doppler probes has a cost implication, with each probe costing around 250–300 Eur. This has to be balanced against the potential reduction in flap failures but also the false positives leading to unwarranted exploration. Implantable Doppler probes only detect flow within the pedicle, and this does not necessarily correlate with perfusion of the entire flap.

11.3.2.4 Laser Doppler Assessment

Laser Doppler flowmetry uses the Doppler shift of laser light reflecting from blood flow as opposed to sound in acoustic Doppler probes and was first shown to be of potential use in free-flap monitoring in 1982 [42]. Laser Doppler flow assessment is a noninvasive and reliable method for assessing tissue perfusion, but is affected by ambient conditions, fluid accumulation under the probe and motion of the patient and even staff within the room. Patient respiration or muscle contraction can lead to falsely elevated values being measured [43]. Despite this limitation, it permits continuous flow monitoring and has led to improvement in flap salvage and overall success rates in some series [43].

Laser Doppler perfusion imaging and laser speckle analysis expands on this method to provide a two-dimensional image of tissue perfusion. A near-infrared laser beam scans over the skin surface of the tissue, penetrating from 0.5 to 2 mm to assess the Doppler shift of reflected light from the blood in the microvasculature. The perfusion measured can be displayed numerically or as a colour-coded image overlayed onto an image taken simultaneously by a digital camera. This has been shown to aid both planning and monitoring of non-buried flaps by identification of areas of poor perfusion [44, 45]. It is as yet unable to prove continuous monitoring due to slow acquisition speeds [46]. The imaging device is the size of a large video camera, easy to use, and although the initial cost is around 70,000 Eur, the only consumable is a sterile cover. Intraoperatively, it can be used to guide final flap design after anastomosis and may prove to be a valuable modality for postoperative monitoring for non-buried flaps.

11.4 Other Monitoring Methods

Other methods for free-flap monitoring that have been reported in small studies include continuous bedside photoplethysmograph waveform monitoring [47], technetium-99m sestamibi scintigraphy [48] perfusion-weighted magnetic resonance imaging [49] and microdialysis to assess flap capillary glucose and lactate levels [50, 51]. While these show some promise, further evidence of improvement in outcomes is required, ideally in the form of clinical trials, before they can be recommended for widespread use.

11.5 Summary

With the large number of free flaps currently described, it is helpful to have reliable methods to help guide the choice of reconstruction for a particular head and neck defect in a particular patient. MRA and thermal imaging assessment are likely to be of increasing utility in the near future in this respect as they are noninvasive, and the latter easily repeatable with a hand-held device. ICG angiography has become a great asset in intraoperative assessment of free-flap perfusion and guidance of design as it demonstrates whole-flap perfusion, rather than simply flow at the pedicle. The current evidence base shows both ICG angiography and laser Doppler assessment of tissue perfusion to be of benefit in improving flap survival. The threshold measurements for viable and non-viable tissue still need clarification for both of these techniques however. It may be that the future ideal monitoring protocol may be a combination of two or more of the methods described in this chapter that will provide continuous assessment of whole-flap perfusion and reliable, timely indication of when salvage surgery is required.

References

1. Chao AH, Meyerson J, Povoski SP, Kocak E. A review of devices used in the monitoring of microvascular free tissue transfers. Expert Rev Med Devices. 2013;10:649–60.
2. Chen HC, Coskunfirat OK, Özkan Ö, Mardini S, Cigna E, Salgado CJ, et al. Guidelines for the optimization of microsurgery in atherosclerotic patients. Microsurgery. 2006;26:356–62.
3. Zhao EH, Nishimori K, Brady J, Siddiqui SH, Eloy JA, Baredes S, et al. Analysis of risk factors for unplanned reoperation following free flap surgery of the head and neck. Laryngoscope. 2018;128(12):2790–5.
4. Allen EV. Thromboangiitis obliterans: methods of diagnosis of chronic occlusive arterial lesions distal to the wrist with illustrative cases. Am J Med Sci. 1929;178:237–44.
5. Asif M, Sarkar PK. Three-digit Allen's test. Ann Thorac Surg. 2007;84(2):686–7.
6. Greenhow DE. Incorrect performance of Allen's test-ulnar-artery flow erroneously presumed inadeguate. Anesthesiology. 1972;37(3):356–7.
7. Hardwicke JT, Osmani O, Skillman JM. Detection of perforators using smartphone thermal imaging. Plast Reconstr Surg. 2016;137(1):39–41.
8. Lutz BS, Wei FC, Ng SH, Chen IH, Chen SHT. Routine donor leg angiography before vascularized free fibula transplantation is not necessary: a prospective study in 120 clinical cases. Plast Reconstr Surg. 1999;103:121–7.
9. Chen Y-W, Yen J-H, Chen W-H, Chen I-C, Lai C-S, Lu C-T, et al. Preoperative computed tomography angiography for evaluation of feasibility of free flaps in difficult reconstruction of head and neck. Ann Plast Surg. 2016;76:S19–24.
10. Thurmüller P, Kesting MR, Hölzle F, Retzgen H, Wolff K-D. Volume-rendered three-dimensional spiral computed tomographic angiography as a planning tool for microsurgical reconstruction in patients who have had operations or radiotherapy for oropharyngeal cancer. Br J Oral Maxillofac Surg. 2007;45(7):543–7.
11. Hingorani A, Ascher E, Markevich N, Kallakuri S, Schutzer R, Yorkovich W, et al. A comparison of magnetic resonance angiography, contrast arteriography, and duplex arteriography for patients undergoing lower extremity revascularization. Ann Vasc Surg. 2004;18:294–301.
12. Mast BA. Comparison of magnetic resonance angiography and digital subtraction angiography for visualization of lower extremity arteries. Ann Plast Surg. 2001;46:261–4.
13. Fukaya E, Saloner D, Leon P, Wintermark M, Grossman RF, Nozaki M. Magnetic resonance angiography to evaluate septocutaneous perforators in free fibula flap transfer. J Plast Reconstr Aesthetic Surg. 2010;63:1099–104.
14. Fukaya E, Grossman RF, Saloner D, Leon P, Nozaki M, Mathes SJ. Magnetic resonance angiography for free fibula flap transfer. J Reconstr Microsurg. 2007;23:205–11.
15. Krag C, Holck S. The value of the patency test in microvascular anastomosis: correlation between observed patency and size of intraluminal thrombus: an experimental study in rats. Br J Plast Surg. 1981;34(1):64–6.
16. Tadros A, Kumar K, Jaffe W, London N, Varma S. Free flap neovascularization: Fact or fiction? Eur J Plast Surg. 2003;26:1–2.
17. Hope-Ross M, Yannuzzi LA, Gragoudas ES, Guyer DR, Slakter JS, Sorenson JA, et al. Adverse reactions due to Indocyanine Green. Ophthalmology. 1994;101:534–41.
18. Raabe A, Beck J, Gerlach R, Zimmermann M, Seifert V, Macdonald RL, et al. Near-infrared indocyanine green video angiography: a new method for intraoperative assessment of vascular flow. Neurosurgery. 2003;52:132.
19. Casey WJ, Connolly KA, Nanda A, Rebecca AM, Perdikis G, Smith AA. Indocyanine green laser angiography improves deep inferior epigastric perforator flap outcomes following abdominal suction lipectomy. Plast Reconstr Surg. 2015;135:491e.

20. Kroll SS, Schusterman MA, Reece GP, Miller MJ, Evans GRD, Robb GL, et al. Timing of pedicle thrombosis and flap loss after free-tissue transfer. Plast Reconstr Surg. 1996;98:1230.
21. Beckler AD, Ezzat WH, Seth R, Nabili V, Blackwell KE. Assessment of fibula flap skin perfusion in patients undergoing oromandibular reconstruction comparison of clinical findings, fluorescein, and indocyanine green angiography. JAMA Facial Plast Surg. 2015;17:422.
22. Schusterman MA, Miller MJ, Reece GP, Kroll SS, Marchi M, Goepfert H. A single center's experience with 308 free flaps for repair of head and neck cancer defects. Plast Reconstr Surg. 1994;93:472.
23. Hidalgo DA, Disa JJ, Cordeiro PG, Hu QY. A review of 716 consecutive free flaps for oncologic surgical defects: refinement in donor-site selection and technique. Plast Reconstr Surg. 1998;102:722.
24. Smit JM, Acosta R, Zeebregts CJ, Liss AG, Anniko M, Hartman EHM. Early reintervention of compromised free flaps improves success rate. Microsurgery. 2007;27:612.
25. Te Chen K, Mardini S, Chuang DCC, Lin CH, Cheng MH, Te LY, et al. Timing of presentation of the first signs of vascular compromise dictates the salvage outcome of free flap transfers. Plast Reconstr Surg. 2007;120:187–95.
26. Van Genechten M, Rahmel B, Batstone MD. Red or white? Use of high colour-rendering index, light-emitting diodes in monitoring of free flaps of the head and neck. Br J Oral Maxillofac Surg. 2015;53:416.
27. Dort JC, Farwell DG, Findlay M, Huber GF, Kerr P, Shea-Budgell MA, et al. Optimal perioperative care in major head and neck cancer surgery with free flap reconstruction. JAMA Otolaryngol Neck Surg. 2017;143(3):292.
28. Machens H-G, Mailaender P, Rieck B, Berger A. Techniques of postoperative blood flow monitoring after free tissue transfer: an overview. Microsurgery. 1994;15:778.
29. Stepnick DW, Hayden RE. Postoperative monitoring and salvage of microvascular free flaps. Otolaryngol Clin N Am. 1994;27:1201.
30. Salgado CJ, Moran SL, Mardini S. Flap monitoring and patient management. Plast Reconstr Surg. 2009;124:e295.
31. Mercer J, De Weerd L, Miland Å, Weum S. Pre-, intra-, and postoperative use of Dynamic Infrared Thermography (DIRT) provides valuable information on skin perfusion in perforator flaps used in reconstructive surgery. Proc Inframation. 2010;184.
32. Schön R, Düker J, Schmelzeisen R. Ultrasonographic imaging of head and neck pathology. Atlas Oral Maxillofac Surg Clin North Am. 2002;10:213.
33. Sekido M, Yamamoto Y, Sugihara T. Arterial blood flow changes after free tissue transfer in head and neck reconstruction. Plast Reconstr Surg. 2005;115:1547.
34. Vakharia KT, Henstrom D, Lindsay R, Cunnane MB, Cheney M, Hadlock T. Color Doppler ultrasound: effective monitoring of the buried free flap in facial reanimation. Otolaryngol Head Neck Surg. 2012;146:372.
35. Khalid AN, Quraishi SA, Zang WA, Chadwick JL, Stack BC. Color Doppler ultrasonography is a reliable predictor of free tissue transfer outcomes in head and neck reconstruction. Otolaryngol Head Neck Surg. 2006;134:635.
36. Swartz WM, Jones NF, Cherup L, Klein A. Direct monitoring of microvascular anastomoses with the 20-mhz ultrasonic doppler probe: an experimental and clinical study. Plast Reconstr Surg. 1988;81:149.
37. Han ZF, Guo LL, Liu LB, Li Q, Zhou J, Wei AZ, et al. A comparison of the Cook-Swartz Doppler with conventional clinical methods for free flap monitoring: a systematic review and a meta-analysis. Int J Surg. 2016;32:109.
38. Schmulder A, Gur E, Zaretski A. 296 Direct monitoring by Cook-Swartz Doppler – a study of 7 years in Free-Flaps operations; macro, micro and re-exploration results in regard to breast reconstructive surgeries. Eur J Cancer Suppl. 2010;8:144.
39. Ferguson REH, Yu P. Techniques of monitoring buried fasciocutaneous free flaps. Plast Reconstr Surg. 2009;123:525.
40. Rosenberg JJ, Fornage BD, Chevray PM. Monitoring buried free flaps: Limitations of the implantable Doppler and use of color duplex sonography as a confirmatory test. Plast Reconstr Surg. 2006;118:109.
41. Unadkat JV, Rothfuss M, Mickle MH, Sejdic E, Gimbel ML. The development of a wireless implantable blood flow monitor. Plast Reconstr Surg. 2015;136:199.
42. Jones BM, Mayou BJ. The Laser Doppler flowmeter for microvascular monitoring: a preliminary report. Br J Plast Surg. 1982;35:147.
43. Clinton MS, Sepka RS, Bristol D, Pederson WC, Barwick WJ, Serafin D, et al. Establishment of normal ranges of laser doppler blood flow in autologous tissue transplants. Plast Reconstr Surg. 1991;87:299.
44. To C, Rees-Lee JE, Gush RJ, Gooding KM, Cawrse NH, Shore AC, et al. Intraoperative tissue perfusion measurement by laser speckle imaging: a potential aid for reducing postoperative complications in free flap breast reconstruction. Plast Reconstr Surg. 2019;143:935e.
45. Brennan PA, Brands MT, Gush R, Alam P. Laser-speckle imaging to measure tissue perfusion in free flaps in oral and maxillofacial surgery: a potentially exciting and easy to use monitoring method. Br J Oral Maxillofac Surg. 2018;56(6):556–8.
46. Schlosser S, Wirth R, Plock JA, Serov A, Banic A, Erni D. Application of a new laser Doppler imaging system in planning and monitoring of surgical flaps. J Biomed Opt. 2010;15:036023. [Erratum appears in J Biomed Opt. 2010 Sep-Oct;15(5):059801].
47. Jones JW, Wiebalck R. Continuous postoperative free-flap monitoring with an EKG-interfaced photoplethysmograph. J Reconstr Microsurg. 1992;8:61.

48. Top H, Sarikaya A, Aygit AC, Benlier E, Kiyak M. Review of monitoring free muscle flap transfers in reconstructive surgery: role of 99mtc sestamibi scintigraphy. Nucl Med Commun. 2006;27:91.

49. Jung EM, Prantl L, Schreyer AG, Schreyer CI, Rennert J, Walter M, et al. New perfusion imaging of tissue transplants with Contrast Harmonic Ultrasound Imaging (CHI) and Magnetic Resonance Imaging (MRI) in comparison with laser-induced Indocyanine Green (ICG) fluorescence angiography. Clin Hemorheol Microcirc. 2009;43:19.

50. Guillier D, Moris V, Cristofari S, Gerenton B, Hallier A, Rizzi P, et al. Monitoring of myocutaneous flaps by measuring capillary glucose and lactate levels: experimental study. Ann Plast Surg. 2018;80:416.

51. Nielsen HT, Gutberg N, Birke-Sorensen H. Monitoring of intraoral free flaps with microdialysis. Br J Oral Maxillofac Surg. 2011;49:521.

New Technologies and Reconstruction of the Temporomandibular Joint (TMJ)

12

Eduardo Sánchez-Jáuregui and Luis Vega

12.1 Introduction

New technologies have totally changed the way we plan surgeries in the cranio-maxillofacial area. In the 3D printing era, customized implants are gaining more and more popularity, and its use in maxillofacial surgery is currently widely spread. Temporomandibular joint (TMJ) replacement has suffered as well the impact of these new technologies. New materials and patient-specific implants provide us much better prosthesis design, with a more accurate surgery and better outcomes in terms of pain, function, and esthetics. New technologies combining 3D imaging, CAD/CAM procedures, and navigation can make possible nowadays to approach complex TMJ reconstruction cases with a high success rate (Fig. 12.1).

Despite these advantages, there is still controversy in the management of TMJ pathology. Furthermore, all the new developments should be studied long term and properly tested.

12.2 History: Materials

History of alloplastic TMJ reconstruction is based on the evolution of the different materials used along the years. Most of these materials has been abandoned since many reports published related problems such as foreign body reaction, heterotopic bone formation, and material fragmentation. On the other hand, TMJ prosthesis evolution has followed for many years the wrong trail of the design and materials used by orthopedics in other joints like the hip, whose load and biomechanics are not comparable to the TMJ.

Currently, three main factors have contributed to achieve more efficient design in the TMJ prosthesis:

- Better knowledge of the TMJ biomechanics
- Better materials (more resistant and long-term stable new alloys and polymers)
- CAD-CAM technology that allow to customize the prosthesis to each single situation

The first published case reporting an alloplastic reconstruction of the TMJ was in 1840 by the neurosurgeon John Carnochan who used a piece of wood for keeping the gap in a joint after an ankylosis resection surgery [1]. The first materials had an interpositional function after ankylosis, condylectomy, or discectomy surgery. Among the multitude of materials used in the past, we

E. Sánchez-Jáuregui (✉)
Department of Oral and Maxillofacial Surgery,
Ramón y Cajal University Hospital, Madrid, Spain
e-mail: eduardo.sanchezjauregui@salud.madrid.org

L. Vega
Department of Oral and Maxillofacial Surgery,
Vanderbilt University Medical Center,
Nashville, TN, USA
e-mail: luis.vega@vumc.org

© Springer Nature Switzerland AG 2021
J. Acero (ed.), *Innovations and New Developments in Craniomaxillofacial Reconstruction*,
https://doi.org/10.1007/978-3-030-74322-2_12

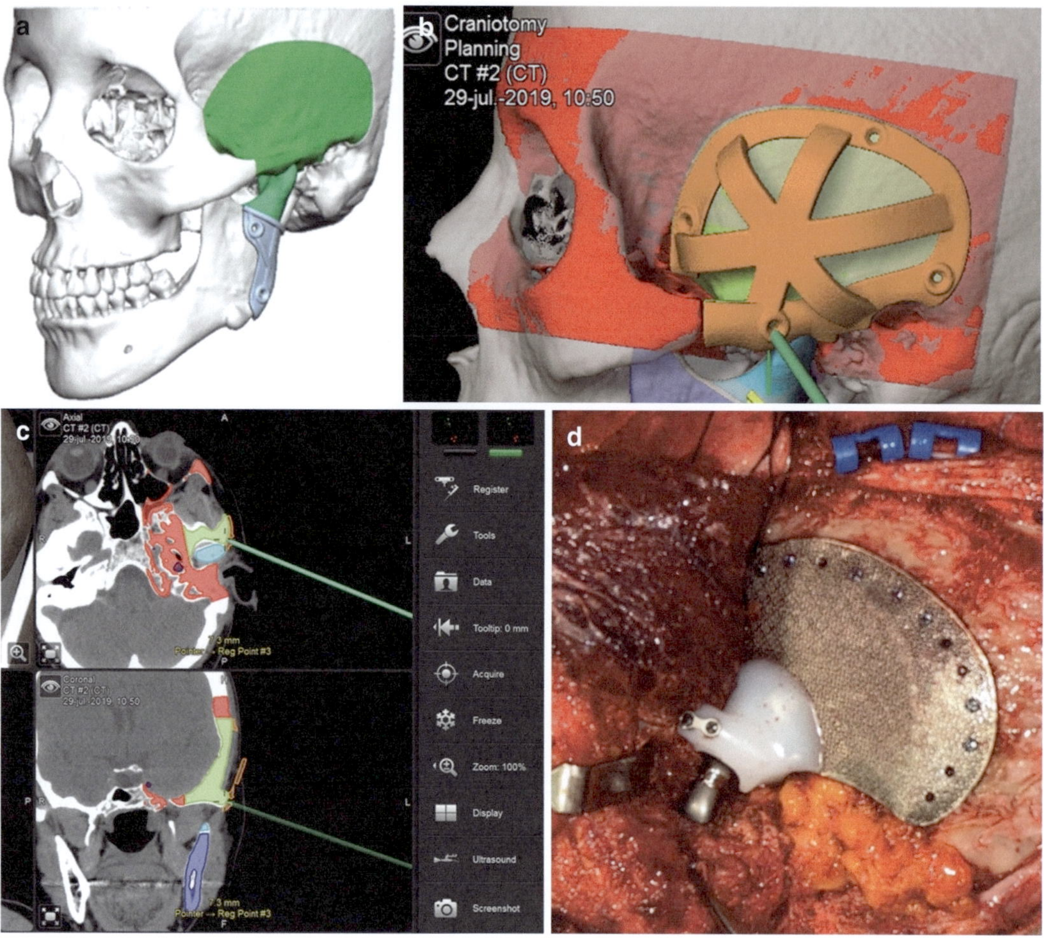

Fig. 12.1 (**a**) Meningioma affecting the temporal bone. Virtual planning of the resection including the glenoid fossa and the mandibular condyle. (**b**) Resection planning downloaded into the navigation system including the cutting guides. (**c**) Navigation-assisted resection. (**d**) Patient-specific implant to repair temporal defect including the TMJ. Intraoperative view

should notice ivory, rubber, gold foil, stainless steel, etc. [2].

However, the real boost of the TMJ prosthesis starts in the middle of the last century with the reports published by some authors; In the 1960s, Robinson publishes stainless steel implant fixed with screws, covering the articular fossa and eminence. Later, this author changed the steel for a silastic sponge (polysiloxane). Silastic was first time used as joint replacement material in 1968, but its use was discontinued some years later (in 1993) because of instability and the production of foreign body reaction. Silastic parti-

cles were even found in histologic study of the regional nodes [3].

In 1963, Christensen published an implant made out of Vitallium (Cr-Co alloy). It was a stock of 44 preformed plates according to the anatomical variations of the fossa and eminence facilitating the surgeon to select the best "fit stock" implant. Two years later, this author published the first total joint replacement using a ramus component made out of vitallium with a covering of polymethylmethacrylate (PMMA) for the condylar head [4]. Polymethylmethacrylate used by Christensen for the condylar head, or by others authors as a cement to get a better prosthesis fixation to the bone, was also abandoned because of its complications such as fragmentation with significant breakage and tissue reaction to wear debris, surrounding tissue infiltration by non-polymerized material, or burning of the tissue secondary to the heat that produced during the polymerization process [5].

In 1972, Kent introduced a new material Teflon (polytetrafluoroethylene) which posteriorly turned in the most unpopular. In the first design, Teflon covered the condylar head, and lately, it was used for the fossa component as well. The material could be enforced with carbon fiber or with aluminum oxide (Proplast I and II) [6]. Teflon was first used with great expectations but also was abandoned in the 1990s due to the adjacent tissue swelling produced by the material fragmentation related to chronic loads, severe bone resorption, and chronic swelling. FDA made a safety alert in 1990 to US oral and maxillofacial surgeons, who were asked to re-examine all patients treated with Proplast or Teflon [7] and finally withdrew Teflon for this purpose.

Since the end of the 1970s until the half of 1980s, several modifications concerning the materials and the prosthesis component design were made; Kiehn, Raveh, Morgan, House, Kummoona, Sonnenburg, etc. reported their results using new materials. Teflon in the articular surface was replaced by a ultra-high molecular weight polyethylene (UHMPE). The high-density polyethylene showed much better biomechanical qualities and a long-term less wear.

In 1989, Techmedica developed a total prosthesis by using first time CAD-CAM technology. A stereolithographic model was printed, and then, a preformed fossa (titanium mesh coated with UHMPE) and ramus (titanium with a vitallium condylar head) were created [8, 9].

Walter-Lorenz developed a stock prosthesis including three different kinds of fossa coated with UHMPE and three different sizes of ramus made out of vitallium and Ti plasma spray for the surface. Long-term studies in a large number of patients lead 10 years later to the FDA approval

for these prosthesis [10]. In 1997, Wolford and Mercuri designed the TMJ Concepts system. Multicentric studies endorsed this system and showed better results in terms of mandibular function, mouth opening, pain decreasing, as well as better quality of life.

In 1996, Chase reinvented Christensen's prosthesis, replacing the PMMA condylar head with a Cr-Co condylar head, creating a "metal on metal" system. This and other systems called "metal on metal" have been subjected to study showing some related problems: cyclic loading of the fossa could lead to micro-motion, fretting corrosion, fatigue, and even fracturing of the fossa, material fatigue, hypersensibility to the metal (elevated body levels of Cr and Cb), etc. [11].

In summary, the evolution of the alloplastic prosthesis has been based on a trial–error process. Despite promising short-term results, the long-term evolution has led to give up some systems. Changes in materials and designs over time can explain why certain systems failed, whereas others are still used today with good long-term results [2].

Some important criteria should be kept in mind in order to select a material to be implanted in the patient bone [12–14]:

1. The material must be biocompatible.
2. Proper fixation to the bone is needed.
3. Osseointegration of the ramus component of the prosthesis.
4. Stiff enough to prevent micromotions, but the elastic modulus must be comparable to that of bone to prevent the shielding of the underlying bone from forces on the implant.
5. The wear resistance of the material (a material with a low wear resistance will develop wear debris).

The future will be based on the development of new coatings and alloys (β-titanium, alumina-toughened, zirconia, etc.), providing implant systems with an elastic modulus closer to bone, with better wear properties and better biocompatibility [15].

12.3 CAD-CAM Technology and Autogenous TMJ Reconstruction

12.3.1 Indications

Although alloplastic implants offer advantages over autogenous replacement of the TMJ, such as avoiding donor site morbidity, decreasing surgical and anesthetic time, and allowing for earlier physical rehabilitation, indications for an autologous reconstruction of the TMJ currently still exist. Growing patients is one of the main indications of this kind of reconstruction due to two main reasons:

1. Mandible bone grows up to 16–18 years old, and the new joint should potentially grow with the child (Fig. 12.2).
2. Life expectancy of a child is higher than those of an adult, and a not-yet resolved problem is related to the average lifetime of an alloplastic TMJ prosthesis.

The most common indications for a TMJ reconstruction in childhood are [16]:

- Ankylosis (secondary to a condylar fracture or an ear infection)
- Rheumatoid diseases
- Congenital aplasia/hypoplasia (hemifacial microsomy)

One of the main advantages of using an autologous graft or flap for the TMJ reconstruction is to permit an adaptative growth or remodeling of the new joint [17].

12.3.1.1 Technical Options

Several techniques have been historically used for an autogenous reconstruction of the TMJ:

1. Sliding ramus osteotomy
2. Costochondral graft
3. Sternoclavicular graft
4. Osteogenic distraction
5. Vascularized free flaps:
   - Fibula flap
   - Second metatarsal free flap

Some of these techniques are rarely used nowadays, but some others are still popular. Osteogenic distraction and vascularized free flaps are in fact the workhorse for autogenous TMJ reconstruction. Both techniques can clearly benefit from CAD-CAM technology [18]. The use of free flaps is discussed in the mandibular reconstruction chapter.

12.3.2 Distraction Osteogenesis in TMJ Reconstruction Technique

Some congenital malformations with a progressive facial asymmetry and malocclusion like the hemifacial microsomy (HFM) are potential candidates to undergo a mandibular distraction, especially those cases with a Pruzansky II in which remains recognizable condyle and fossa. The aim of the osteogenic distraction is to lengthen the mandibular ramus allowing the condyle to reach the fossa, thus correcting the asymmetry and also improving the occlusion.

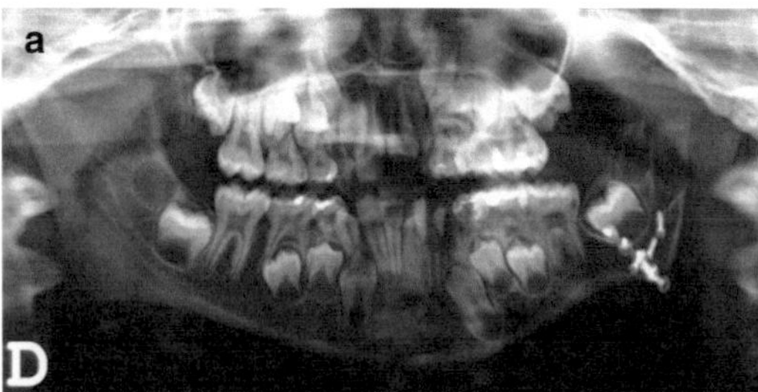
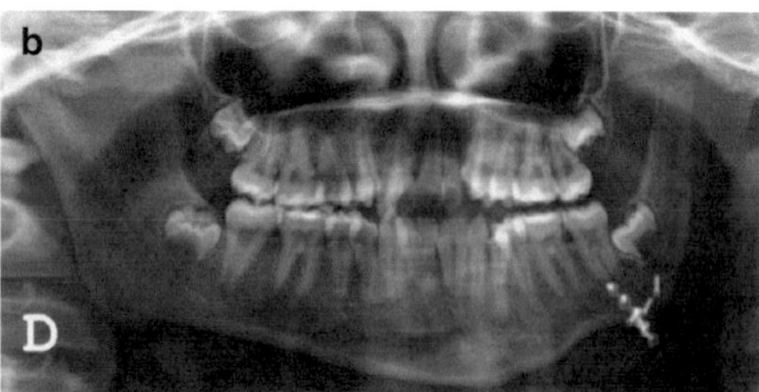

Fig. 12.2 (**a**) Postoperative panoramic radiography of a 5-year-old female with a costochondral graft after a TMJ ankylosis resection. (**b**) Seven years follow-up radiological control. Notice the growth of the graft comparing with the immediate postop panoramic

The use of computer-assisted surgery in osteogenic distraction can be considered in:

Preoperative virtual planning: A thin-cut craniofacial CT is performed, and then fused with the intraoral dental scan (Fig. 12.3a–d). DICOM files are uploaded to a specific software in order to plan the virtual surgery. Next step is to decide the distraction vector which is

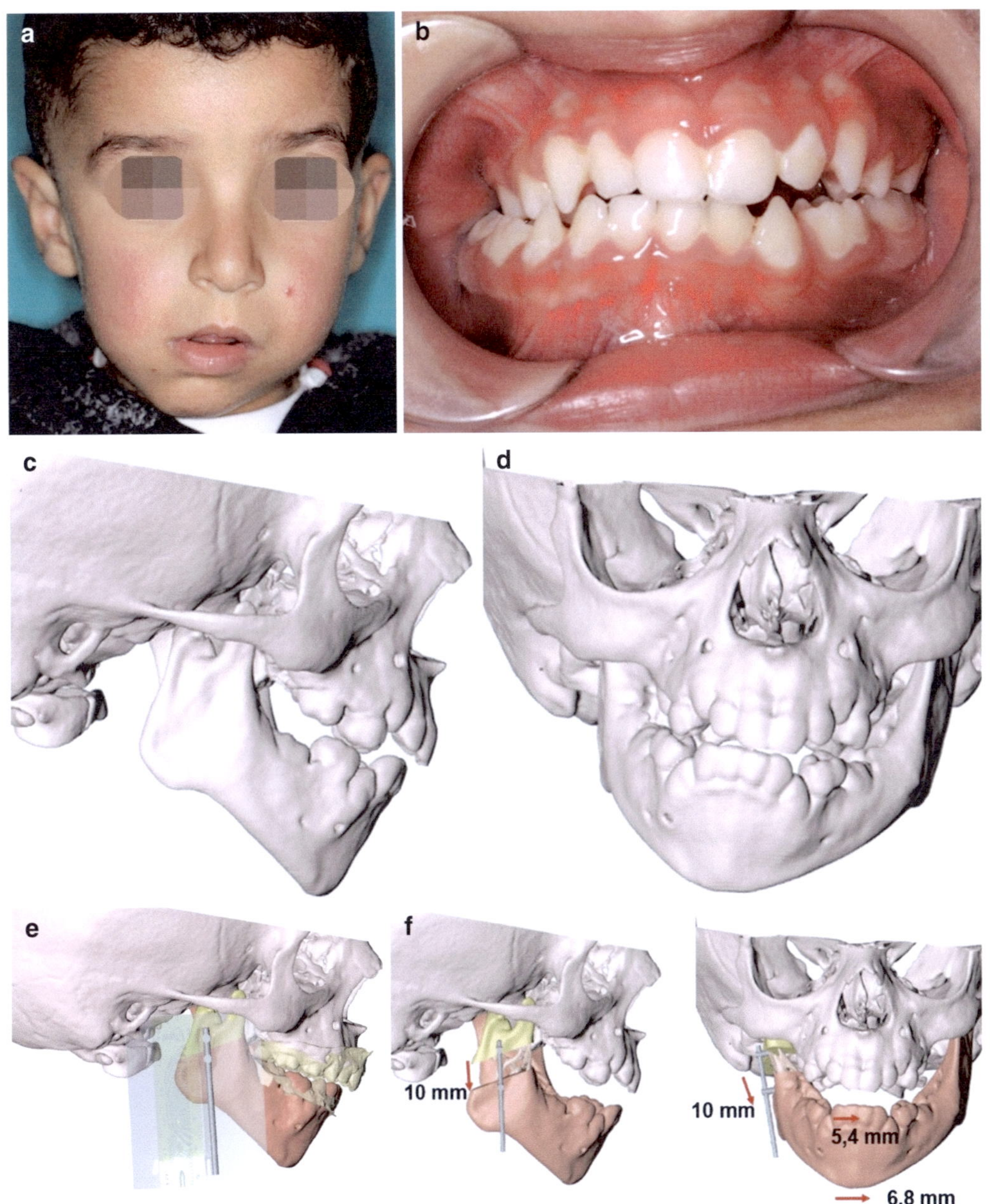

Fig. 12.3 (**a**) Preoperative aspect of a 4-year-old male with a right HFM. (**b**) Occlusion prior to the surgery. Inferior incisor midline deviated to the right with a left open bite. (**c**) Preoperative CT, lateral view: TMJ hipoplasia (Pruzansky IIb). (**d**) Preoperative CT, frontal view: Severe chin deviation to the right coincident with the dental midline deviation. (**e**) STL file with distractor device placed in the desired position to achieve the planned vector. (**f**) Measurements of the mandible virtual movement and the gap created in the osteotomy. (**g**) Virtual design of the ramus osteotomy avoiding the second molar bud. (**h**) Customized cutting and drilling guide placed in the outer cortex of the ramus with a dental reference. (**i**) 2 months postop radiological control. (**j**) Sixmonths postop facial appearance. Notice the improvement of the facial symmetry (**k**) Final occlusion

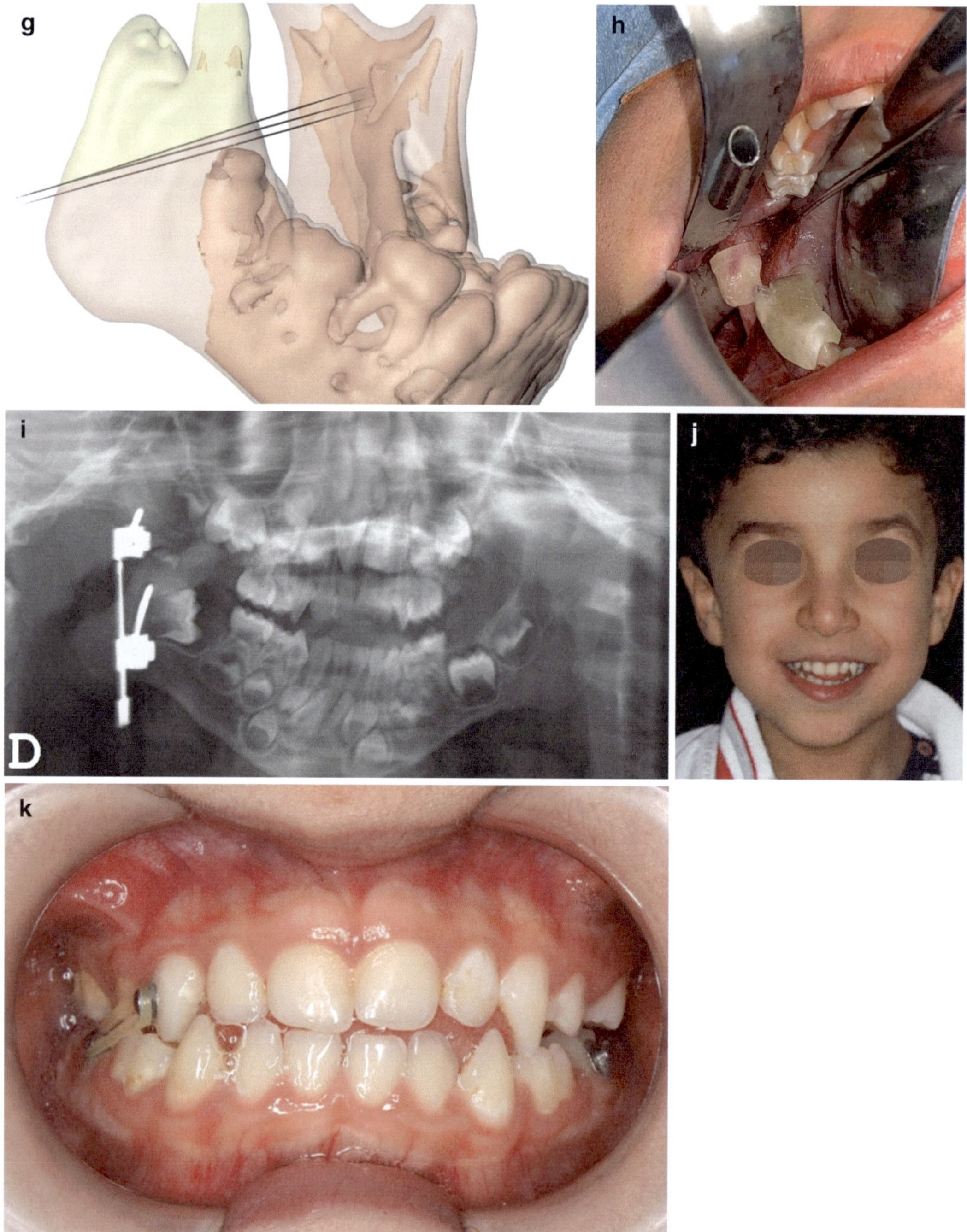

Fig. 12.3 (continued)

defined by the pin distractor location and the osteotomy design. A STL file with the distractor device is also uploaded to the software (Fig. 12.3e).

The planning software allows us to stablish the vector of the distraction regarding the necessary mandible movement. The osteotomy and the position of the distractor device can be virtually designed (Fig. 12.3f) [19]. The osteotomy height and angulation is stablished according to the vector but also avoiding the teeth and the inferior alveolar nerve (Fig. 12.3g).

3D printing: A cutting and a drilling guide is designed to assist the surgeon to perform the osteotomy and the holes for the pins according to the virtual plan [20]. Mandibular ramus surface lacks anatomical landmarks, so the location of the guide could be difficult to establish. At this point, a dental reference is very helpful to ensure the right position of the customized guide (Fig. 12.3h).

12.3.2.1 Surgical Technique

The technique may vary according to the type of distractor to be used. In our hands, the simple the vector and the distractor, the better outcome and easy management. By using an extraoral distractor, the surgical approach is limited to an intraoral incision to expose the ramus in order to perform the osteotomy. Pins of the distractor are placed through a transbuccal way being inserted in the holes previously drilled with the customized guide. Finally, an intraoperative activation is made to ensure the correct movement of the distractor.

12.3.2.2 Follow-Up

There are no variations in the phases and rhythm of distraction. Radiological recordings are made to analyze the gap created and to ensure the correct distraction process (Fig. 12.3i). Pins are removed without need of anesthesia within 6–8 weeks after finishing the distraction.

Orthodontic support is helpful in the management of these patients, not only during the distraction but also in the consolidation phase. In order to keep the new occlusion, elastics are often placed for several weeks (Fig. 12.3j, k).

12.4 Alloplastic TMJ Reconstruction

12.4.1 Indications

The history of alloplastic TMJ reconstruction has been surrounded by noteworthy controversy as reviewed previously in this chapter; however, they currently represent a safe and predictable way to restore the TMJ and its surroundings [10,

21–23]. Indications and contraindications of this type of reconstruction can be seen in Table 12.1. Custom and stock prosthesis are available, and a comparison between both the systems can be seen in Table 12.2. Two established systems have been approved by the United States Food and Drug Administration (FDA): TMJ Concepts custom-made prosthesis (Ventura, California) and the Zimmer Biomet stock prosthesis (Jacksonville, Florida) which is available worldwide. Long-term data outcomes on these two

Table 12.1 Indications and contraindications for alloplastic total TMJ reconstruction

Indications
Congenital and developmental disorders (condylar agenesis, condylar hyperplasia)
Neoplasia
Severe degenerative disease
Severe inflammatory disease
Posttraumatic deformities
Ankylosis
Previous failed autogenous reconstructions
Previous failed alloplastic reconstructions
Contraindications
Growing patients (relative)
Uncontrolled systemic disease
Psychiatric instability
Active infection
Allergy to prosthetic components
Uncontrolled parafunction

Table 12.2 Comparison between stock and custom-made total TMJ prostheses

Stock prosthesis	Custom-made prosthesis
Make fit	Made to fit
Lower cost	Higher cost
Shorter treatment timeframes	Longer treatment timeframes
Removal of bone	No or minimal removal of bone
More difficult to obtained primary stability	Easier to obtain primary stability
Potential micromovement	No micromovement
Placement versatility	Less placement versatility
Potential for longer surgical time	Potential for less surgical time
Limited use for large or difficult anatomical defects	Great for large or difficult anatomical defects

systems represent the bulk of the knowledge on alloplastic TMJ reconstruction (TMJR); however, emerging new systems globally are providing further scientific contributions. Advances in 3D printing have allowed the inception of some of these systems, and like all new technologies, new questions have arisen about the safety of 3D printed metallic medical devices especially considering the complex history of alloplastic TMJ replacements. The use of 3D printed metallic devices bring important biomechanical concerns that need further research:

1. **Porosity control.** The more pores are in the material, lower the density, making it more prone to fracture under loading.
2. **Density control.** While operating under cyclic stress, density will determine whether or not the part will fail under pressure.
3. **Residual stress control.** Variable thermal changes during 3D printing can lead to residual stress resulting in potential deformation of the device.
4. **Cracking and warping.** It occurs when the melted metal cools down after printing. Cracking may also occur if the powder material was not properly melted.
5. **Post processing surface roughness.** 3D printed devices are commonly printed with rough surfaces that require additional post-processing that could damage the integrity of the device.

With regard to the issue of wear with 3D printed TMJ replacements, it depends on the bearing surface materials. Most of the 3D printed TMJ devices have all-titanium alloy ramus/condyle components which in orthopedic hips and knees joint replacements are not utilized as titanium alloy has poor wear properties when functioning against polyethylene. However, we seem to be able to get away with that bearing coupling for TMJR due to the exponentially lower functional loads presented to the TMJ (Mercuri, personal communication). How these 3D printed TMJ devices will perform long-term has yet to be determined. Characteristics of some of worldwide systems are illustrated in Table 12.3 [24].

For the purpose of this chapter, our discussion is based on our experience with the TMJ Concepts custom-made prosthesis and the Zimmer Biomet stock prosthesis as examples of both approaches to TMJ alloplastic reconstruction. Diagnosis and management protocols of the primary process for which the alloplastic TMJ replacement is indicated is outside of the scope of this chapter. At the same time, it is important to remind the readers that due to the intricate nature of these etiologic factors, ancillary techniques such as virtual surgical planning, preoperative embolization, ultrasonic osteotomes, 3D printing cutting guides, and intraoperative imaging and navigation are to be considered [25–33] (Fig. 12.4).

12.4.2 Stock vs Custom-Made Prosthesis

12.4.2.1 Stock Prosthesis

Stock prosthesis concept is based on a stock device in which the patient has to "make fit" to the prosthesis. In the above-mentioned Zimmer Biomet system, the mandibular ramus component is made of a cobalt-chrome alloy with a roughened titanium plasma coating on the host bone side. It comes in three different lengths: 45, 50, 55 mm; two widths: standard and narrow; and two different condylar angulations: straight and off set. It has a fossa component made completely of ultra-high molecular weight polyethylene with a standard base with a flange that varies in three sizes (small, medium, large) (Fig. 12.5). This component has the potential disadvantage that to be adapted it requires the removal of bone from the eminence and glenoid fossa to create a flat surface (Fig. 12.6). On the other hand, the system has the great advantage that it is readily available to use without any manufacture delays. Advances in planning and surgical technique with this type of prosthesis have been reported in the literature. Virtual surgical planning has been done by incorporating a virtual model of the stock TMJ prosthesis allowing the creation of cutting and positional guides to help with the placement of the prosthetic components [34–39]. Modifications of the surgical technique include fossa bone graft

Table 12.3 Total alloplastic temporomandibular replacement systems currently being produced or developed worldwide

Country	System	Stock	Custom	Fossa	Ramus/condyle	Start
Australia	OMX Solutions		X	All UHMWPE	3D printed Ti alloy (DMLS)	2012
Australia	OrthoTiN		X	Metal-backed UHMWPE	Forged Ti alloy	2017
Belgium	CADskills		X	Ti alloy—UHMWPE	3D printed Ti alloy—DLC-coated condyle	2017
Brazil	Bioconect		X	Metal-backed UHMWPE	3D printed CoCrMo condyle Ti alloy ramus (DMLS)	2016
Brazil	PROMM		X	All UHMWPE	3D printed CoCrMo condyle Ti alloy ramus (DMLS)	2015
Brazil	Engimplan		X	Metal-backed UHMWPE	3D printed CoCrMo condyle Ti alloy ramus (DMLS)	2016
Brazil	CPMH		X	Metal-backed UHMWPE	3D printed CoCrMo condyle Ti alloy ramus (DMLS)	2018
Brazil	Genovesi		X	PEEK LT1 20% Ba	PEEK LT1 20% Ba	2018
Brazil	Enterprises Artfix		X	All UHMWPE	CoCrMo condyle Ti alloy ramus	2018
Brazil	Osteomed		X	Ti-backed UHMWPE	CoCrMo condyle Ti alloy ramus	2018
China	Yang system		X	All UHMWPE	3D printed all Ti alloy (SLM)	2017
Germany	Rotec	X		All UHMWPE	CoCr condyle and ramus	2008
Italy	Sintac		X	Ti-backed UHMWPE	3D printed Ti alloy ramus (DMLS)	2018
Lithuania	OrthoBaltic		X	All UHMWPE	3D printed Ti alloy ramus (DMLS)	2018
Netherlands	Groningen		X	Ti alloy-backed UHMWPE	Zr condyle 3D printed Ti alloy ramus (DMLS)	2018
South Africa	Butow	X		Ti nitride alloy	Ti nitride alloy	1994
UK	Dundee		X	None	CoCr	2014
USA	TMJ Concepts		X	cpTi mesh-backed UHMWPE	CoCrMo condyle Ti alloy ramus	1999
USA	Zimmer Biomet	X	X	All UHMWPE	CoCr condyle and ramus	2000

Modified from: Elledge R, Mercuri LG, Attard A, Green J, Speculand B. Review of emerging temporomandibular joint total joint replacement systems. *Br J Oral Maxillofac Surg*. 2019;57(8):722–728; with permission

UHMWP ultra-high molecular weight polyethylene, *Ti* titanium, *cpTi* commercially pure titanium, *CoCrMo* cobalt chrome molybdenum, *PEEK* polyether ether ketone, *DMLS* direct metal laser melting, *DLC* diamond-like carbon, *SLM* selective laser melting

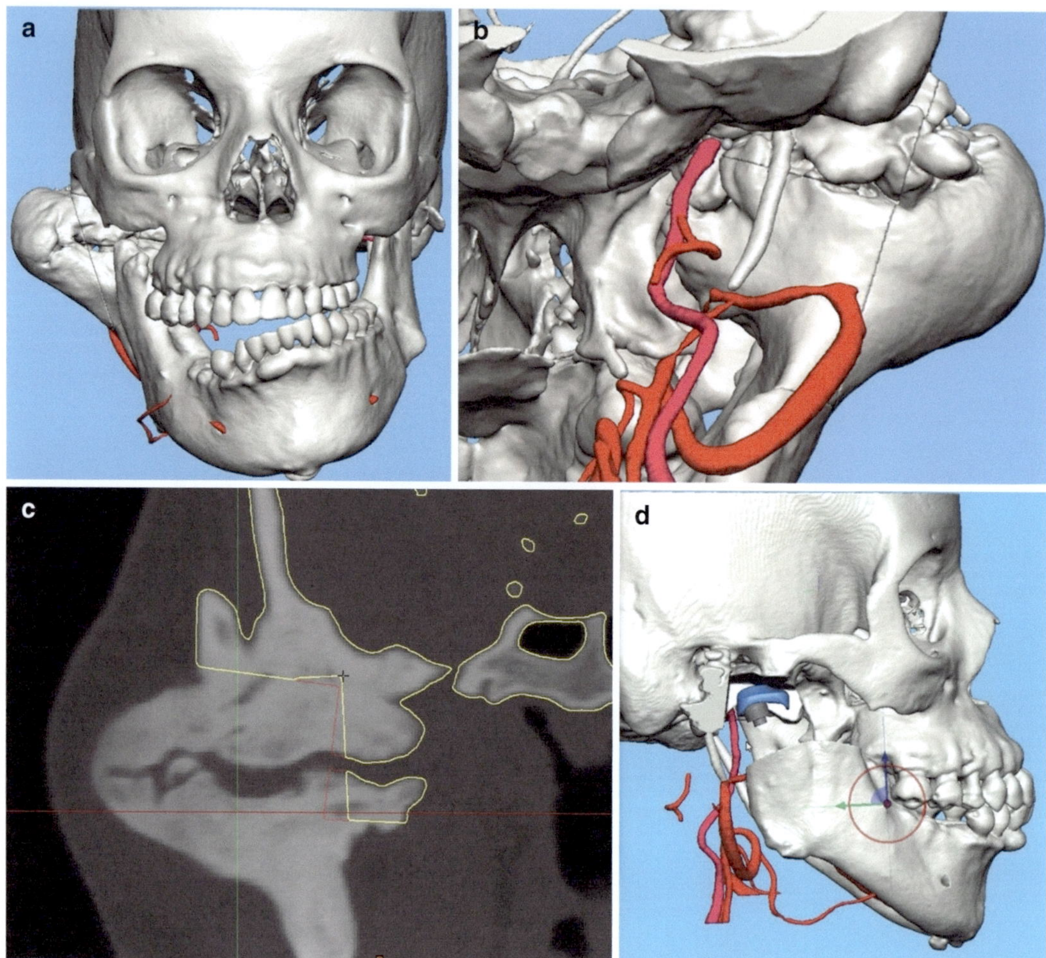

Fig. 12.4 Preoperative virtual planning of a 48-year-old female with severe right TMJ ankylosis showing. (**a**) Frontal view 3D CT scan reconstruction showing a large right TMJ ankylotic mass with mandibular asymmetry. (**b**) Posterior view 3D CT scan reconstruction showing the relation of internal carotid (fuchsia) and maxillary (red) arteries with the ankylotic mass. Proposed osteotomies marked in gray. Case will require preoperative embolization. (**c**) CT scan view showing the proposed osteotomies to create the necessary space for a custom-made TMJ fossa prosthesis. (**d**) Lateral view 3D CT scan reconstruction showing the final gap arthroplasty with a virtual fossa and condyle. A sagittal osteotomy has been done on the left side to properly reposition the mandible into the correct occlusion. (**e–g**) Frontal and lateral views 3D CT scan reconstruction of the proposed ankylotic mass osteotomies

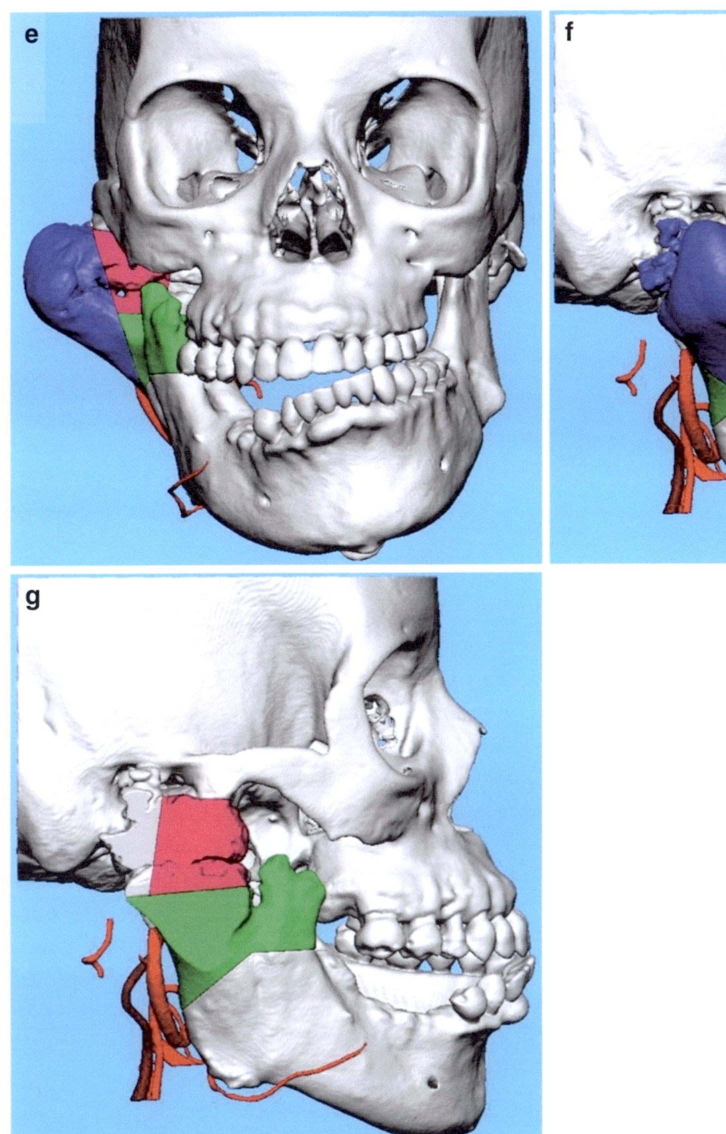

Fig. 12.4 (continued)

to stabilize the fossa component, salvage of the residual disk, and harvesting of fat from the retromandibular approach [40, 41].

Studies by Abramowicz and Brown have demonstrated that stock prosthesis could have been utilized in a great variety of situations in which custom-made prosthesis were done. Still, stock prostheses have the disadvantage that they have a limited application in patients where a substantial vertical and/or horizontal mandibular movement is indicated (concomitant correction of dentoskeletal deformities) or in cases with a significant congenital or acquired deformity or loss of the native anatomy [42, 43].

12.4.2.2 Custom-Made Prosthesis

A customized TMJ prosthesis has the distinct characteristic that it is a "made to fit" device that allows for great versatility in complex TMJ reconstructions [44]. Efforts to classify extended

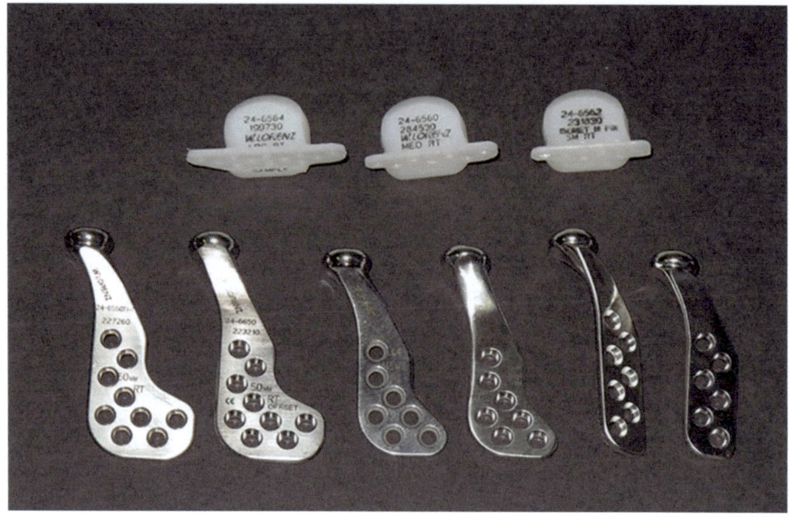

Fig. 12.5 Zimmer Biomet stock TMJ prosthesis. Note that the fossa base is flat and has the same size; what changes is the size of the flange. Standard (larger foot plate) and narrow mandibular components

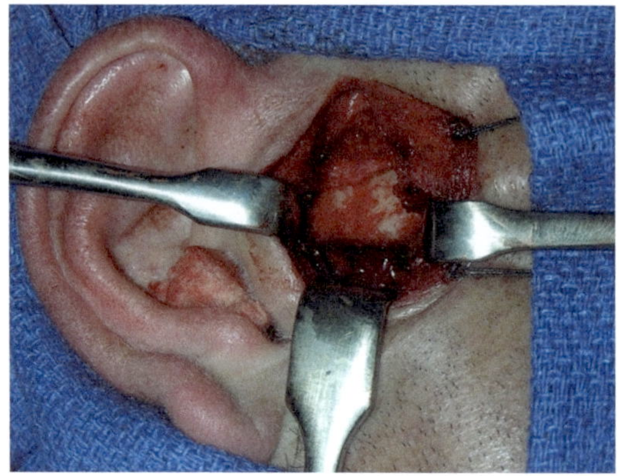

Fig. 12.6 Flatten mandibular fossa after removal of eminence with a power rasp. Site prepared for a stock fossa component

alloplastic TMJ/mandibular reconstructions have been described in the literature [45, 46]. The mandibular component of the TMJ Concepts prosthesis has a body made of machined alloyed titanium with a condylar head of chrome-cobalt-molybdenum (Cr-Co-Mb) alloy. The fossa component has a titanium mesh backing with an ultra-high molecular weight polyethylene articulating surface (Fig. 12.7). The biggest disadvantage of this prosthesis is the time required for its construction.

The process for construction of this type of device starts with a thin-cut maxillofacial CT scan that is used for the construction of a virtual model. If necessary, in selective cases such as concomitant correction of dentoskeletal deformities, neoplasm resection, and pathological or traumatic reconstruction, virtual surgical planning is then performed [47–51]. A stereolithographic model is then constructed. This model is then further studied to determine if any osteotomies are to be made to achieve the necessary clearance to the placement of the prosthetic parts. A minimum 13–15 mm of clearance is necessary between the lowest portion of the mandibular eminence to the sigmoid notch. A wax-up is done in the stereolithographic model. The prosthesis is then manufactured after the surgeon has approved the prosthetic design.

12.4.3 Computer-Assisted Surgery

The use of computer-assisted surgery in alloplastic TMJ reconstruction has the following steps:

Preoperative virtual planning: By obtaining a thin-cut maxillofacial CT scan and dental records (intraoral scan), a virtual hybrid model can be fabricated in which accurate bony and dental surfaces can be obtained. This model will allow for better visualization and understanding of defects, neoplasms, deformities, or discrepancies for which the alloplastic TMJ replacement is indicated. Once proper analysis and diagnosis have been done, a virtual surgical planning can be carried out. Virtual condylectomies are done

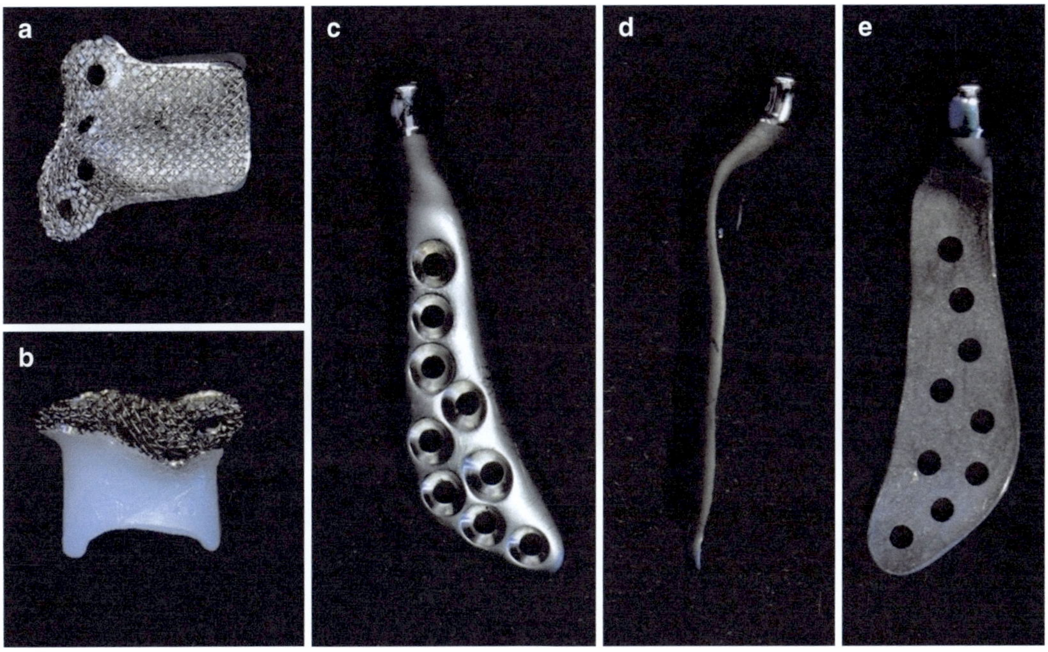

Fig. 12.7 TMJ Concepts custom-made prosthesis: mandibular fossa component. (**a**) Titanium mesh that articulates with bone from the mandibular fossa. (**b**) Lateral view of the fossa. Note the posterior ledge in the block of the ultra-high molecular weight polyethylene. Mandibular component (**c**) Front view. Polished surface. (**d**) Coronal view. Note the significant angle between the ramus and the condyle. (**e**) Back view. Unpolished surface

to assure the proper space required for the prosthesis components. Cases of dentoskeletal deformities have the occlusion and the jaws moved to their ideal position. Neoplasms, bony ankylosis, or failed previous reconstructions can be virtually resected. Cutting guides and positional aides can be designed. Although not available in the USA due to FDA regulations, a virtual TMJ prosthesis can be incorporated or designed to reestablish the lost anatomy.

3D printing: Virtual hybrid, dental, verification, or any other kind of anatomical model can be printed to aid at the time of surgery. Splints, cutting, and positional guides could also be printed in different types of materials that range from plastics to metal. Additionally, as described before, new emerging systems are able to 3D print alloplastic TMJ replacements (Fig. 12.8).

Virtual intraoperative navigation: Once the preoperative virtual planning was defined, the digital information can be exported to a navigator. With the virtual intraoperative navigator, surgeons can establish a comparison between the images on the monitor's screen and the actual bone.

Validation of the techniques: Postoperative imaging is obtained and fused to the preoperative virtual plan to determine the level of accuracy of the procedure.

12.4.4 Surgical Technique

The need of one or two reconstructive stages as well as the different surgical sequences for the placement of the prosthesis depends on the primary process for which the alloplastic TMJ replacement is indicated as well as surgeon's preference and experience. The basic technique consists of:

1. **Nasal intubation.** The size, position, and lack of mobility of the mandible put this patient population on a higher risk for a difficult airway. Preoperative discussion of the airway requirements with the anesthesia

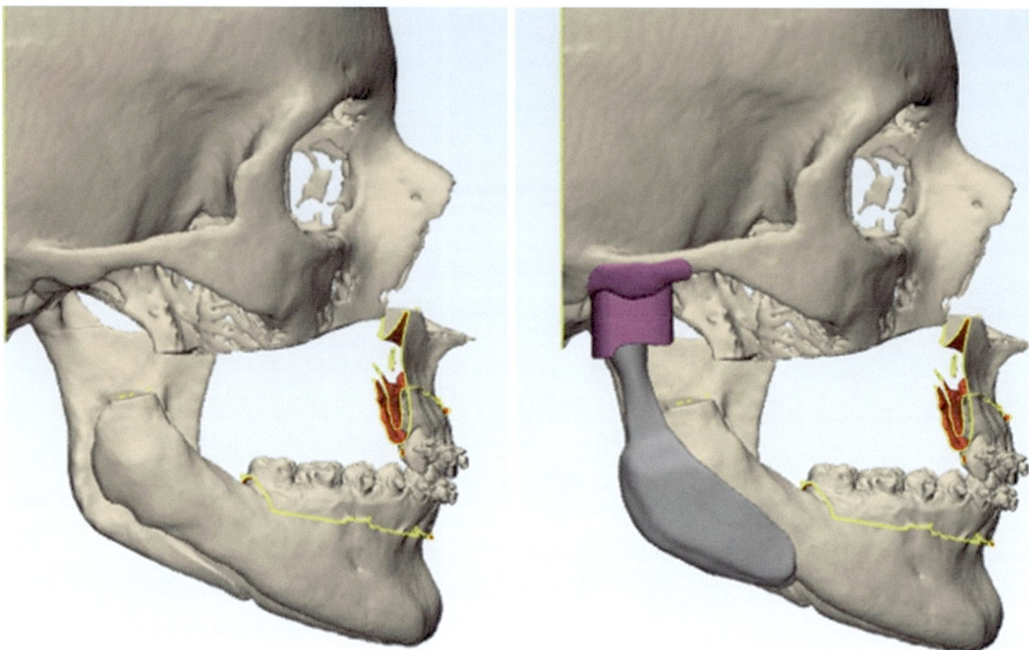

Fig. 12.8 Sequela of osteomyelitis after orthognathic procedure. Virtual planning of a custom-made TMJ prosthesis

team is therefore of paramount importance. Advance techniques such as awake nasofiberoptic or retrograde intubation should be required.

2. **Establishment of maxillomandibular fixation.** Depending on the case and surgeon's preference, the establishment of maxillomandibular fixation could be done prior to prepping and draping the patient. This will decrease the chance of saliva contamination by minimizing the need of intraoperative intraoral maneuvers. In certain circumstances such as bony ankylosis cases, the establishment of MMF is not done until the mandible has been released. Furthermore, some surgeons will wait until the condylectomy has been carried out to put the patient in MMF.

3. **Sterile prep and drape.** Sterility is extremely important to avoid contamination and potential infection of the prosthesis. The patient is instructed to wash their hair the day of surgery. The external auditory canals are checked preoperatively to rule out any ear infections. The patient is then prepped and then draped in standard sterile fashion avoiding, if possible, having residual hair in the surgical field. The mouth, the nose, and the endotracheal tube are isolated by covering them with transparent dressings. An ear wick with antibiotic ointment is placed in the external auditory canal. Antisialagogues should be considered as an adjuvant to decrease the salivary flow while performing the surgery.

4. **Mandibular fossa approach.** The mandibular fossa approach is done via a preauricular, endaural, or modifications to these approaches. The approach depends on the primary etiology to which the reconstruction is indicated, the size of the fossa prosthesis to be utilized, and surgeon's preference. Skin is incised, dissection is carried out through the different layers until the zygomatic arch is reached. Care is taken to avoid injury to the temporal branch of the facial nerve which runs in the temporoparietal fascia, subperiosteal dissection is performed exposing the lateral border of mandibular fossa and eminence. Medial dissection of the fossa is not done until the condylectomy is done.

5. **Neck approach.** The neck approach also depends on the primary etiology for the TMJ alloplastic reconstruction, size of the mandibular/ramus prosthetic component, and surgeon's preference. Approaches vary from standard sub- or retromandibular to facelift, parotidectomy or even apron type of approaches.

6. **Communication of both approaches.** Once the fossa and the mandibular ramus have been exposed, through the neck approach, blunt dissection is carried out with a long clamp such as tonsillar clamp until both approaches are communicated. A Penrose drain can be placed to help with retraction of the tissues in between both approaches.

7. **Condylectomy with or without coronoidectomy.** Condylectomy can be carried out in two different manners: (1) *Through the preauricular region*, in this method, the mandibular condyle is cut using a fissure bur or piezosurgery. Additional removal of bone inferiorly in the ramus can be performed by manipulating the mandible posteriorly and superiorly, allowing exposure of the bone to be cut through the preauricular region. It is important to mention that using this technique means that the patient is not placed in maxillomandibular fixation until the condylectomy is done. If necessary, a coronoidectomy can be carried out through this approach. (2) *Through the neck region*, in this technique, an oblique cut is done from the sigmoid notch to the posterior border of the mandible with an angled oscillating saw. Similarly, the coronoid is cut by doing an oblique cut from the sigmoid notch to the anterior border of the ramus. Using this procedure in ankylosis cases requires a combined method: the inferior cut is done through the neck as described above, then the condylar head is cut into smaller pieces through the preauricular region.

8. **Fossa preparation and placement of the fossa component.** With the condyle removed, the mandibular fossa and eminence are easily accessible. Any soft tissues covering these surfaces is excised as well as any residual remnant of the articular disk. Typically, a medial bleeding is expected after removal of the disk, but it is easily controlled with local hemostatic agents. Cases with a custom-made fossa rarely require removal of bone. Cases with a stock fossa are the opposite and most certain will require some bone removal. The most typical approach is to use a power rasp to flatten the bone to provide the proper primary stability to the fossa implant (Fig. 12.6). An elegant modification of this technique includes the use of the eminence as a graft in the mandibular fossa. Once primary stability of the fossa implant has been corroborated, the implant is fixated with at least four screws (Fig. 12.9).

9. **Preparation and placement of the mandibular condyle component.** In cases of stock prosthesis, the angle region where the masseter muscle attaches and the most superior portion of the posterior border of the mandible just shy from the condylectomy are commonly areas that need to be flattened to provide primary stability to the mandibular component. The narrow mandibular component has the advantage in comparison to the standard component that it fits very well posteriorly to the inferior alveolar nerve avoiding a potential injury while securing the prosthesis (Fig. 12.10). The ramus rarely needs bone removal; when using a custom-made prosthesis, still some surgeons opt to flatten the mandibular ramus in the stereolithographic model. This is done to allow more versatility of placement specially in cases in which a dentoskeletal deformity is to be corrected, and no proper dental records were available due to the patient's inability to open their mouth.

10. **Condylar position.** The condylar head should be placed centered on the fossa bearing in the medial/lateral direction and seated in the most posterior portion of the fossa, in the case of the custom-made prosthesis against the posterior ledge (Fig. 12.11). To facilitate this placement, the vertical position of the prosthesis is achieved by securing one of the superior screws of the mandibular

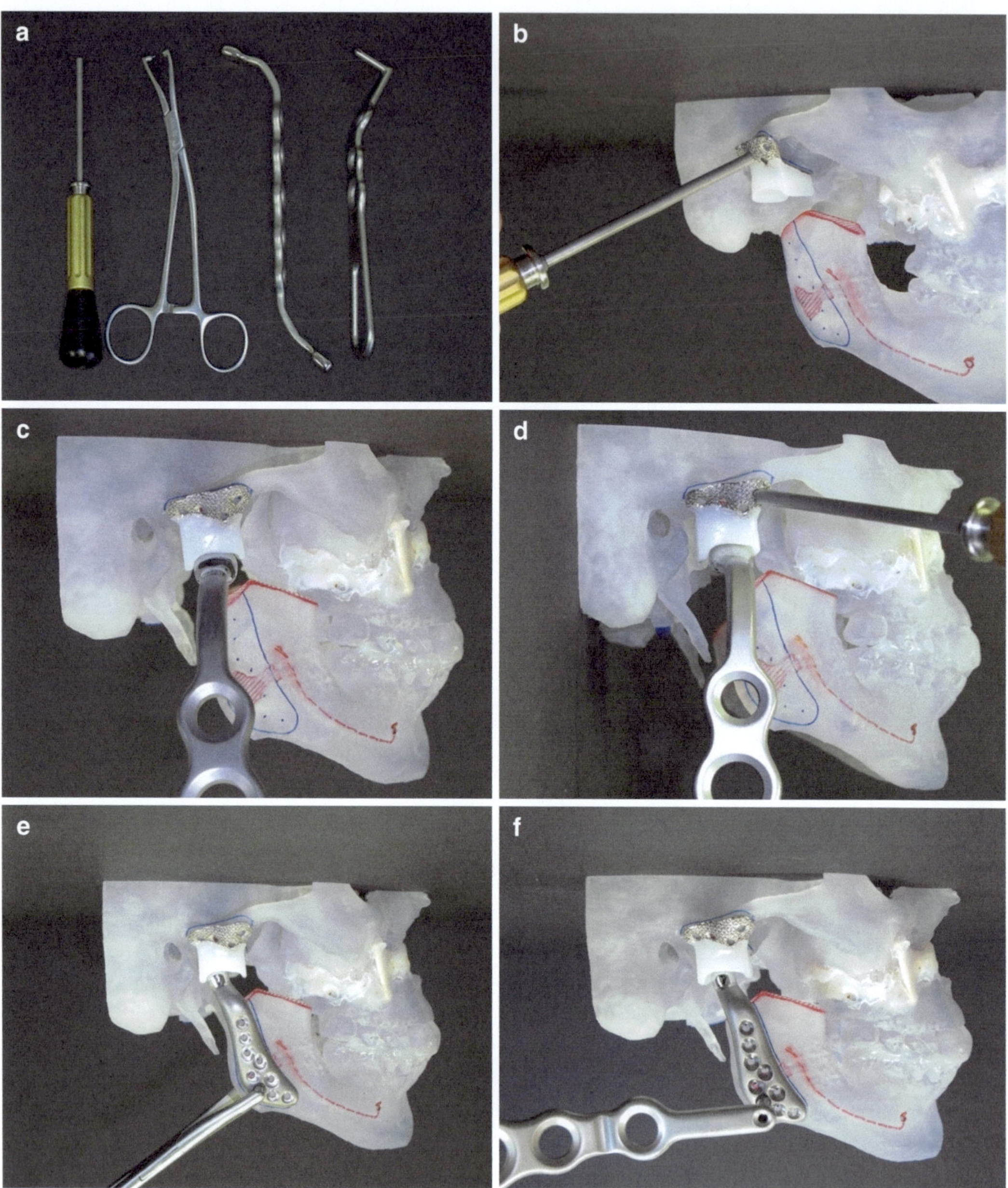

Fig. 12.9 TMJ Concepts instrumentation, prosthesis, and sequence of placement. (**a**) TMJ instruments, fossa pusher, mandibular component clamp, fossa seater, drill trocar. Once the fossa is placed: (**b**) The fossa pusher is used to adapt the fossa prosthesis flange to the zygomatic arch. (**c**) The fossa seater is used to push the fossa superi-orly avoiding any gaps between the prosthesis and the mandibular fossa. (**d**) Both instruments are used together to place the screws. (**e**) Mandibular component clamp helping to stabilize the prothesis to the ramus. (**f**) Drill trocar use the protect the surrounding soft tissues and to help the proper angulation of the drill bit

component first. Next, the inferior portion of the prosthesis is slightly rotated anteriorly to allow seating to the condylar in the most posterior position. This position is then secured with the placement of another screw in the anterior/lower portion of the prosthesis. If indicated, fat grafts can be implanted around the condylar head.

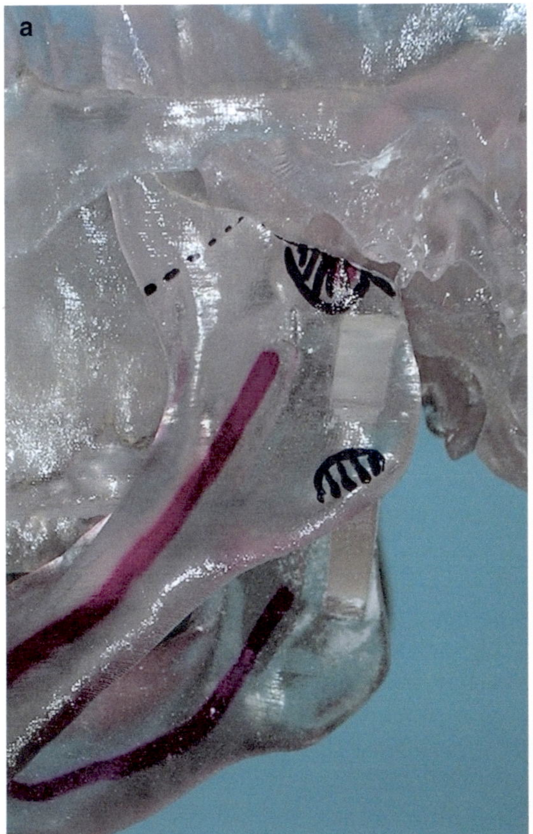
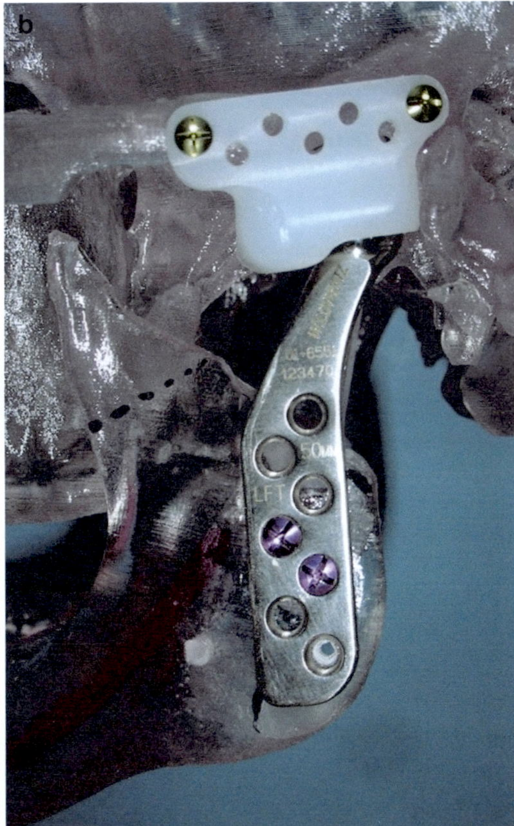

Fig. 12.10 (**a**) Typical areas of interference (angle region and posterior border closer to the mandibular osteotomy) for the placement of the stock mandibular component. (**b**) Narrow mandibular component nicely adapted behind the infraalveolar nerve

11. **Check occlusion.** Maxillomandibular fixation is released. Occlusion is checked. Maximum interincisal opening is recorded and if this is limited, considered further dissection of the medial pterygoid muscles or coronoidectomies if they were not done previously.
12. **Closure.** The wounds are copiously irrigated, and layered closure is achieved. The external auditory canals are inspected to rule out any unnoticed perforations, and the patient is placed on guiding elastics.

In bilateral cases, both joints are accessed and prepared before the placement of the prosthesis, as this will facilitate their placement. Needleless to say sterility is paramount to avoid contamination and potential infection of the prosthesis [52].

12.4.4.1 Postoperative Care of Alloplastic TMJ Reconstruction

The postoperative care should focus in avoiding dislocation. Head dressings or guiding elastics can be used for this purpose. Physical therapy with a TheraBite or similar device must start as early as possible. One week of antibiotics is recommended, and diet is advanced as tolerated [53].

12.5 Outcomes and Complications

Long-term outcome studies with the described custom-made and stock prosthesis have shown that they are safe and predictable option when alloplastic reconstruction of the TMJ is indicated.

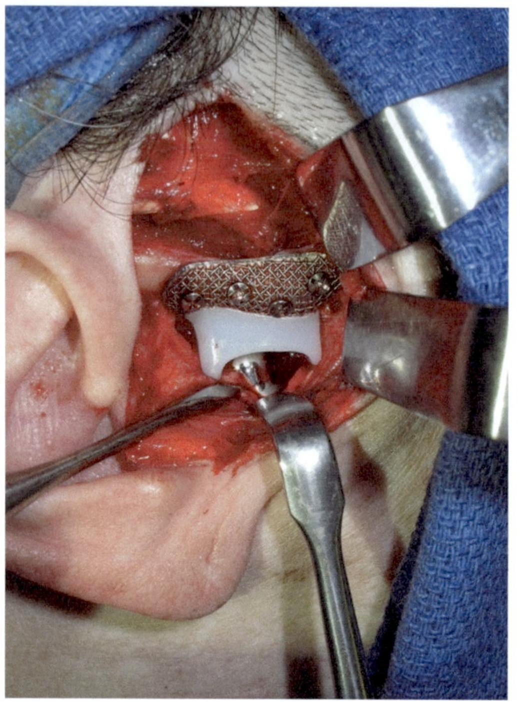

Fig. 12.11 Clinical picture of the proper placement of the fossa and the condylar head within the fossa in a superior and posterior position touching the posterior ledge

Improvements of quality of life, with increase of mandibular range of motion, improvement of diet, and decrease of pain have been reported in the literature [3, 8, 10, 54–66] (Figs. 12.12, 12.13, and 12.14).

Intraoperative complications are rare and include excessive bleeding that requires intraoperative embolization, external auditory canal perforation, inability to properly place the prosthesis. Immediate postoperative complications include TMJ dislocation, malocclusion, permanent or temporary injury to the temporal branch and/or marginal mandibular nerves. Infections could occur within days of implantation or years after surgery. They are difficult to diagnose and to treat. The literature reports an incidence that ranges from 1.6 to 4.5% for TMJ alloplastic prosthesis infections (Fig. 12.15). True mechanical hardware failure due to wear or broken components is rare and is more common to encounter heterotopic bone formation (2%) or patients with hyper sensibility to metals. Several protocols for the management of these complications have been reported in the literature [67–76].

Fig. 12.12 TMJ reconstruction using stock TMJ prosthesis. A 48-year-old female involved in a motor vehicle collision in which she sustained a mandibular symphysis and bilateral subcondylar fractures. She was treated with open reduction and internal fixation of the symphysis fracture and closed reduction with 4 weeks of maxillomandibular fixation (MMF) for the subcondylar fractures. As soon as she was released from MMF, she developed a significant malocclusion with retrusion of her mandible. After significant physical therapy, neither her occlusion nor mandibular position changed. She was referred to the author for further evaluation and treatment 6 months after her original injury. After clinical and radiographical evaluation, it was determined that the patient had mandibular retrognathia and widening with subsequent malocclusion due to loss of vertical support from the subcondylar fractures and the improperly reduced symphysis fracture. Due to the small size of the condyles and location of the fractures, a decision was made to reconstruct the area with alloplastic TMJ prostheses. Stock Zimmer Biomet prostheses were selected because the patient did not want to wait several months for a custom-made prosthesis to be manufactured. An additional mandibular midline osteotomy was also indicated to properly reestablish the width of the mandible. (**a, b**) Posttraumatic preoperative frontal and lateral clinical views showing mandibular retrognathia. (**c**) View of the posttraumatic occlusion showing a significant Class II malocclusion. (**d, e**) Posttraumatic panoramic and lateral cephalometric radiographs showing small and malpositioned bilateral condyles and mandibular retrognathia. (**f–h**) Posttraumatic 3D CT reconstructions showing the small, malpositioned bilateral condyles as well as widening of the mandible due to the improper reduction. (**i, j**) Postoperative frontal and lateral clinical views showing a normal mandibular position. (**k**) View of the postoperative occlusion showing a normal occlusion. (**l, m**) Postoperative panoramic and lateral cephalometric radiographs showing narrow Zimmer Biomet TMJ prostheses, new mandibular symphysis hardware, and normalized anteroposterior position of the mandible

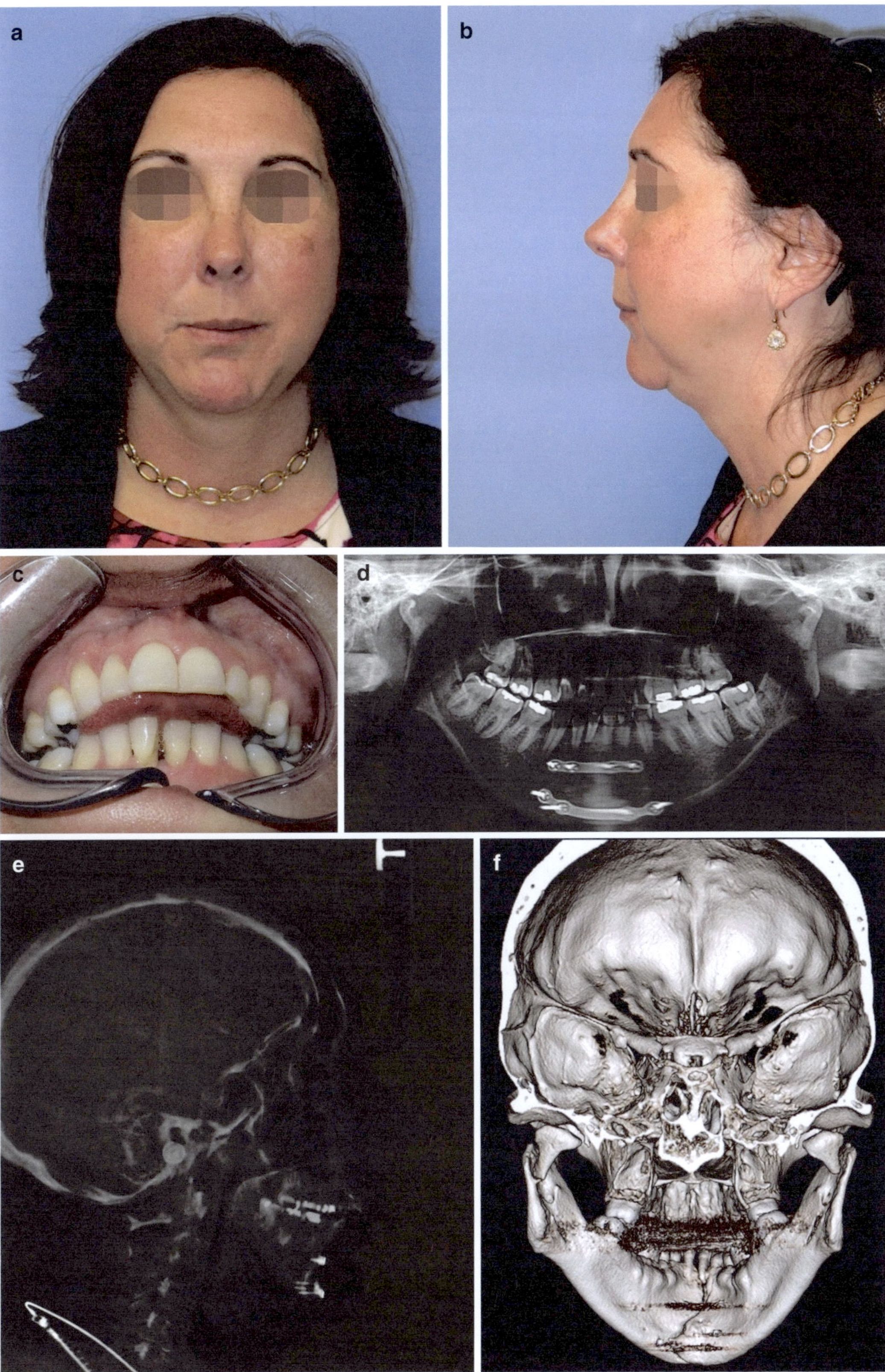

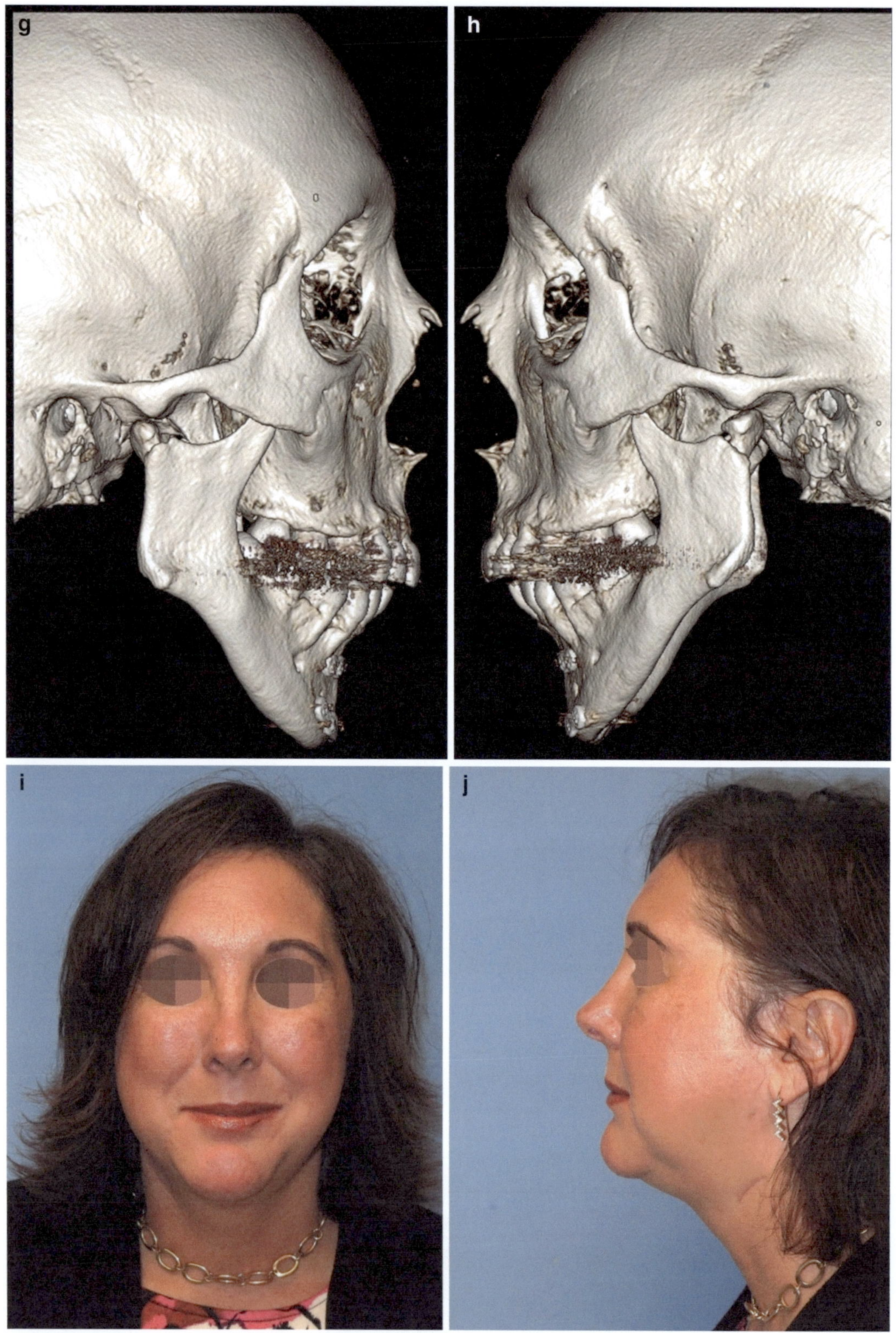

Fig. 12.12 (continued)

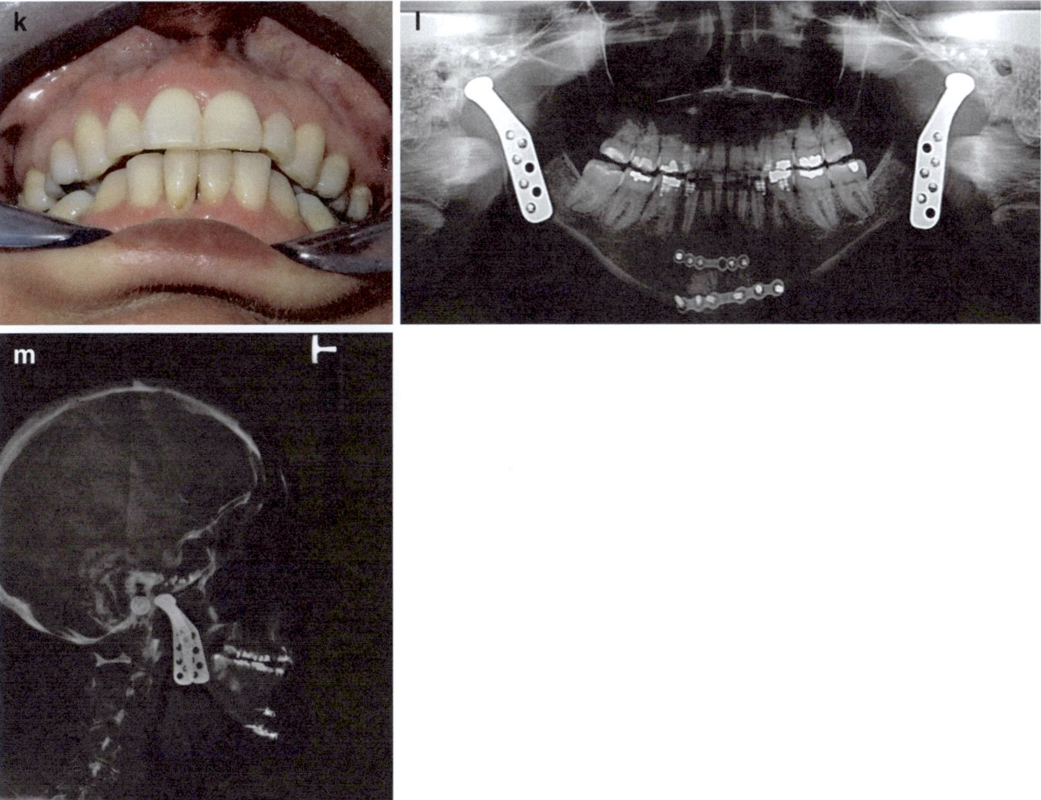

Fig. 12.12 (continued)

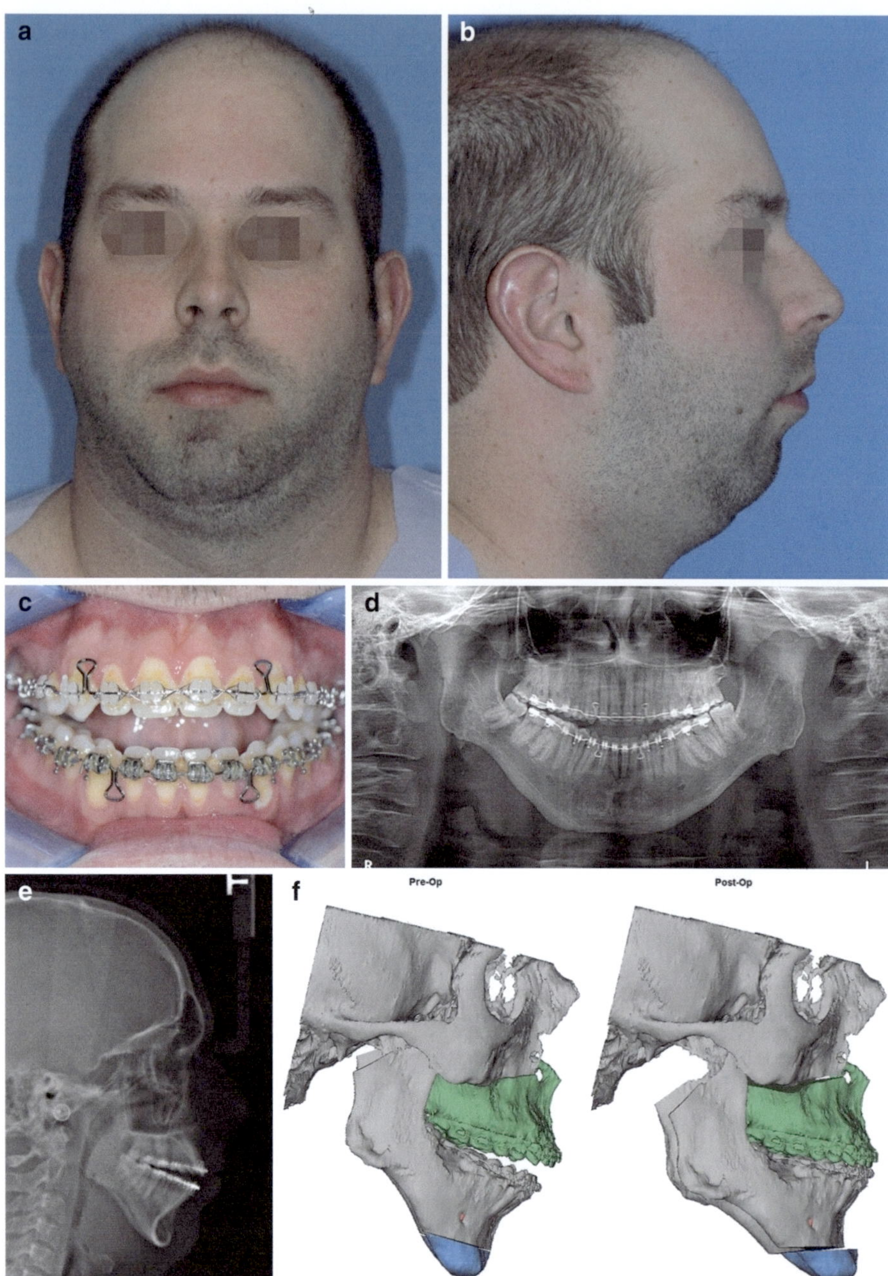

Fig. 12.13 Combined orthognathic and TMJ reconstruction using custom-made TMJ Concepts prosthesis. A 29-year-old male with a history of idiopathic condylar resorption resulting in a significant dentoskeletal discrepancy (anterior open bite with mandibular retrognathia). After clinical and radiographical evaluation, a decision was made to perform a counterclockwise rotation of the maxillomandibular complex by doing a combined orthognathic (Le Fort I, genioplasty) and a custom-made alloplastic TMJ reconstruction. (**a**, **b**) Preoperative frontal and lateral clinical views showing significant mandibular retrognathia. (**c**) Preoperative view of the occlusion showing an anterior open bite. (**d**) Preoperative panoramic radiograph showing severely reabsorbed con-dyles. (**e**) Preoperative lateral cephalometric radiograph showing an anterior open bite, mandibular retrognathia and small airway. (**f**) Pre and postoperative views of the virtual surgical planning showing the counterclockwise rotation of the maxillomandibular complex. (**g**, **h**) View of the custom-made prostheses. (**i**, **j**) Postoperative frontal and lateral clinical views showing significant improvement of facial harmony. (**k**) Postoperative view of the occlusion showing correction of the anterior open bite. (**l**) Postoperative panoramic radiograph showing proper placement of the custom-made TMJ prostheses. (**m**) Postoperative lateral cephalometric radiograph showing correction of the dento-skeletal discrepancy and improvement of the airway size

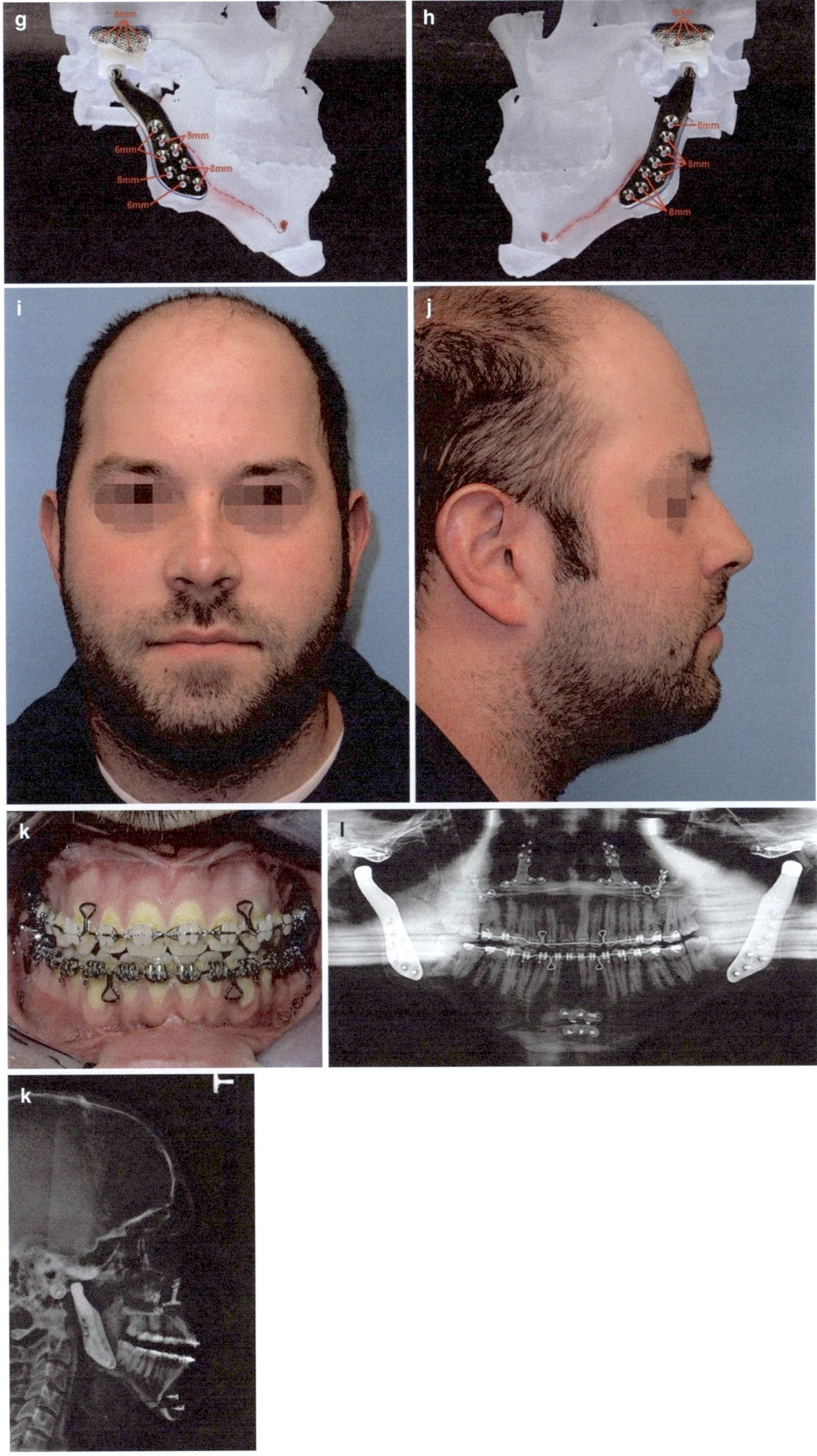

Fig. 12.13 (continued)

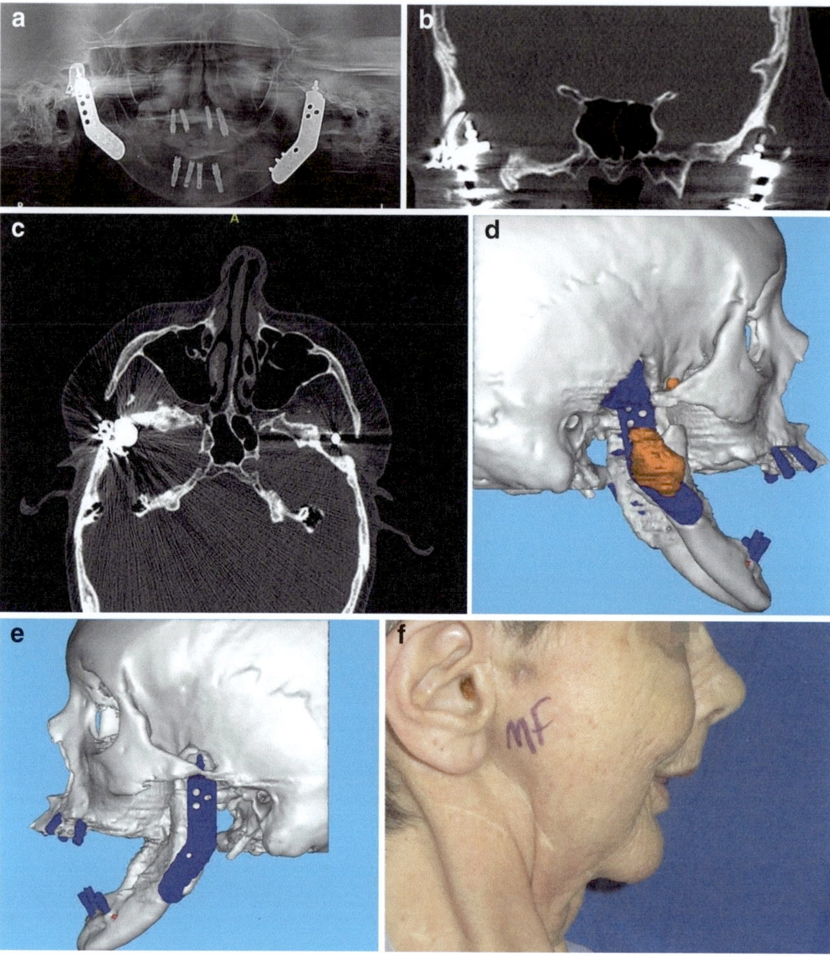

Fig. 12.14 Reconstruction of the base of the skull and mandibular defects with a custom-made TMJ prostheses. A 66-year-old female with a long history of failed TMJ surgeries that included a Kent-Vitek prostheses. She had them replaced with bilateral total TMJ Christensen prosthesis in the early 1990s. She presented to our clinic due to pain increase, worse dysfunction, and a new right preauricular cutaneous fistula. After clinical and radiographical evaluation, it was determined that the patient had bilateral TMJ prostheses failure with the right prosthesis displaced into the middle cranial fossa. A neurosurgical consultation was obtained. A decision was made to approach the case in two stages. The first stage consisted in a join approach with neurosurgery with removal of bilateral TMJ prostheses with exploration of the middle cranial fossa defect. Counterclockwise rotation of the mandible stabilized with modified Gunning splints. The second stage consisted of placement of the extended TMJ custom-made prosthesis to cover the base of the skull defect and to reconstruct the TMJ and missing mandible. (**a–c**) Preoperative imaging demonstrating bilateral TMJ Christensen prostheses failure with the right prosthesis displaced into the middle cranial fossa.

(**d, e**) Preoperative 3D CT scan reconstructions demonstrating the failed hardware with resulting mandibular retrognathia. (**f**) Preoperative lateral clinical picture showing mandibular retrognathia and the area of the preauricular cutaneous fistula. (**g**) Intraoperative view of the failed right TMJ prosthesis. (**h**) Modified gunning splints in place. (**i, j**) Postoperative 3D CT scan reconstructions demonstrating the removal of the hardware and the new position of the mandible being held by the gunning splints. (**k, l**) Right lateral view of the stereolithographic model showing the base of the skull defect and the custom-made prosthesis. (**m, n**) Left lateral view of the stereolithographic model showing the zygomatic arch defect and the custom-made prosthesis. (**o**) Intraoperative view of the right base of skull defect. (**p**) Right custom-made. TMJ prosthesis in place. (**q**) Left custom-made TMJ prosthesis in place. (**r**) Postoperative coronal CT scan view demonstrating the coverage of the base of the skull defect by the fossa prosthesis. (**s**) Postoperative panoramic radiograph showing proper placement of the bilateral custom-made TMJ replacements. (**t**) Postoperative lateral clinical picture showing normalize mandibular position

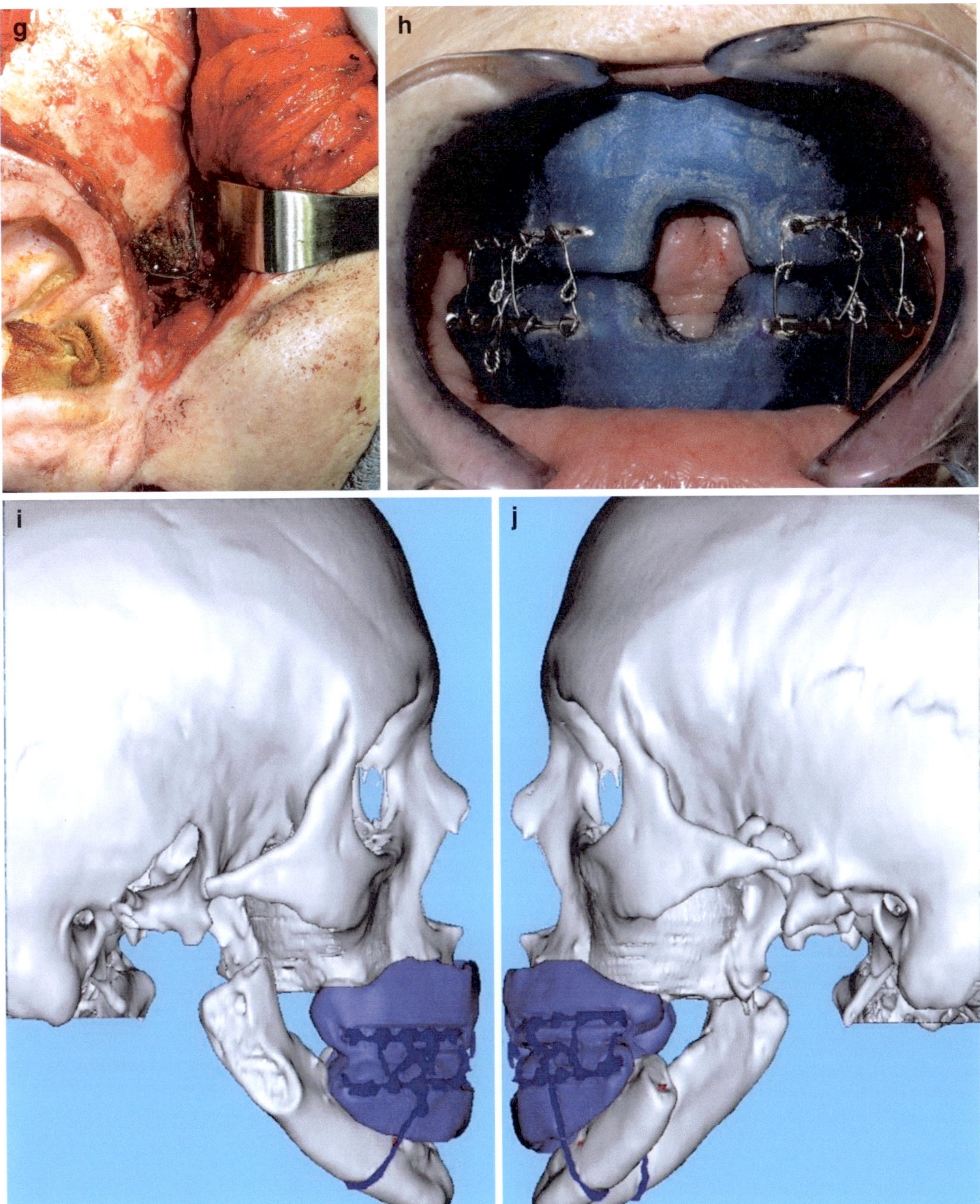

Fig. 12.14 (continued)

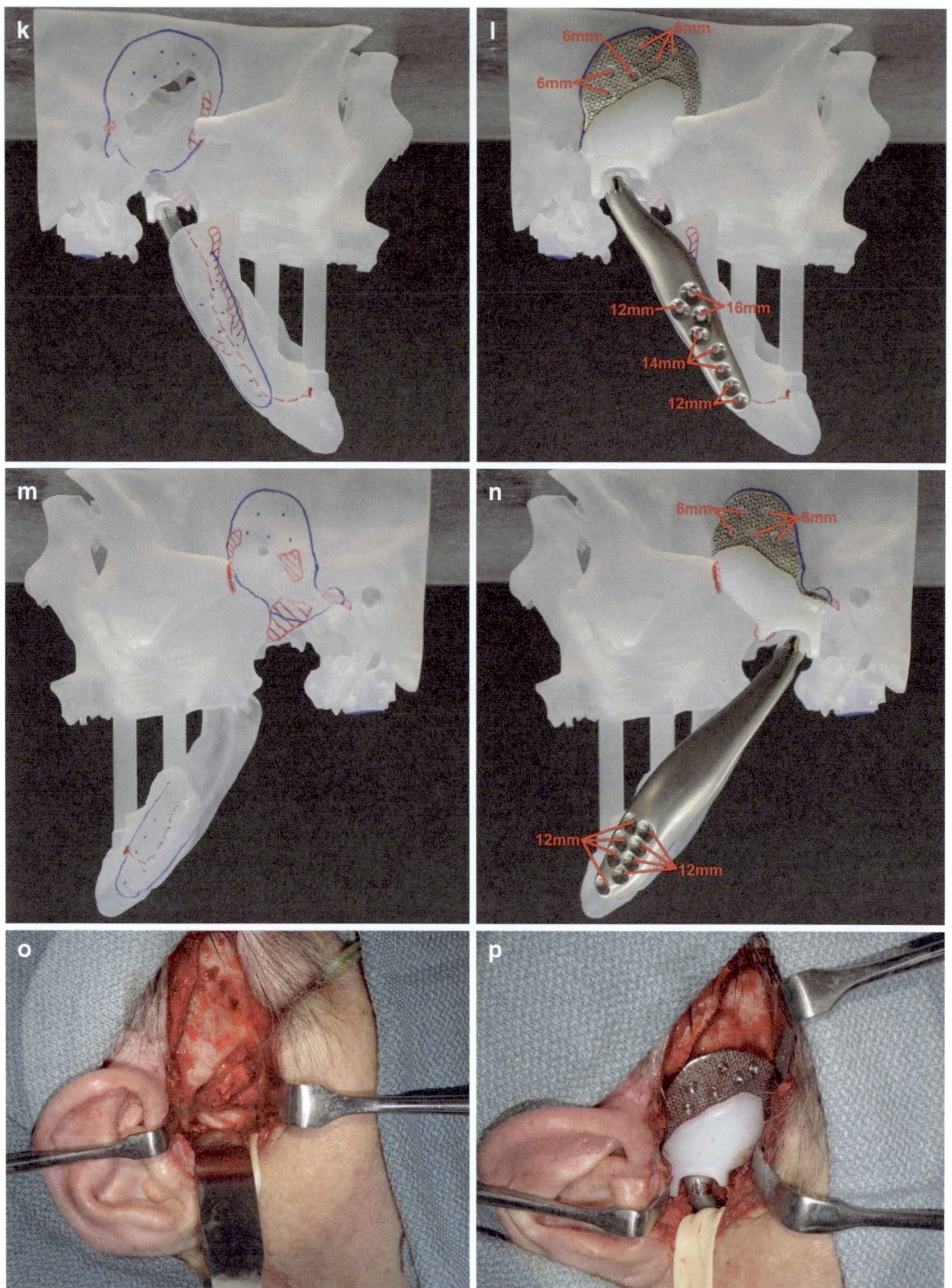

Fig. 12.14 (continued)

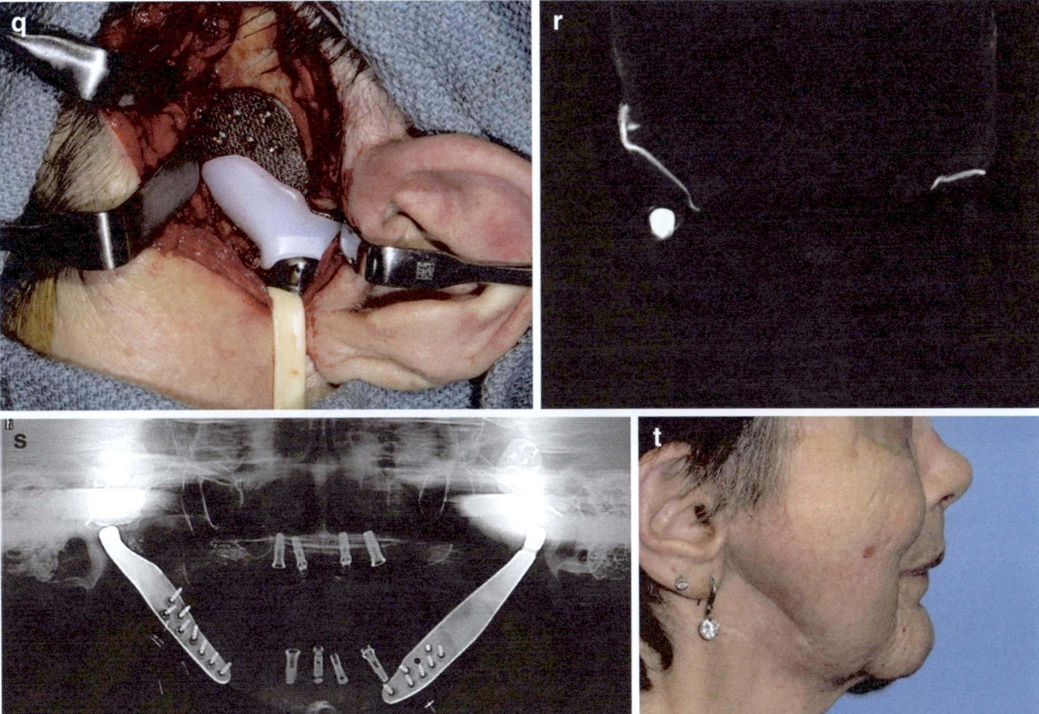

Fig. 12.14 (continued)

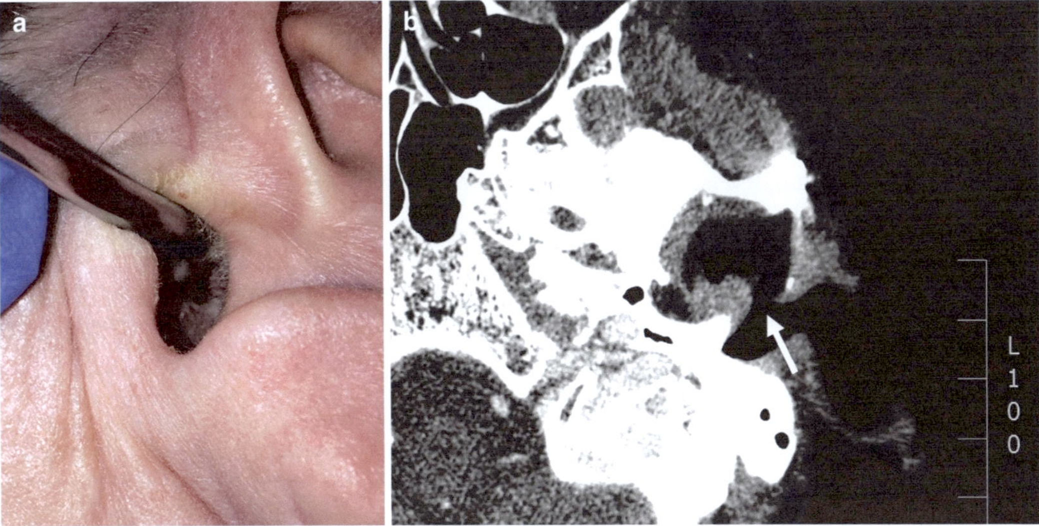

Fig. 12.15 Infected prosthesis. (**a**) Clinical view of a fistula in the anterior portion of the external auditory canal. (**b**) Axial CT Scan view demonstrating the fistula. Note the emphysema in the fossa region

References

1. Mercuri LG. Temporomandibular joint re-placement: past, present and future material considerations. In: TMS 2014 supplemental proceedings; 2014. p. 181–90.
2. De Meurechy N, Mommaerts MY. Alloplastic temporomandibular joint replacement systems: a systematic review of their history. Int J Oral Maxillofac Surg. 2018;47:743–54.
3. Mercuri LG, Giobbie-Hurder A. Long-term outcomes after total alloplastic temporomandibular joint reconstruction following exposure to failed materials. J Oral Maxillofac Surg. 2004;62:1088–96.
4. Driemel O, Braun S, Müller-Richter UD, Behr M, Reichert TE, Kunkel M, Reich R. Historical development of alloplastic temporomandibular joint replacement after 1945 and state of the art. Int J Oral Maxillofac Surg. 2009;38:909–20.
5. Mercuri LG. Measurement of the heat of reaction transmitted intracranially during polymerization of methylmethacrylate cranial bone cement used in stabilization of the fossa component of an alloplastic temporomandibular joint prosthesis. Oral Surg Oral Med Oral Pathol. 1992;74:137–42.
6. Kent JN, Misiek DJ, Akin RK, Hinds EC, Homsy CA. Temporomandibular joint condylar prosthesis: a ten year report. J Oral Maxillofac Surg. 1983;41:245–54.
7. Spagnoli D, Kent JN. Multicenter evaluation of temporomandibular joint proplast–teflon disk implant. Oral Surg Oral Med Oral Pathol. 1992;74:411–21.
8. Mercuri LG, Wolford LM, Sanders B, White RD, Hurder A, Henderson W. Custom CAD/CAM total temporomandibular joint reconstruction system. Preliminary multicenter report. J Oral Maxillofac Surg. 1995;53:106–15.
9. Van Loon JP, de Bont LG, Boering G. Evaluation of temporomandibular joint prostheses. Review of the literature from 1946 to 1994 and implications for future prosthesis designs. J Oral Maxillofac Surg. 1995;53:984–96.
10. Giannakopoulos HE, Sinn DP, Quinn PD. Biomet microfixation temporomandibular joint replacement system: a 3 year follow-up study of patients treated during 1995 to 2005. J Oral Maxillofac Surg. 2012;70(4):787–96.
11. Wolford LM. Autologous fat grafts placed around temporomandibular joint (TMJ) total joint prostheses to prevent heterotopic bone. In: Shiffman MA, editor. Autologous fat transfer: art, science, and clinical practice. Berlin: Springer; 2010. p. 361–82.
12. Wolford LM. Factors to consider in joint prosthesis systems. Baylor Univ Med Cent Proc. 2006;19:232–8.
13. Baier RE, Meyer AE. TMJ TJR biomaterials. In: Mercuri LG, editor. Temporomandibular joint total joint replacement (TMJ TJR): a comprehensive reference for researchers, materials scientists, and Surgeons. New York: Springer; 2016. p. 29–39.
14. Anderson JM, Rodriguez A, Chang DT. Foreign body reaction to biomaterials. Semin Immunol. 2008;20:86–100.
15. Kurtz SM, Kocagöz S, Arnholt C, Huet R, Ueno M, Walter WL. Advances in zirconia toughened alumina biomaterials for total joint replacement. J Mech Behav Biomed Mater. 2014;31:107–16.
16. Sidebottom AJ. Alloplastic or autogenous reconstruction of the TMJ. J Oral Biol Craniofac Res. 2013;3:135–9.
17. Kaban LB, Bouchard C, Troulis MJ. A protocol for management of temporomandibular joint ankylosis in children. J Oral Maxillofac Surg. 2009;67(9):1966e1978.
18. Khadka A, Hu J. Autogenous grafts for condylar reconstruction in treatment of TMJ ankylosis: current concepts and considerations for the future. Int J Oral Maxillofac Surg. 2012;41:94–102.
19. Zheng LW, Ma L, Shi XJ, Zwahlen RA, Cheung LK. Comparison of distraction osteogenesis versus costochondral graft in reconstruction of temporomandibular joint condylectomy with disc preservation. J Oral Maxillofac Surg. 2011;69(2):409e417.
20. Sun H, Li B, Zhao Z, Zhang L, Shen S, Wang X. Error analysis of a CAD/CAM method for unidirectional mandibular distraction osteogenesis in the treatment of hemifacial microsomia. Br J Oral Maxillofac Surg. 2013;51(8):892–7.
21. Mercuri LG. Alloplastic temporomandibular joint replacement: rationale for the use of custom devices. Int J Oral Maxillofac Surg. 2012;41(9):1033–40.
22. Mercuri LG, Swift JQ. Considerations for the use of alloplastic temporomandibular joint replacement in the growing patient. J Oral Maxillofac Surg. 2009;67(9):1979–90.
23. Keyser BR, Banda AK, Mercuri LG, Warburton G, Sullivan SM. Alloplastic total temporomandibular joint replacement in skeletally immature patients: a pilot survey [published online ahead of print, 2020 Feb 26]. Int J Oral Maxillofac Surg. 2020;S0901-5027(20)30050-3. https://doi.org/10.1016/j.ijom.2020.02.001
24. Elledge R, Mercuri LG, Attard A, Green J, Speculand B. Review of emerging temporomandibular joint total joint replacement systems. Br J Oral Maxillofac Surg. 2019;57(8):722–8.
25. Susarla SM, Peacock ZS, Williams WB, Rabinov JD, Keith DA, Kaban LB. Role of computed tomographic angiography in treatment of patients with temporomandibular joint ankylosis. J Oral Maxillofac Surg. 2014;72(2):267–76.
26. Alderazi YJ, Shastri D, Wessel J, et al. Internal maxillary artery preoperative embolization using n-butyl cyanoacrylate and pushable coils for temporomandibular joint ankylosis surgery. World Neurosurg. 2017;101:254–8.
27. Hossameldin RH, McCain JP, Dabus G. Prophylactic embolisation of the internal maxillary artery in patients with ankylosis of the temporomandibular joint. Br J Oral Maxillofac Surg. 2017;55(6):584–8.

28. Jose A, Nagori SA, Virkhare A, Bhatt K, Bhutia O, Roychoudhury A. Piezoelectric osteoarthrectomy for management of ankylosis of the temporomandibular joint. Br J Oral Maxillofac Surg. 2014;52(7):624–8.

29. Spinelli G, Valente D, Mannelli G, Raffaini M, Arcuri F. Surgical management of ankyloses of the temporomandibular joint by a piezoelectric device. J Craniomaxillofac Surg. 2017;45(4):441–8.

30. Schmelzeisen R, Gellrich NC, Schramm A, Schön R, Otten JE. Navigation-guided resection of temporomandibular joint ankylosis promotes safety in skull base surgery. J Oral Maxillofac Surg. 2002;60(11):1275–83.

31. Malis DD, Xia JJ, Gateno J, Donovan DT, Teichgraeber JF. New protocol for 1-stage treatment of temporomandibular joint ankylosis using surgical navigation. J Oral Maxillofac Surg. 2007;65(9):1843–8.

32. Jones R. The use of virtual planning and navigation in the treatment of temporomandibular joint ankylosis. Aust Dent J. 2013;58(3):358–67.

33. Newman MF, Lee DG, Lecholop MK. Protocol for single-stage bilateral temporomandibular joint replacement using intraoperative navigation in patients with ankylosis. J Oral Maxillofac Surg. 2018;76(7):1418–23.

34. Chandran R, Keeler GD, Christensen AM, Weimer KA, Caloss R. Application of virtual surgical planning for total joint reconstruction with a stock alloplast system. J Oral Maxillofac Surg. 2011;69(1):285–94.

35. Bai G, He D, Yang C, Chen M, Yuan J, Wilson JJ. Application of digital templates to guide total alloplastic joint replacement surgery with Biomet standard replacement system. J Oral Maxillofac Surg. 2014;72(12):2440–52.

36. Gerbino G, Zavattero E, Berrone S, Ramieri G. One stage treatment of temporomandibular joint complete bony ankylosis using total joint replacement. J Craniomaxillofac Surg. 2016;44(4):487–92.

37. Hu Y, Zhang L, He D, et al. Simultaneous treatment of temporomandibular joint ankylosis with severe mandibular deficiency by standard TMJ prosthesis. Sci Rep. 2017;7:45271.

38. Xu X, Ma H, Jin S. One-stage treatment of Giant condylar osteoma: alloplastic total temporomandibular joint replacement aided by digital templates. J Craniofac Surg. 2018;29(3):636–9.

39. Rhee SH, Baek SH, Park SH, Kim JC, Jeong CG, Choi JY. Total joint reconstruction using computer-assisted surgery with stock prostheses for a patient with bilateral TMJ ankylosis. Maxillofac Plast Reconstr Surg. 2019;41(1):41.

40. Zhang S, Liu H, Yang C, Zhang X, Abdelrehem A, Zheng J, et al. Modified surgical techniques for total alloplastic temporomandibular joint replacement: one institution's experience. J Craniomaxillofac Surg. 2015;43(6):934–9.

41. Bai G, Yang C, He D, Zhang X, Abdelrehem A. Application of fossa bone graft to stabilize stock total joint prosthesis in temporomandibular joint surgery. J Craniomaxillofac Surg. 2015;43(8):1392–7.

42. Abramowicz S, Barbick M, Rose SP, Dolwick MF. Adaptability of stock TMJ prosthesis to joints that were previously treated with custom joint prosthesis. Int J Oral Maxillofac Surg. 2012;41(4):518–20.

43. Brown ZL, Sarrami S, Perez D. Will they fit? Determinants of the adaptability of stock TMJ prostheses where custom TMJ prostheses were utilized. Int J Oral Maxillofac Surg. 2020; https://doi.org/10.1016/j.ijom.2020.05.009.

44. Westermark A, Hedén P, Aagaard E, Cornelius CP. The use of TMJ concepts prostheses to reconstruct patients with major temporomandibular joint and mandibular defects. Int J Oral Maxillofac Surg. 2011;40(5):487–96.

45. Vega L, Meara D. Mandibular replacement utilizing TMJ TJR devices. In: Mercuri LG, editor. Temporomandibular joint total joint replacement – TMJ TJR. New York: Springer; 2016. p. 165–83.

46. Elledge R, Mercuri LG, Speculand B. Extended total temporomandibular joint replacements: a classification system. Br J Oral Maxillofac Surg. 2018;56(7):578–81.

47. Wolford LM. Computer-assisted surgical simulation for concomitant temporomandibular joint custom-fitted Total joint reconstruction and orthognathic surgery. Atlas Oral Maxillofac Surg Clin North Am. 2016;24(1):55–66.

48. Ruiz Valero CA, Duran-Rodriguez G, Solano-Parra N, Castro-Núñez J. Immediate total temporomandibular joint replacement with TMJ concepts prosthesis as an alternative for ameloblastoma cases. J Oral Maxillofac Surg. 2014;72(3):646.e1–12.

49. Sarlabous M, Psutka DJ. Treatment of mandibular Ameloblastoma involving the mandibular condyle: resection and concomitant reconstruction with a custom hybrid total joint prosthesis and iliac bone graft. J Craniofac Surg. 2018;29(3):e307–14.

50. Farzad P. A case of an extensive keratocystic odontogenic tumor in the mandible reconstructed with a custom-made total joint prosthesis. Craniomaxillofac Trauma Reconstr. 2018;11(2):131–7.

51. Dantas JFC, Nogueira Neto JN, Sarmento VA, Campos PSF. Temporomandibular joint reconstruction after condylar fracture complication related to osteosynthesis material. Int J Oral Maxillofac Surg. 2018;47(1):137–9.

52. Mercuri LG. Patient-fitted ("custom") alloplastic temporomandibular joint replacement technique. Atlas Oral Maxillofac Surg Clin North Am. 2011;19(2):233–42.

53. Mercuri LG, Psutka D. Perioperative, postoperative, and prophylactic use of antibiotics in alloplastic total temporomandibular joint replacement surgery: a survey and preliminary guidelines. J Oral Maxillofac Surg. 2011;69(8):2106–11.

54. Wolford LM, Pitta MC, Reiche-Fischel O, Franco PF. TMJ concepts/Techmedica custom-made TMJ total joint prosthesis: 5-year follow-up study. Int J Oral Maxillofac Surg. 2003;32(3):268–74.

55. Mercuri LG, Edibam NR, Giobbie-Hurder A. Fourteen-year follow-up of a patient-fitted total temporomandibular joint reconstruction system. J Oral Maxillofac Surg. 2007;65(6):1140–8.
56. Mercuri LG, Ali FA, Woolson R. Outcomes of total alloplastic replacement with periarticular autogenous fat grafting for management of reankylosis of the temporomandibular joint. J Oral Maxillofac Surg. 2008;66(9):1794–803.
57. Wolford LM, Mercuri LG, Schneiderman ED, Movahed R, Allen W. Twenty-year follow-up study on a patient-fitted temporomandibular joint prosthesis: the Techmedica/TMJ concepts device. J Oral Maxillofac Surg. 2015;73(5):952–60.
58. Westermark A. Total reconstruction of the temporomandibular joint. Up to 8 years of follow-up of patients treated with Biomet(®) total joint prostheses. Int J Oral Maxillofac Surg. 2010;39(10):951–5.
59. Leandro LF, Ono HY, Loureiro CC, Marinho K, Guevara HA. A ten-year experience and follow-up of three hundred patients fitted with the Biomet/Lorenz microfixation TMJ replacement system. Int J Oral Maxillofac Surg. 2013;42(8):1007–13.
60. Sanovich R, Mehta U, Abramowicz S, Widmer C, Dolwick MF. Total alloplastic temporomandibular joint reconstruction using Biomet stock prostheses: the University of Florida experience. Int J Oral Maxillofac Surg. 2014;43(9):1091–5.
61. Johnson NR, Roberts MJ, Doi SA, Batstone MD. Total temporomandibular joint replacement prostheses: a systematic review and bias-adjusted meta-analysis. Int J Oral Maxillofac Surg. 2017;46(1):86–92.
62. Gerbino G, Zavattero E, Bosco G, Berrone S, Ramieri G. Temporomandibular joint reconstruction with stock and custom-made devices: indications and results of a 14-year experience. J Craniomaxillofac Surg. 2017;45(10):1710–5.
63. Kanatsios S, Breik O, Dimitroulis G. Biomet stock temporomandibular joint prosthesis: long-term outcomes of the use of titanium condyles secured with four or five condylar fixation screws. J Craniomaxillofac Surg. 2018;46(10):1697–702.
64. Zou L, Zhang L, He D, Yang C, Zhao J, Ellis E 3rd. Clinical and radiologic follow-up of Zimmer Biomet stock total temporomandibular joint replacement after surgical modifications. J Oral Maxillofac Surg. 2018;76(12):2518–24.
65. Gonzalez-Perez LM, Gonzalez-Perez-Somarriba B, Centeno G, et al. Prospective study of five-year outcomes and postoperative complications after total temporomandibular joint replacement with two stock prosthetic systems. Br J Oral Maxillofac Surg. 2020;58(1):69–74.
66. Gupta B, Ahmed N, Sidebottom AJ. Quality of life outcomes one year after replacement of the temporomandibular joint using a modified SF36 questionnaire. Br J Oral Maxillofac Surg. 2020;58(3):304–8.
67. McKenzie WS, Louis PJ. Temporomandibular total joint prosthesis infections: a ten-year retrospective analysis. Int J Oral Maxillofac Surg. 2017;46(5):596–602.
68. Granquist EJ, Bouloux G, Dattilo D, et al. Outcomes and survivorship of biomet microfixation total joint replacement system: results from an FDA Postmarket study [published online ahead of print, 2020 Apr 23]. J Oral Maxillofac Surg. 2020;S0278-2391(20)30427-4.
69. Machoň V, Levorová J, Hirjak D, et al. Evaluation of complications following stock replacement of the temporomandibular joint performed between the years 2006 and 2015: a retrospective study [published online ahead of print, 2020 Apr 23]. Oral Maxillofac Surg. 2020. https://doi.org/10.1007/s10006-020-00840-z
70. Gakhal MK, Gupta B, Sidebottom AJ. Analysis of outcomes after revision replacement of failed total temporomandibular joint prostheses. Br J Oral Maxillofac Surg. 2020;58(2):220–4.
71. Mercuri LG, Anspach WE. Principles for the revision of total alloplastic TMJ prostheses. Int J Oral Maxillofac Surg. 2003;32(4):353–9.
72. Mercuri LG. Microbial biofilms: a potential source for alloplastic device failure. J Oral Maxillofac Surg. 2006;64(8):1303–9.
73. Wolford LM, Rodrigues DB, McPhillips A. Management of the infected temporomandibular joint total joint prosthesis. J Oral Maxillofac Surg. 2010;68(11):2810–23.
74. Mercuri LG. Avoiding and managing temporomandibular joint Total joint replacement surgical site infections. J Oral Maxillofac Surg. 2012;70(10):2280–9.
75. Mercuri LG, Saltzman BM. Acquired heterotopic ossification of the temporomandibular joint. Int J Oral Maxillofac Surg. 2017;46(12):1562–8.
76. Mercuri LG, Caicedo MS. Material hypersensitivity and alloplastic temporomandibular joint replacement. J Oral Maxillofac Surg. 2019;77(7):1371–6.

New Developments in Pediatric Cranio-Maxillofacial Reconstruction

13

Marta Redondo, Ana Isabel Romance, and Gregorio Sánchez-Aniceto

13.1 Introduction

Computer-assisted surgery in cranio-maxillofacial pediatric reconstruction can help us to reduce operating time, predict and avoid possible complications, and obtain more accurate and predictable results. However, there are some disadvantages such as the learning curve, the pre-operative work, time burden, and high cost.

In this chapter, we will go through the most common craniofacial deformities that affect the pediatric population, checking how we can improve our results with the help of new technologies. Also an update on the impact of the new technologies in the reconstruction of the mandible in pediatric patients will be included.

13.2 Craniosynostosis

Simple craniosynostosis demands corrective surgery for functional and esthetic outcomes. Although there are many surgical techniques described for their correction, most of them involve cranial vault expansion and improve the skull morphology and symmetry. However, our results may vary due to different reasons such as

2D planning inaccuracy, surgeon's experience, and subjective assessment or the inability to evaluate our results intraoperatively.

For the more complex cases, there are some tools available to achieve more predictable results. Although hand-made templates have been used during many years, the biggest change has come with virtual planning. Average cranial vault models appropriate for each age have been designed in a way that we can overlap them to our patient's skull and virtually plan the osteotomies to be performed and remodeling to be done so as to adapt it to the norm. For that purpose, a recent CT scan from the patient is needed. Cutting and positioning guides can be obtained from our planning software and used during surgery to show us where to make the osteotomies and where to place the bone segments obtained [1] (Figs 13.1 and 13.2).

Intraoperative navigation can also be used to check that we achieve our goals, both in primary and secondary cases of craniosynostosis. Figure 13.3 shows the preoperative planning with Brainlab® software of the ideal position of the cranial vault and orbits in a case of plagiocephaly, the intraoperative control under navigation, and the postoperative control.

In recent years, augmented reality (AR) has become more popular and has already arrived to the medical field. Although this tool has not been included in the current practice yet, one of its multiple applications could be craniofacial surgery, where it can be used to overlay the deep

M. Redondo (✉) · A. I. Romance
G. Sánchez-Aniceto
Maxillofacial Surgery Department,
12 de Octubre University Hospital, Madrid, Spain
e-mail: gsaniceto@meytel.net

© Springer Nature Switzerland AG 2021
J. Acero (ed.), *Innovations and New Developments in Craniomaxillofacial Reconstruction*,
https://doi.org/10.1007/978-3-030-74322-2_13

">

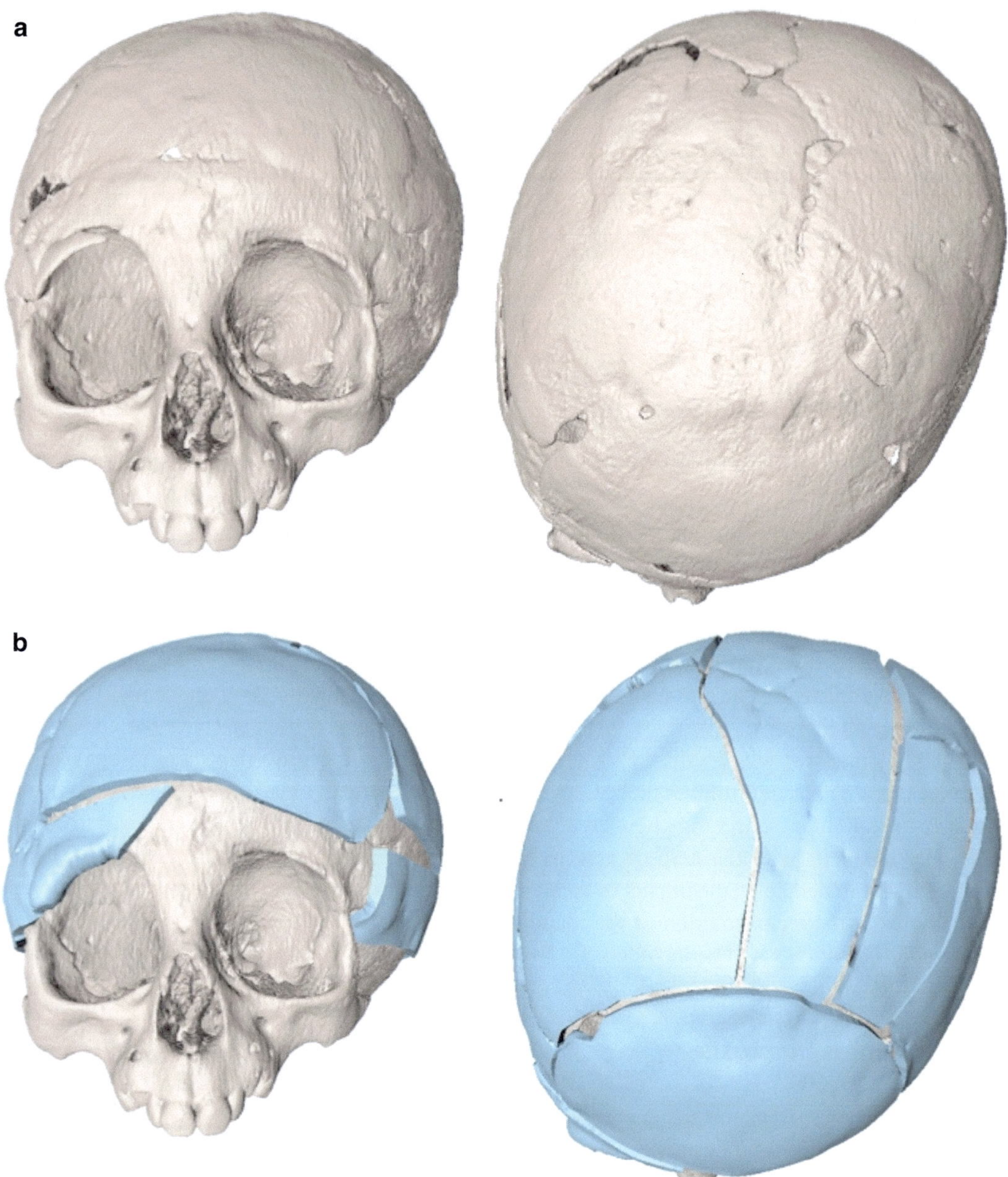

Fig. 13.1 Virtual planning in patient with complex craniosynostosis for secondary surgery. (**a**) Preoperative frontal and superior view of the asymmetric skull. (**b**) Cutting guides designed. (**c**) Final position of bone segments

c

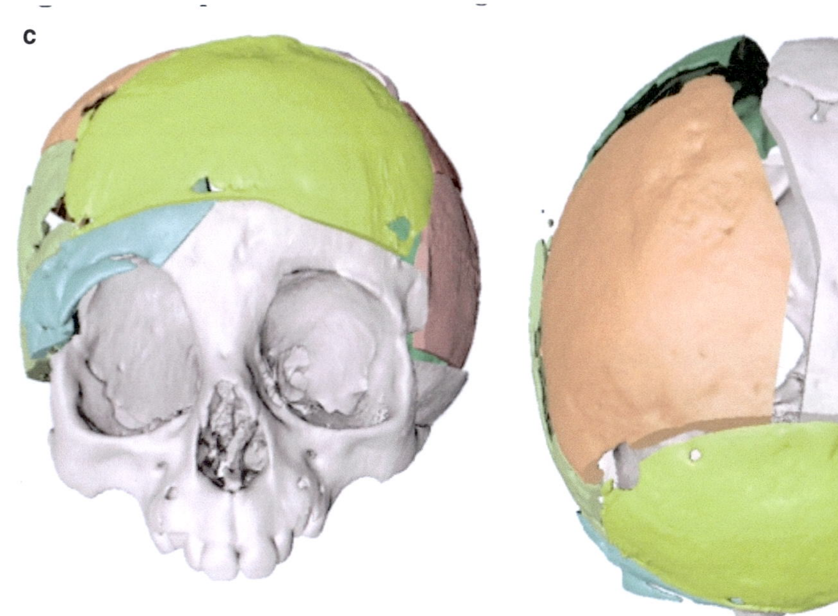

Fig. 13.1 (continued)

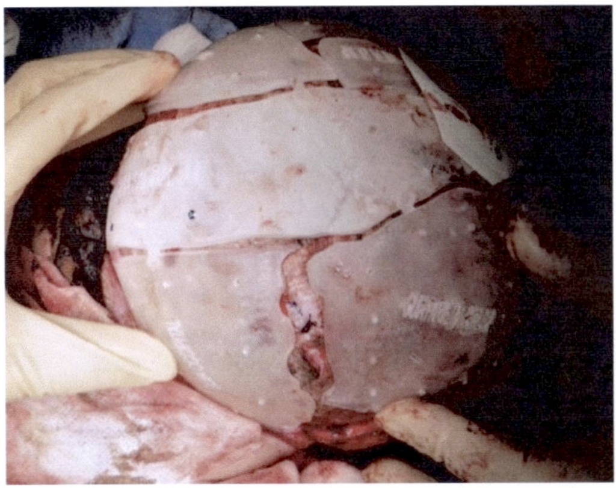

Fig. 13.2 Cutting guides placed during the surgery

anatomic structures in the surgical field in real time. In craniosynostosis surgery, it has been employed after the virtual planning to mark the osteotomies and accurately position the bone segments to make sure the plan is fulfilled. With AR, the surgeon is able to see the virtual image overlaid to the patient in real time.

Han et al. conducted a study using AR in seven plagiocephaly patients. CT scans were performed postoperatively to judge the surgical outcomes.

They conclude that the AR system can be applied to plagiocephaly procedures contributing to obtain reliable and accurate results via a precise osteotomy [2].

13.3 Multiple and Syndromic Craniosynostosis

It is not uncommon for these patients to undergo more than one surgical procedure during their growing period. Frequently when they need a monobloc or midface advancement, because of their condition and previous procedures, patients affected by syndromic cranyosinostosis usually present with an abnormal cranial vault, multiple bone defects, and presence of osteosynthesis material. Even a ventriculoperitoneal shunt (VPS) can be present. Fixation of a rigid external device for a monobloc or midface distraction can lead to serious complications such as VPS malfunction or infection, cranial vault fracture or brain damage. Custom designed and printed rigid external devices (KLS martin®) that will specifically fit in the patient avoiding bone defects, VPS

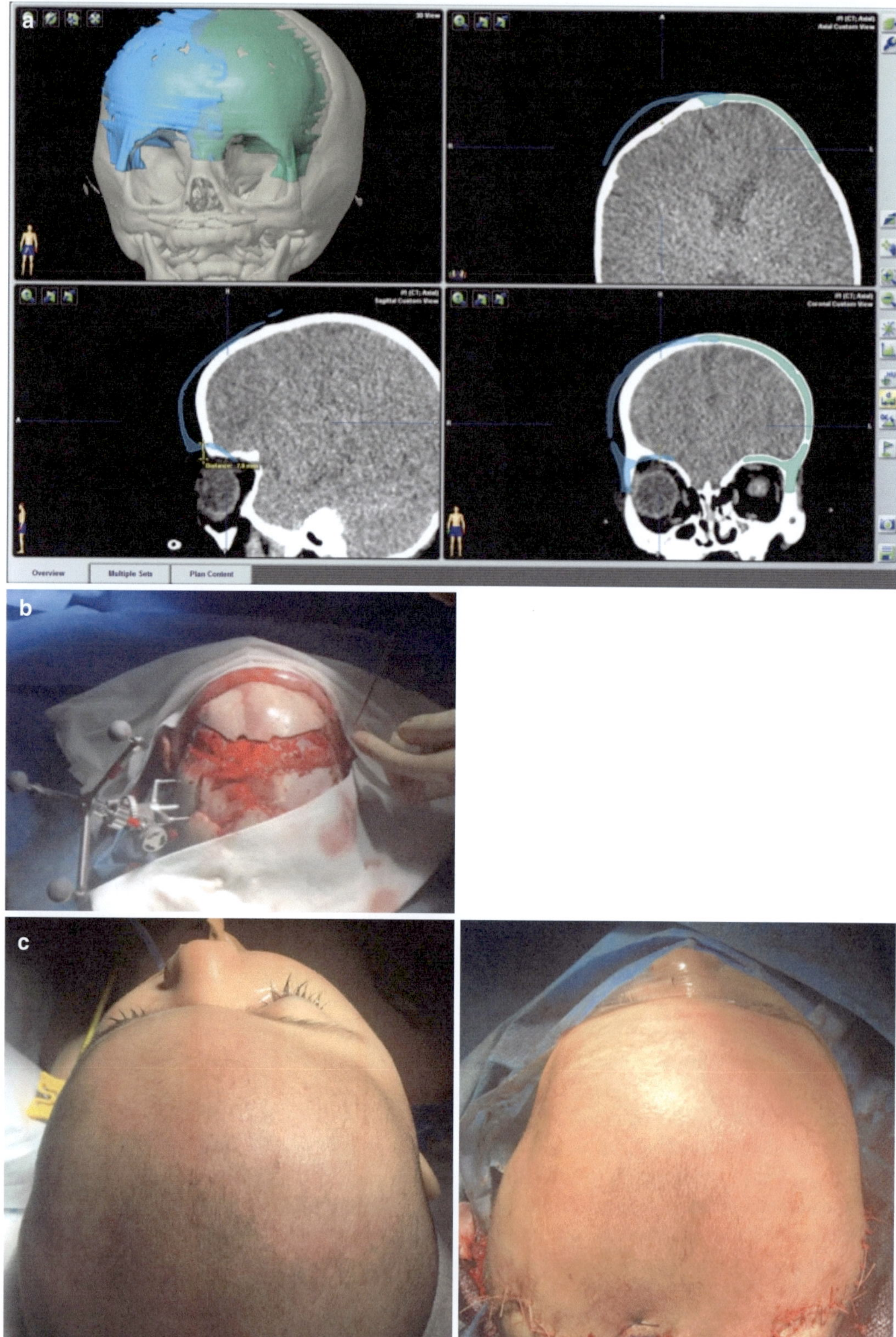

Fig. 13.3 Nine-month-old plagiocephaly. (**a**) Preoperative plan remodeling the skull vault and the supraorbital bandeau with Brainlab® software. (**b**) Intraoperative navigation to check our results. (**c**) Pre- and postoperative pictures of the patient

and adapting to the altered anatomy, can prevent complications related to the placement and fixation of the device [3, 4]. Preoperatively, a customized star-shaped plate is designed, and we can also predict the length of the screws to be used according to the bone thickness (Fig. 13.4).

If additional procedures like orbital dystopia correction are needed, a virtual planning and preparation of 3D printed cutting and positioning guides can also be produced if needed (Fig. 13.5).

13.4   Clefts

Technological advancements can also be useful in the management of patients with cleft lip and palate. Zheng et al. [5] obtained very good results applying 3D printed molding plates with a nasal hook for the presurgical nasoalveolar molding using a laser scanning machine.

Distraction osteogenesis of the maxilla is not unusual in cleft patients when a big advancement is needed and scarred soft tissues can lead to a relapse. For this purpose, internal distraction devices can be designed with custom-made plates and cutting guides, as well as pre-bent plates for surgery, using a stereolithographic model of the patient.

13.5   Mandibular Deformities

13.5.1 Mandible Distraction

In the pediatric population, mandible distraction can be indicated in multiple syndromes or conditions being the most common Pierre Robin sequence, craniofacial microsomia, or Treacher Collins syndrome. Some cases may need unilateral and other bilateral distraction, and the vectors may vary depending on the abnormal anatomy and functional requirements of the patient. In the most complicated cases, due to the severity of mandible hypoplasia, the sequelae of previous interventions, or even the teeth buds, a 3D virtual plan can help to design the osteotomy and the distraction vector (Fig. 13.6).

13.5.2 Mandible Reconstruction and Orthognathic Surgery in Pediatric Patients

On many occasions, patients with unilateral or bilateral mandible hypoplasia will need an orthognathic surgery procedure at the end of skeletal growth in order to achieve functional occlusion, facial harmony, symmetry and to increase upper airway volume. 3D planning in orthognathic

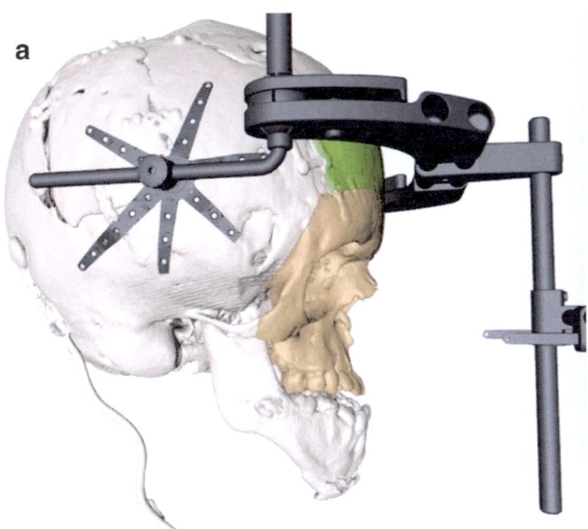
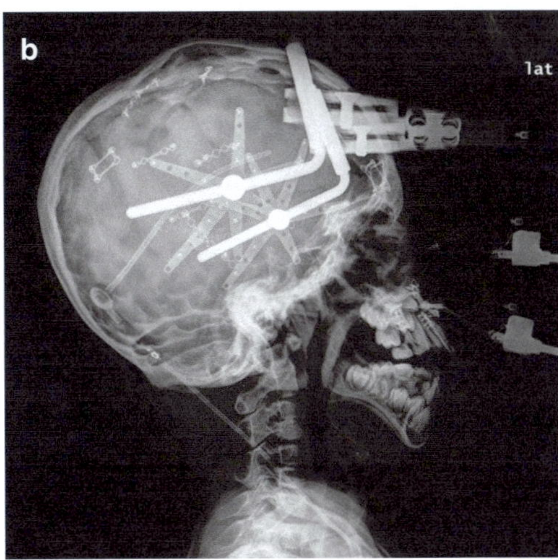

Fig. 13.4 (**a**) Custom-made rigid external device with star-shaped plate in patient with Crouzon syndrome and several previous surgeries. (**b**) Lateral radiograph in consolidation phase. (**c**) Pre- and postoperative results. (*c1*) Frontal view. (*c2*) Lateral view

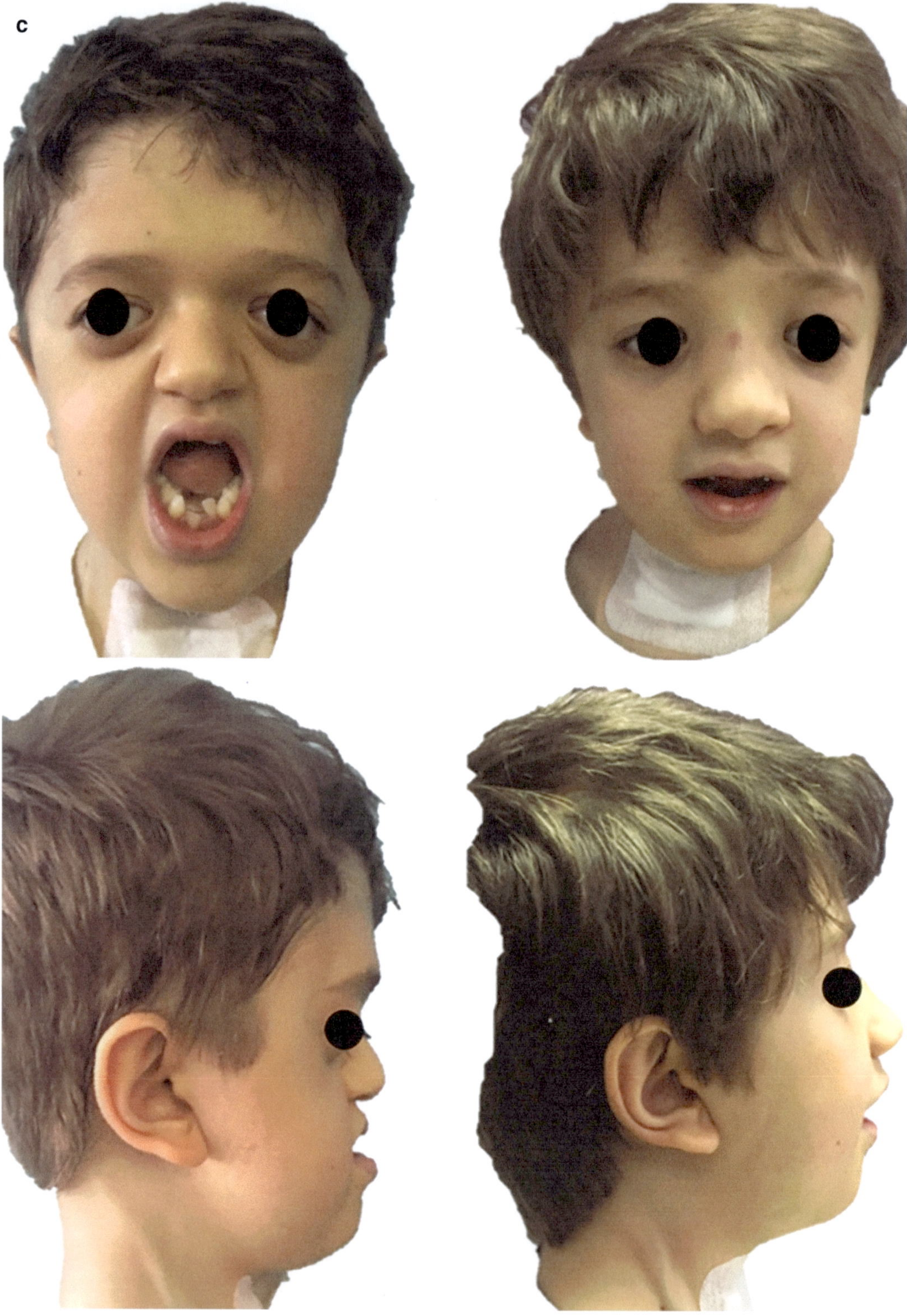

Fig. 13.4 (continued)

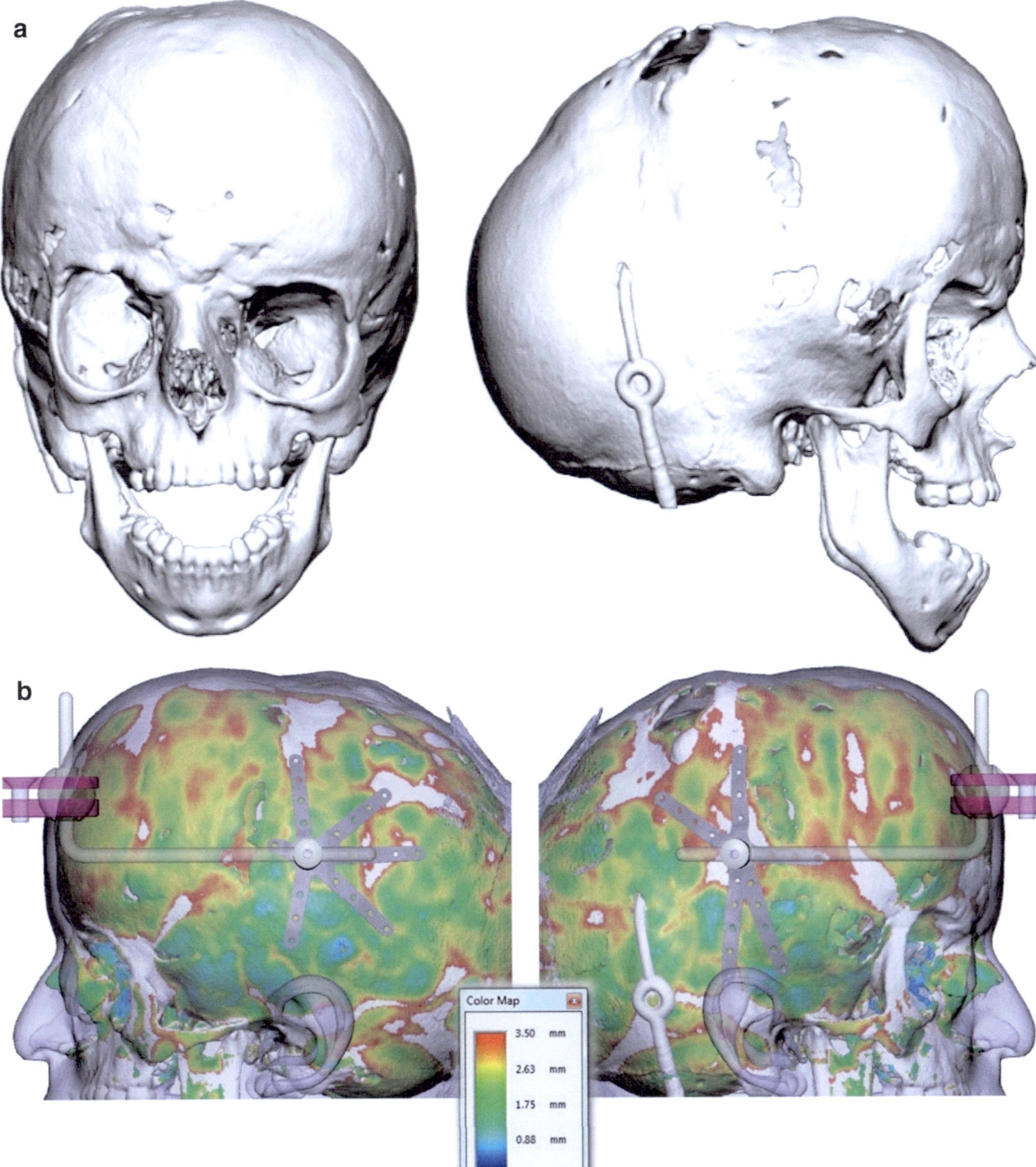

Fig. 13.5 (**a**) Syndromic craniosynostosis needing monobloc advancement and correction of right orbital dystopia and retrusion. Observe the VPS, bone defects and altered anatomy. (**b**) Custom-made star-shaped plate design and bone thickness analysis. (**c**) Positioning guide for the correction of the orbital asymmetry. (**d**) Pre and post top view

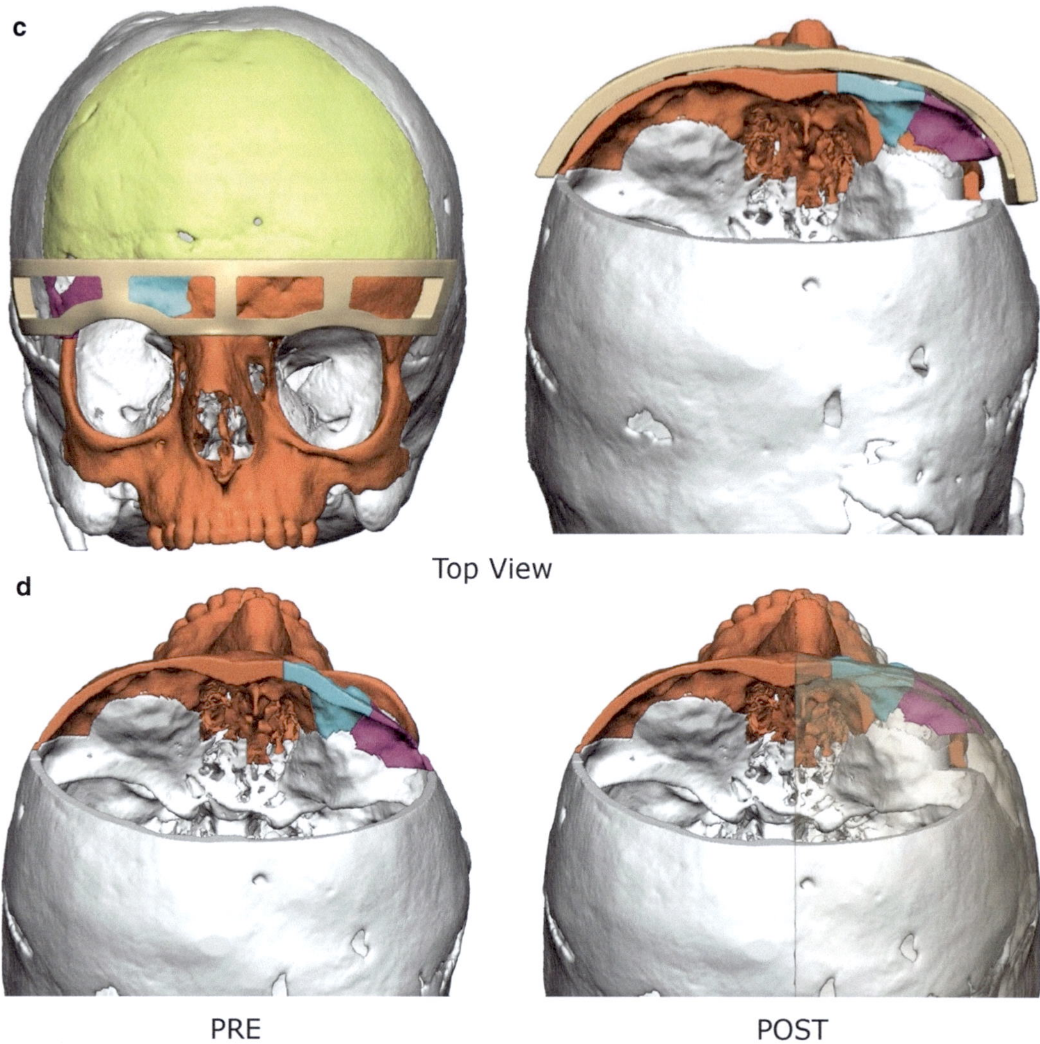

Fig. 13.5 (continued)

surgery has been a common practice for the past 10 years, and it has proven to be significantly better than 2D planning, especially in facial asymmetries and in syndromic patients, where we can plan and predict our results in a far more accurate way.

In severe mandibular malformations, reconstruction of the temporomandibular joint (TMJ) can be needed in addition to the orthognathic procedure. Use of bone grafts or microvascular flaps for TMJ reconstruction in children have been indicated by different authors, although in recent years there is a rising trend to use TMJ prostheses [6]. This tendency is based on the more predictable and stable functional and esthetic results that can be achieved using TMJ prosthesis while avoiding donor site morbidity. Due to the abnormal anatomy of these patients with the absence of established pattern, which leads to a great variability, the gold standard in TMJ reconstruction should be the use of CAD/CAM-customized TMJ prosthesis (Fig. 13.7).

Complex asymmetries frequently need a genioplasty which can also be planned virtually. Use of CAD/CAM cutting guides and customized fixation miniplates can contribute to a more predictable result in these situations. Genioplasty can be postponed as a second operation in cases of TMJ reconstruction in order to avoid communication of the intraoral approach with the prosthesis and to obtain more accurate final results (Fig. 13.8).

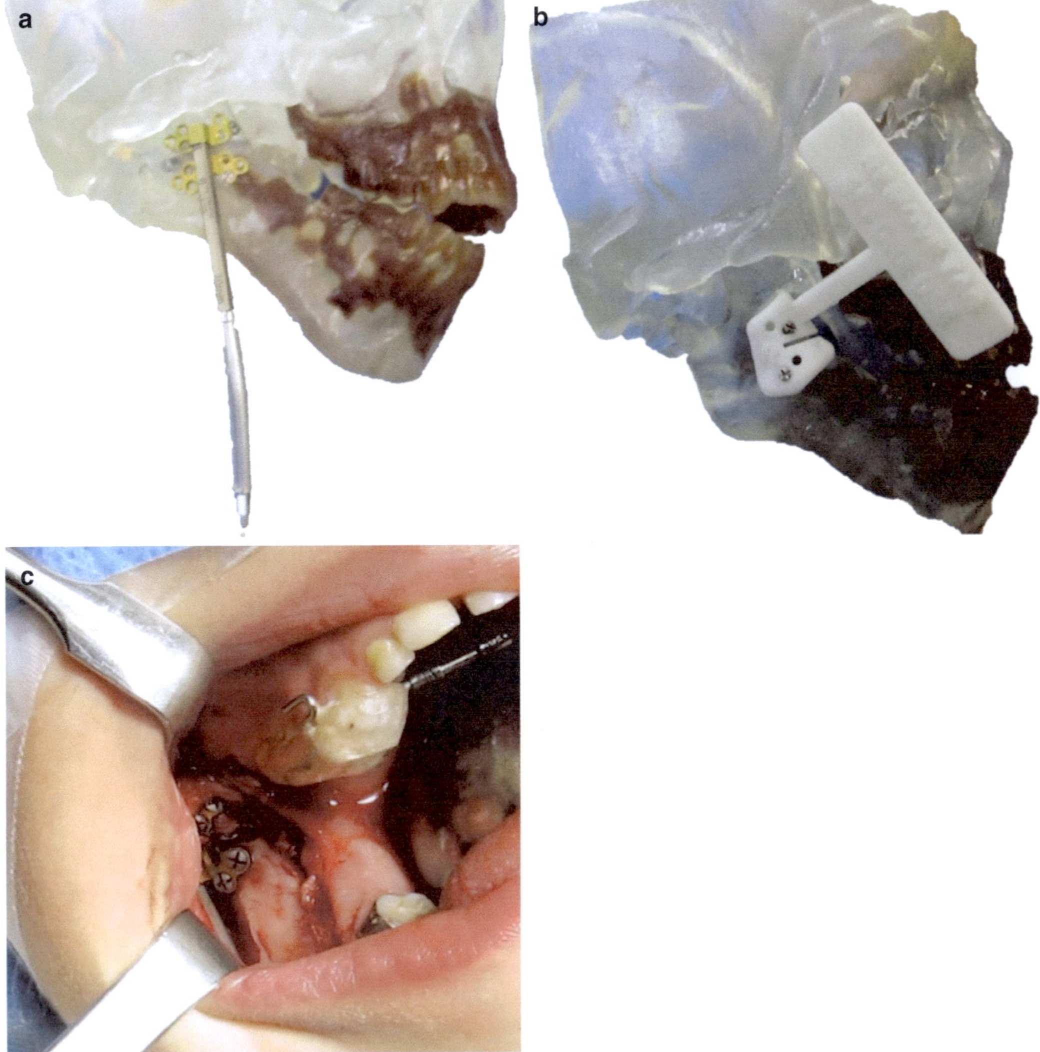

Fig. 13.6 Patient suffering right unilateral craniofacial microsomia. (**a**) Stereolithograpihc model of the skull where we plan the osteotomy and shape the distraction device. Notice the teeth buds. (**b**) Cutting guide for the surgery. (**c**) Intraoperative picture after the internal device is fixed

13.5.3 Mandible Defects After Tumor Resection

Tumor resection in pediatric patients is not as frequent as in adults, but in these cases mandible can need to be repaired. Indication of a bone graft or a microvascularized flap will depend on the size of the defect and the age and characteristics of the pediatric patient. In these situations, virtual planning of the resection and reconstruction can contribute like in adult patients to achieve a better and more predictable outcome, while reducing intraoperative time (Fig. 13.9).

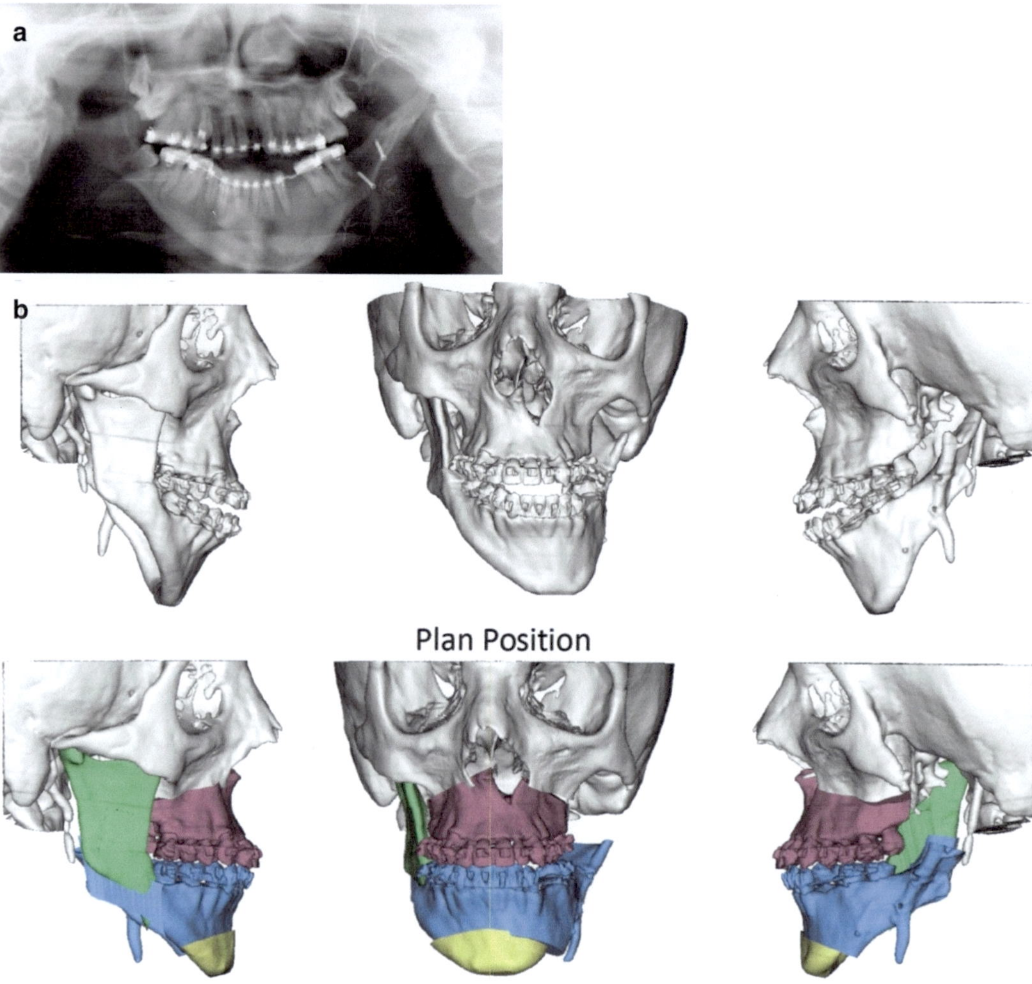

Fig. 13.7 (**a**) Patient with craniofacial microsomia, who had undergone mandible reconstruction with fibula flap and posterior distraction osteogenesis (**b**) Orthognathic 3D plan. (**c**) TMJ prosthesis design (TMJ Concepts®). Notice we know the length of the screws so as not to damage teeth or nerve canal. (**d**) Pre- and postoperative occlusion. (**e**) Pre- and postoperative frontal view of the patient. (**f**) Immediate postoperative OPG

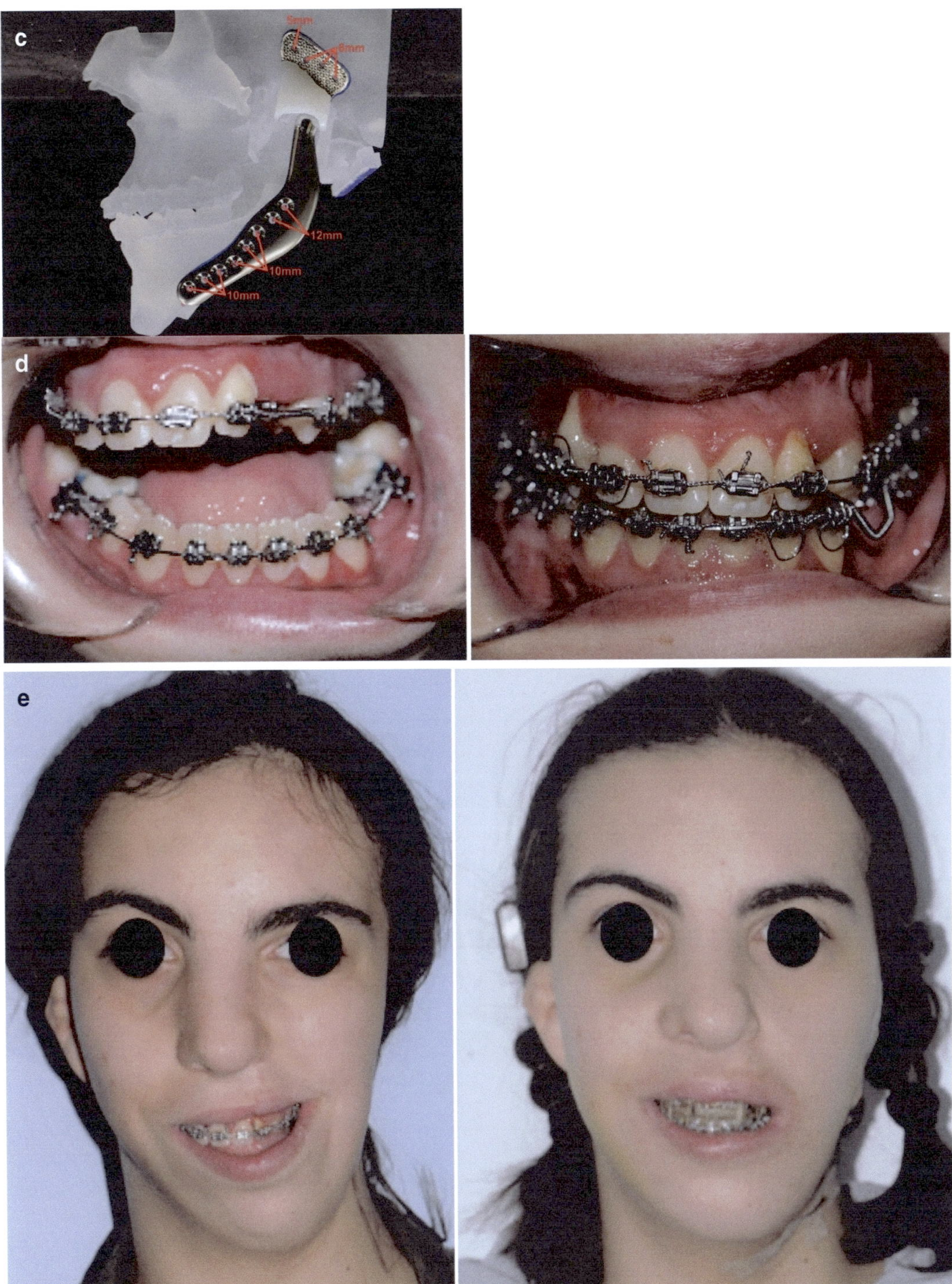

Fig. 13.7 (continued)

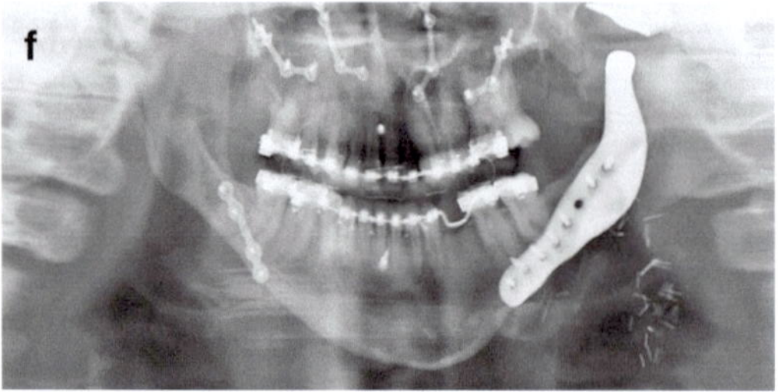

Fig. 13.7 (continued)

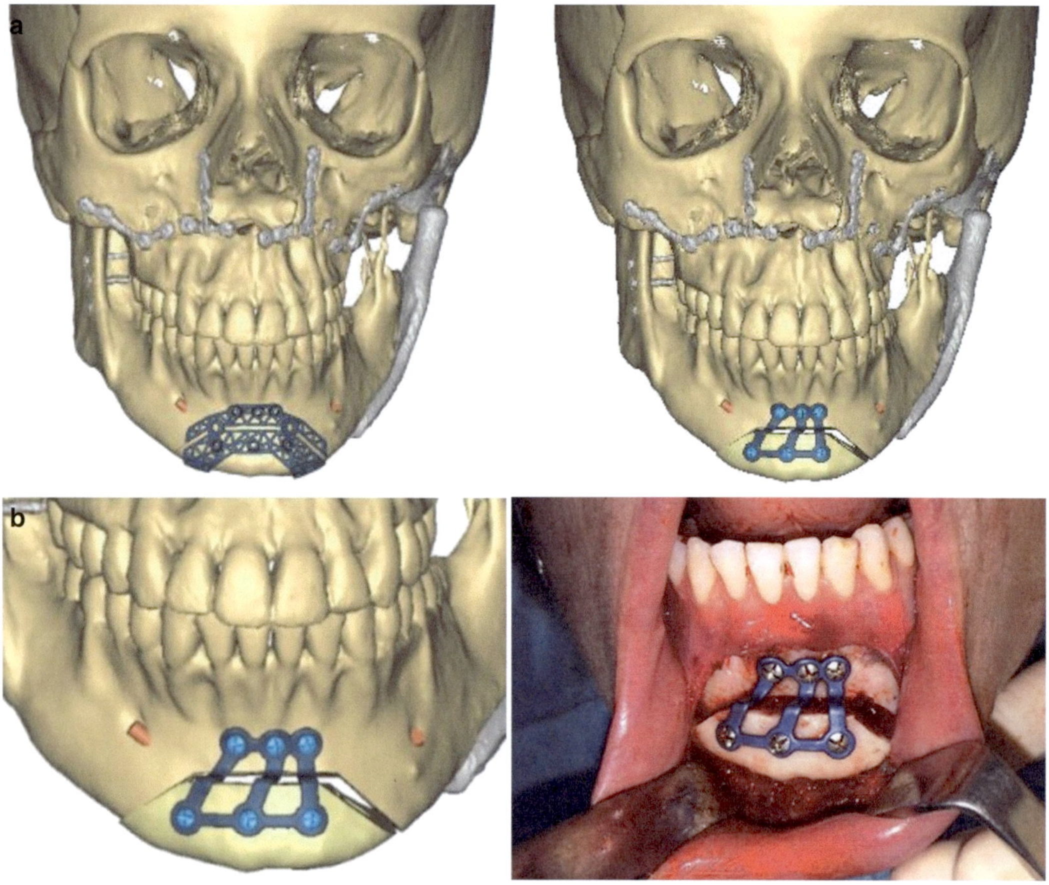

Fig. 13.8 (**a**) Virtual plan for genioplasty with cutting guide and a patient-specific plate in girl with craniofacial microsomia who had undergone an orthognathic surgery and TMJ reconstruction with custom-made prosthesis. (**b**) Virtual plan and surgery. Notice the proximity of the osteotomy to the mandible component of the prosthesis

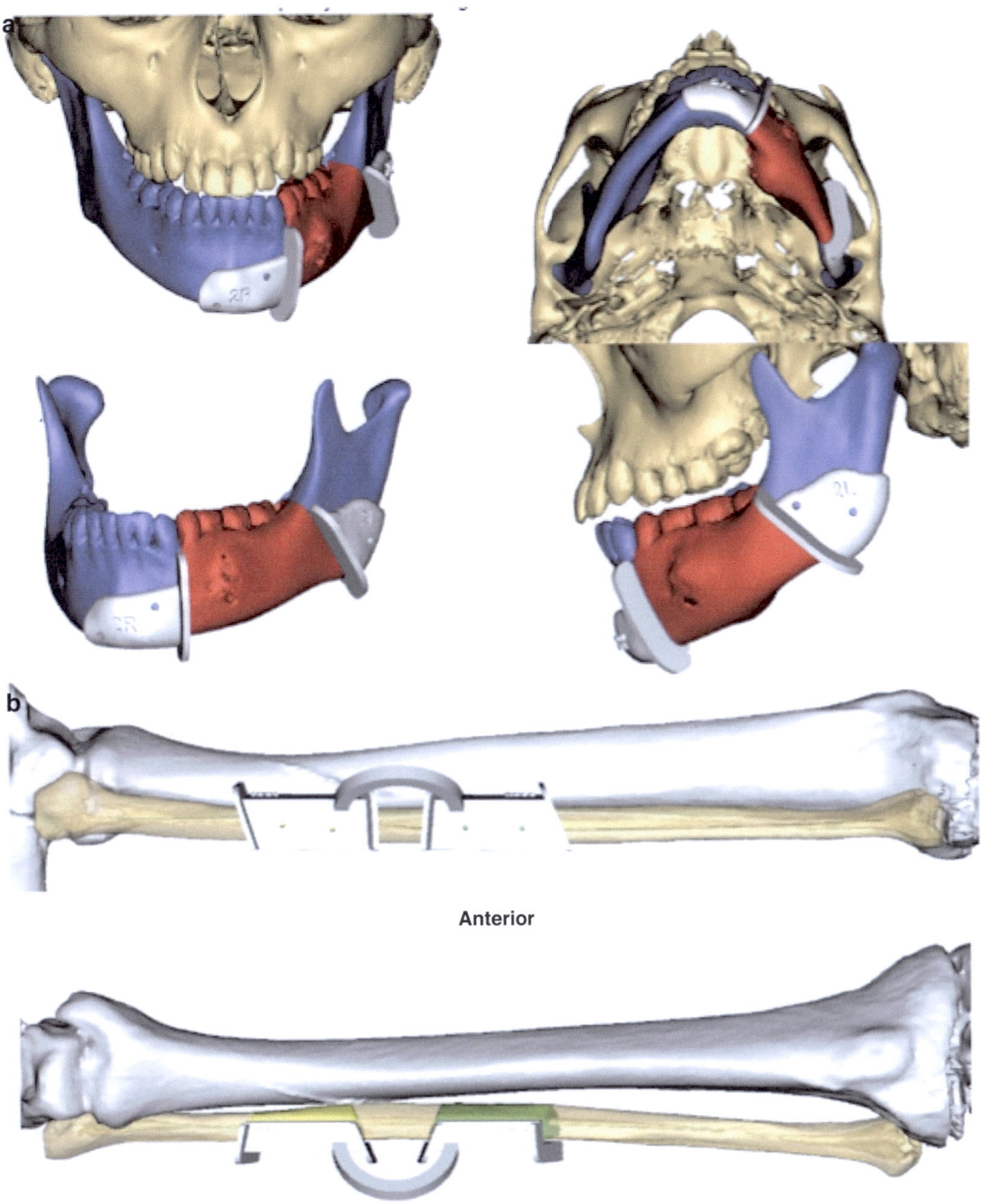

Fig. 13.9 (**a**) Ten-year-old patient with aggressive juvenile ossifying fibroma. Virtual design of the cutting guides to resect the tumor using Materialise® software. (**b**) Cutting guides for the fibula flap. (**c**) Design of the fibula flap placed with a "double barrel" technique for better esthetic and functional outcomes facilitating the dental rehabilitation in the future. (**d**) Postoperative OPG. Titanium plates were previously bent over a stereolithographic model of the reconstructed mandible

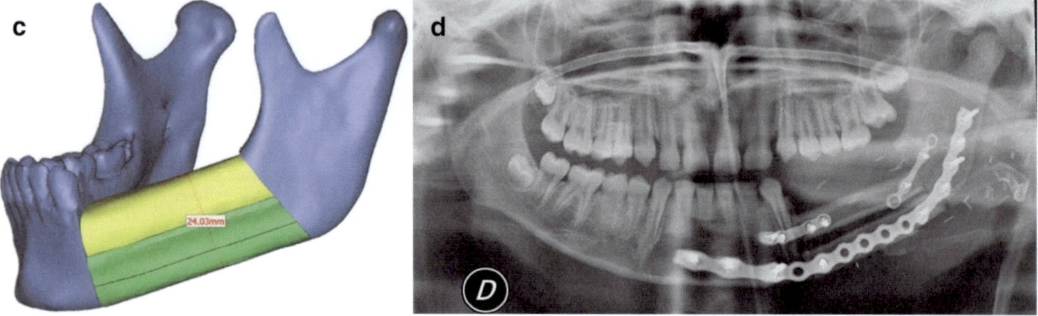

Fig. 13.9 (continued)

13.6 New Technologies in the Management of Fibrous Dysplasia

When complete resection of the pathological bone is not possible in cases affected by fibrous dysplasia because of the location or the severe sequelae that would cause a complete resection, remodeling of the excess of bone till symmetry is achieved can be performed. For this purpose, previous planning with the navigation software designing a mirror image of the healthy side can be done in order to design the surgical objective. Intraoperative navigation can contribute to check if the planned goal has been achieved (Fig. 13.10).

Finally, concerning the use of the new technologies in pediatric malformations of reconstruction, it is also interesting to mention that 3D surface imaging with **stereophotogrammetry** has become more popular in the last years especially for soft tissue analysis. This technique in some occasions can be a less invasive alternative than a CT for postoperative control (Fig. 13.11).

As a final thought, in a world where we are often overwhelmed by the many options that new technologies bring us, we should always apply common sense and use them in an efficient way to optimize our resources. Never forget as Albert Einstein once said, "The human spirit must prevail over technology."

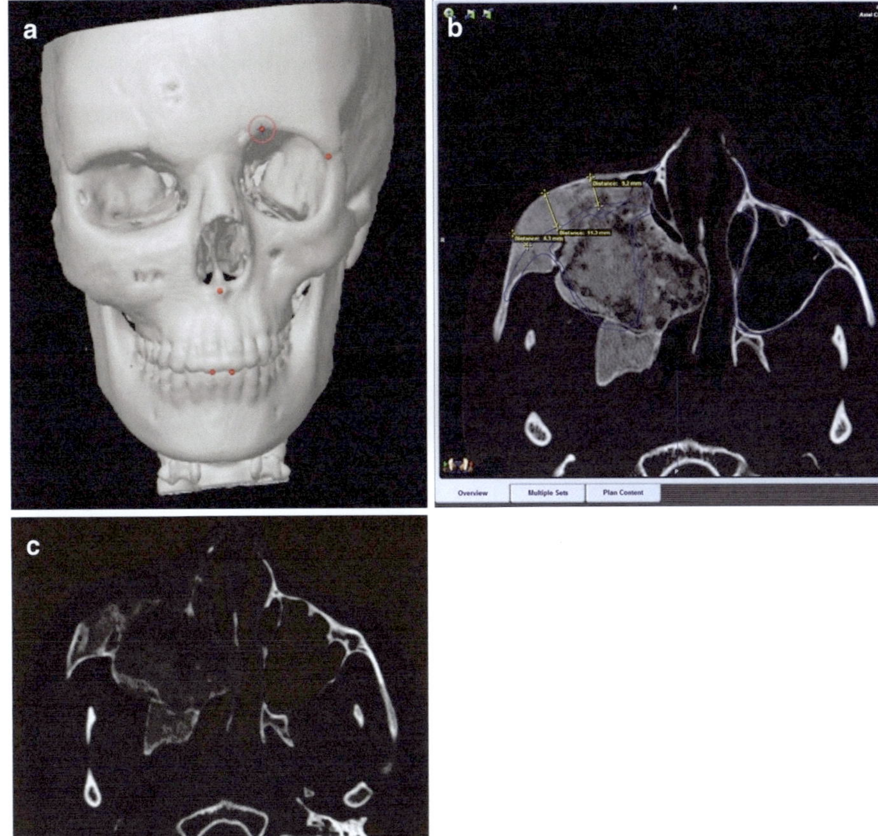

Fig. 13.10 (**a**) Teenage girl with fibrous dysplasia affecting the right side. (**b**) Mirroring of the healthy side, which is our goal for the affected site. Virtual plan using Brainlab®. (**c**) Postoperative CT showing better symmetry after remodeling of the lesion

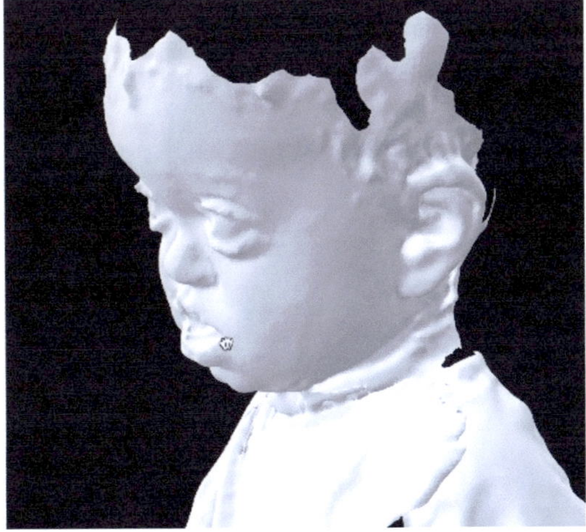

Fig. 13.11 3D surface imaging using Vectra® Camera of a patient with syndromic craniosynostosis

References

1. Chim H, Wetjen N, Mardini S. Virtual surgical planning in craniofacial surgery. Semin Plast Surg. 2014;28(3):150–8.
2. Han W, Yang X, Wu S, et al. A new method for cranial vault reconstruction: augmented reality in synostotic plagiocephaly surgery. J Craniomaxillofac Surg. 2019;47(8):1280–4.
3. Recuero G, Romance AI, Rivero A, Redondo M, Hinojosa J, Pascual B. Monobloc and Le-Fort III distraction in syndromic craniosynostosis using a computer designed RED II halo type distractor. IJOMS. 2015;44:64.
4. Merino F, Santás M, García Recuero I, Redondo M, Sanchez Aniceto G, Romance A. Complication rates following a monobloc advancement using distration osteogenesis with customized distractors. IJOMS. 2019;48:6.

5. Zheng J, He H, Kuang W, Yuan W. Presurgical naso-alveolar molding with 3D printing for a patient with unilateral cleft lip, alveolus, and palate. Am J Orthod Dentofac Orthop. 2019;156(3):412–9.
6. Garcia Recuero I, Fernandez A, Romance A, Redondo M, Sáncaz Aniceto G. The use of computer-aided design/computer-aided manufacturing temporomandibular joint prosthesis and orthognathic surgery in patients with craniofacial anomalies. IJOMS. 2017;46:229.

Federico Biglioli

14.1 Introduction

Facial paralysis is a devastating pathology, affecting 1/65 people during their lifetime. Most of the cases are unilateral, while bilateral ones are rare, generally related to Moebius syndrome, neurological pathologies, brain surgery complications.

The great part of patients suffer of Bell's palsy, a frequent condition probably due to herpes virus infection or physical distress. The majority of Bell's palsy population recovers completely, while 30% has residual deficits of different entity, and less than 1% never recover. That implies a great number of people needing treatment to improve their situation. Other causes of paralysis are malignant tumors of the parotid gland and benign lesions of the facial nerve canal, cranial base and neurosurgical procedures, developmental and congenital cases, traumas, ictus, cerebral hemorrhages, and several neurological conditions.

Facial palsy carries a great degree of psychological suffering because of the evident worsening of the aspect. Among functional deficits, lack of corneal lubrication is the most serious one, often leading to reduced visual acuity because of cornea thickening. Other clinical aspects are summarized in Table 14.1.

Table 14.1 Monolateral facial palsy deficits

Morphological	Functional
Asymmetry of the face	Absence of blinking leading to corneal lesions
Loss of forehead wrinkles	Partial/complete reduction of lacrimal glad production leading to corneal lesions
Eyebrow ptosis	Upper visual field constriction
Partial covering of the pupil by the upper lid	Reduced nasal breathing
Lagophthalmos	Phonatory deficits
Ectropion	Masticatory deficits and cheek biting
Flattening of naso-labial sulcus	
Cheek tissues ptosis	
Medial collapse of the nasal wing	
Asymmetry of the oral rhyme	
Smoothing of neck wrinkles	

14.2 Clinical Examination

Anamnesis must evaluate general conditions, possible neurological causes or other clinical situations that could cause the facial nerve deficit (tumors, metastasis, trauma, others). It is fundamental to assess timing of onset of the paralysis. If it takes place in less than 72 h, given the exclusion of a cerebral accident, the most probable cause is Bell's palsy. A cerebral CT scan is generally accomplished, but it may also be postponed

F. Biglioli (✉)
Maxillofacial Surgery Unit, San Paolo Hospital,
University of Milan, Milan, Italy
e-mail: federico.biglioli@unimi.it

© Springer Nature Switzerland AG 2021
J. Acero (ed.), *Innovations and New Developments in Craniomaxillofacial Reconstruction*,
https://doi.org/10.1007/978-3-030-74322-2_14

3 months only for those who do not show any clinical sign of recovery. For those with a slow onset of the paralysis, along several months, the presence of a malignant lesion of the parotid gland or a benign lesion of the facial nerve canal must always be ascertained. If a neurological disease is ruled out, ecographies and MRI of the parotid gland must be repeated several times up to 2 years in order to find a possible malignant lesion binding the nerve in the parotid gland or a little benign lesion growing into the facial nerve canal determining its compression. Moreover, a high-definition CT scan with contrast may individualize a little neuroma/schwannoma of the facial nerve or the geniculate ganglium determining compression of the VII cranial nerve (cn).

The facial nerve function must be evaluated precisely, paying attention to any detail. It must be assess the orientation and the position of natural wrinkles, their number, depth, and direction, because that is related to mimetic muscles tone at rest. The examination may proceed top to bottom: first is evaluated the front, then the eyebrows, upper lids, orbital rim, lower lid, cheek and naso-labial sulcus, nasal ala (generally collapsed medially because of trasversus nasi deficit), oral rim, chin, submandibular area, and neck. All those tissues are collapsed, much more in older and skinny people, generally less in fat ones because denser tissues tend to mantain their appearance. Children generally do not have an evident deficit of the symmetry at rest because of their tonic and elastic tissues. For those with a paralysis lasting several months to years, orbicularis oris atrophy is particularly evident at the lateral third of the lips.

The second part of examination must rule out any detail of movements. It is fundamental to listen what the patient knows about the condition, because her/his attention to particulars is often high and may direct out attention to little but significant signs of reduced facial nerve function.

Watching the patient while talking let us observe eyelids blinking (often inhibited while staring at him/her during examination) and lip movements. We may then ask the patient to produce several preordinate movements, with different efforts: upper eyebrows elevation, lid closure, smiling, kissing (it is also important to observe

mentalis muscle function), and lower teeth exposure (to ascertain depressor angulis oris, depressor labii, mentalis, and platisma function).

14.2.1 Documentation and Classification

The face at rest and during all movements must be recorded by pictures and videos. The last ones being more reliable of the dynamic part of the examination. Photographic documentation of the patient has absolutely to be dated and repeated over time in order to better understand variations of facial nerve function.

Patient may be classified according to several classifications going from famous House–Brackmann system, to Sunnybrook and others [1, 2]. All have pros and odds; those classifications have the advantage to be very well known but miss to consider some details. The biggest lack for a surgeon is that they apply better to a facial paralysis but are poorly fitted for a post-surgical patient evalutation. Objective classification systems well fitted for those patients have been proposed, but the lack of uniformity limits partly their spread among the scientific community [3]. In order to overcome that problem, the eFACE classification system taking account of all facial districts at rest and during movements has been developed [4]. That may be applied easily to pre- and postoperative situations and its rapid spread among surgeons is fundamental to compare results and speak a common language [5]. The main criticism to this classification is the absence of evaluation of movements according to emotions (ex. smiling because of a joke). The use of motor sources other than the facial nerve stimulates cerebral adaptation with different timing and end-levels for each patient [6]. For example, when utilizing the masseteric nerve, smiling needs to be coupled at the beginning to clenching the teeth. After this first period, smiling may be produced voluntarily by giving an impulse different from clenching the teeth, just by willing to smile. The next step is an automatic smile, without the need to give a voluntary impulse to the muscles. That is often called spontaneous in scientific literature, confusing it with a smile given involuntarily during an empathic moment or laughing because of fun: let us call the last that "emotional" smiling. While the cerebral adaptation may reach the goal of automatic smiling, emotional smiling is a chimera if a neural source other than the facial nerve is used.

Exercising with the guidance of a dedicated physiotherapist helps much to obtain cerebral adaptation, but it is extremely rare to observe an emotional laugh and almost impossible to see an empathic smile (because due to a lighter neural stimulus). Indeed that is achievable with discrete consistency by facial reanimation surgery, but only utilizing the branch of contralateral healthy facial nerve for zygomatic muscles. The stimulus may be driven from one side of the face to the other via a cross-face sural nerve graft.

14.3 Treatment

Facial palsy treatment is very specific and requires a dedicated team including microsurgeon, neurologist, physiotherapist/speech therapist, psychologist as the main professionals.

14.3.1 Physiotherapy

The goal of physiotherapy during the period of recovery after a facial paralysis is to favor the spontaneous processes of functional recovery of the nerve by implementing the function of mimetic musculature, expressiveness, inside of a communicative dimension [7, 8]. It therefore includes functional exercises aimed at smile recovery, and manual treatment of muscles and connective tissues to increase vascularization and trophism. Patients are also encouraged to exercise alone at home.

It is important that the patient activates a motility linked to the stage of neuronal recovery achieved. Therefore, during the first phase of complete denervation, when voluntary muscle contraction is not yet present, it is advisable to avoid stimulating facial activity pending the appearance of the first movements.

Bearing in mind that every action needs a multisensory integration and the brain conceives movement not in terms of activation of single muscles, but rather as a set of finalized gestures, it is more effective to reproduce gestures that imitate certain expressions rather than aimless. In fact, the observation of an action is the basis of learning through imitation.

In the event that functional recovery presents the typical defects such as paresis, hypertone at rest and synkinesis, exercises are aimed at correcting them by promoting brain adaptation, the correct recruitment of the musculature, and limiting the evidence of the acquired defect.

It is advisable to avoid intense voluntary contractions and electrostimulation to inhibit and control synkinesis and hypertone at rest. So the patient must accomplish exercises to increase the perception of direction and amplitude of movements. Other practice is done to release muscular tension, while some exercises are intended to raise awareness of the key points of the face like eyes and corner of the mouth. Finally, some exercises enhance recognition of shapes, sizes, and surfaces, comparing the right and left sides.

Decontracting massages promote muscle relaxation, but their result is limited by the reestablishment of the contracture if the basic signal of the facial nerve is not corrected by the use of botulinum toxin or appropriate microsurgical techniques.

It is important that during the voluntary movements, the healthy contralateral part does not prevail, which would inhibit the correct recruitment of the fibers reinnervated on the paralyzed side. It is therefore necessary to educate the patient to have the right timing, pulling the corners of the mouth during smiling. Therefore, if the paretic movement is not still particularly evident, the patient is taught to reduce the same movement on the sound side to reach a better dynamic symmetry. Obviously that is not sufficient to restore the fullness of mimicry, but still favors the camouflage of the acquired deficits.

In operated patients, physiotherapy is aimed at optimizing the use of what has been done in the operating room. For example, if the masseteric nerve is the new motor source to smile, special exercises are devised to promote cerebral adaptation in order to obtain the fullest and most natural result possible. Patient must carry out the exercises daily at home and monitor every little improvement with videos and photos and functional skills, to quantify progress. Rehabilitation is however very long and the alternation of periods of improvement to periods with no appreciable results is expected. During this period, the patient must be followed and supervised at least once every month in order to increase control of the movements and avoid being demoralized.

It is therefore essential to provide psychological support at all stages of the treatment. A higher mood helps the synergy between physiotherapist and patient to obtain greater results. When self-confidence is increased by a good static and dynamic appearance, the patient feels more motivated to perform facial movements in an open environment, without feeling embarrassed like when suffering from paralysis and self-inhibiting their mimicry. As a matter of fact, an improvement in the esthetic aspect and in the execution of the movements is a stimulus to use the musculature again and, therefore, to exercise it more. Each patient has his own personality and it is therefore important that the physiotherapist develops an empathic relationship to encourage collaboration.

Finally, it is fundamental that physiotherapist and surgeon have a full harmony and exchange of informations to know exactly what has been done in the operating room and to improve the rehabilitative potential.

14.3.2 Botulinum Toxin Treatment

Botulinum neurotoxin A (BTX A) is a valid tool in the treatment of light to medium abnormal facial movements following spontaneous recovery of facial paralysis [9]. The toxin is extracted and purified from various toxins produced by the bacterium *Clostridium* and used to treat several pathologies where it is useful to inhibit synaptic cholinergic transmission and reduce muscular or neurovegetative hyperactivity.

In case of erroneous recovery from facial paralysis, BTX A is injected on the affected side to partially correct erroneous movements related to synkinesis phenomena, due to an anomalous regrowth of axons through the facial nerve branching (aberrant re-innervation). Even the contralateral healthy side must sometimes be treated to simultaneously reduce mirror movements and achieve dynamic facial symmetry.

The inhibitory action of botulinum toxin on the neuromuscular plaque is reversible and has an action duration of 3–6 months; it then tends to decay by the action of the regeneration of neural arborizations. New synaptic buttons take place from the neighboring terminations to those blocked by BTX A, leading to the restoration of nerve transmission and the consequent recovery of muscular function. The administration of the toxin may be done under electromyographic control (EMG) or, in some cases, ultrasound (EcoTG). The scrupulous EMG analysis of the single submuscular units and the identification of hyperactivity allow to be very selective in the inoculation of the muscles to be treated by utilizing cannula needle electrodes connected to an electromyograph; sometimes, the association of EMG and high-frequency probes EcoTG can be useful in the evaluation of anatomical variants or residual muscular trophism. The toxin can be injected with micro-doses to reduce muscle hypertonicity or to partially antagonize the most evident synkinesis. Micro-doses may also paralyze the muscle depressor of the lower lip (DLL) on the healthy side to symmetrize it when the DLL of the paralyzed side does not recover spontaneously.

Experience in the field of neurology and esthetic medicine may give an extra gear in the use of botulinum toxin dedicated to the treatment of facial paralysis.

14.3.3 Facial Reanimation Surgery

Reanimation surgery requires a deep knowledge of the matter, a microsurgical training, and the ability to apply several different techniques because the treatment must be individualized obligatorily.

There are three important key points to take into account while treating facial palsy: timing of intervention, the combined use of static and dynamic procedures, and the mixture of quantitative stimuli (powerful ones, given by the masseteric, hypoglossus, deep-temporalis, spinal nerves, and others) with qualitative stimuli (the natural ones, driven by the homolateral or the contralateral facial nerve branches). All technical solutions should be chosen according to the deficits and desires of the person, sometimes devising individual solutions. Moreover, it is important to remember that surgery is a handiwork, and results may be different when the same techniques are applied by different surgeons.

14.3.3.1 Immediate Facial Nerve Reconstruction

There are clinical situations requiring immediate facial nerve repair: those are typically related to severing of the trunk or its branches because of a trauma or during surgery. The last one being a decision made to obtain a radical resection of a tumor or due to an unintentional cut [10].

If the nerve is simply cut without loss of substance, the two extremities may be repaired accomplishing a direct neurorrhaphy under microscope magnification [11]. After gently juxtaposing the two neural stumps, the epineural layer is sutured tension-free by few 10/0 or 11/0 non-reabsorbable stitches. The spontaneous axoplasmatic fluid will then be able to accomplish partial neural repair. Its rate of progression is considered to be 1 mm per day, but it slows down significantly at the anastomotic site. The exact speed of the fluid cannot be predicted, and it seems to vary according to age, quality of the neurorrhaphy, vascularization of the recipient site, axonal count of the donor nerve and others. At the end, a great discrepancy of time for the onset of first mimetic muscle contraction is observed, generally between 2 and 8 months. Neural repair continues up to several years, the main part being among the first 24 months. The result is generally high quality though never equal to prior to facial nerve severing.

This type of repair might not be suited for injuries of the intracranial course of the facial nerve; its structure at this site is more similar to toothpaste than to a peripheral nerve, making microsurgical reconstruction less effective.

If a part of the facial nerve is missing, a direct neurorrhaphy of the two stumps is impossible and a cable graft must be utilized. Autologous nerve grafting is the gold standard, the two most common sources being the suralis and the great auricular, though several others might be used whether being sensitive or motor nerves; the most commonly used graft sources are the great auricular nerve, the sural nerve, the medial and lateral antebrachial cutaneous nerves, the cervical plexus branches, and the superficial radial nerve [12–14]. Choosing which nerve to harvest is related to the caliber and length of the branch of the facial nerve to reconstruct and the donor site morbidity.

At present, autologous nerve graft is the gold standard. Because of the importance to obtain the best functional recovery, cryopreserved or decellularized nerves, and collagen tube substitutes are not the first reconstructive choice for facial nerve reconstruction.

Finally, there are two typical situations requiring the sacrifice of all extra-cranial facial nerve branching: surgical removal of a malignant parotid tumor involving the facial nerve and extended parotidectomy to treat pleomorphic adenoma recurrences after several prior surgeries. In those cases, it is mandatory to reconstruct immediately the facial nerve to obtain the best facial palsy correction [15]. In fact, immediate facial nerve reconstruction leads to the best functional result compared to delayed reconstructions, because of a higher axonal regenerative potential and because the mimetic muscles are subjected to a short non-stimulated period reducing their degeneration toward fibrous-fatty metaplasia. It is advisable to add a fascia lata graft set from the nasolabial sulcus to the infraorbital rim to suspend soft tissues of the middle third of the face because a perfect tone at rest of mimetic muscles after the reconstruction is not guaranteed. Also, in case of failure of neural regeneration through the grafted nerve, the soft tissues suspension allows at least to obtain a good symmetry of the face at rest.

If postoperative radiotherapy is expected because of treating a high-grade tumor, its negative influence on a traditional nerve graft is controversial [16]. Several authors assert that positive results may be obtained also in those cases with traditional nerve grafting [17]. In order to improve the chances of a good recovery of facial nerve function, some authors proposed the use of free vascularized nerve flaps, eventually coupled with a cutaneous component of the flap [18–20]. On the contrary, most of authors agree on utilizing a traditional nerve graft to substitute facial nerve branching with several options: sural nerve, lateral antebrachial cutaneous nerve, medial antebrachial cutaneous nerve, the nerve to the vastus lateralis, and the great auricular nerve [17, 21]. The most utilized donor nerve, the suralis, carries an undeniable drawback: there are one, at the most two, significant lateral branches. That limits the number of distal facial nerve branches to be reconstructed, also antagonized by an evident mismatch of caliber between the suralis and distal facial nerve branches. On the contrary, the caliber of the suralis and that one of the trunk of the facial nerve are similar, matching easily for a good neurorrhaphy. The second must-used graft is the great auricular nerve: it has few very tiny distal branches and its caliber is considerably lesser than the trunk of the facial nerve, making its use relatively inadequate for facial nerve branching substitution. Its popularity for this purpose is due mainly to its contiguity to the parotid gland and low morbidity of harvesting. On the contrary, its presence closer to the tumor might suggest not to use it because of oncological reasons.

The most fitted nerve for substituting facial nerve branching is the thoracodorsal nerve [22, 23] because its branching is really similar, and calibers of the trunk and distal branches of the two nerves coincide much (Scheme 14.1, Figs. 14.1 and 14.2). Up to eight distal branches

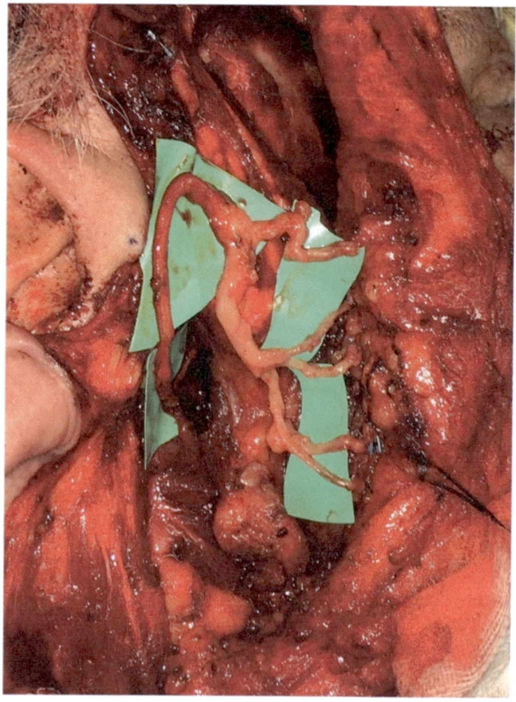

Fig. 14.1 The facial nerve branching reconstructed by the thoracodorsal nerve

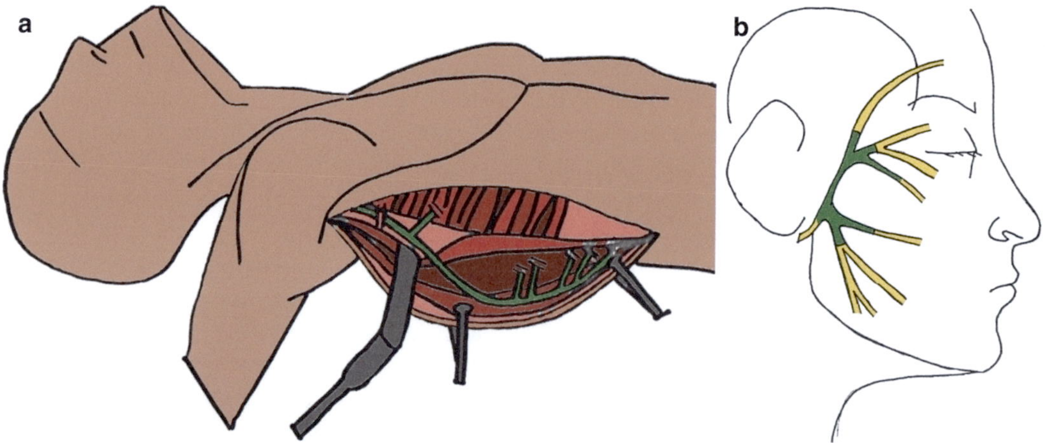

Scheme 14.1 The thoracodorsal nerve (green) harvested (**a**) to substitute the entire extracranial facial nerve branching (**b**)

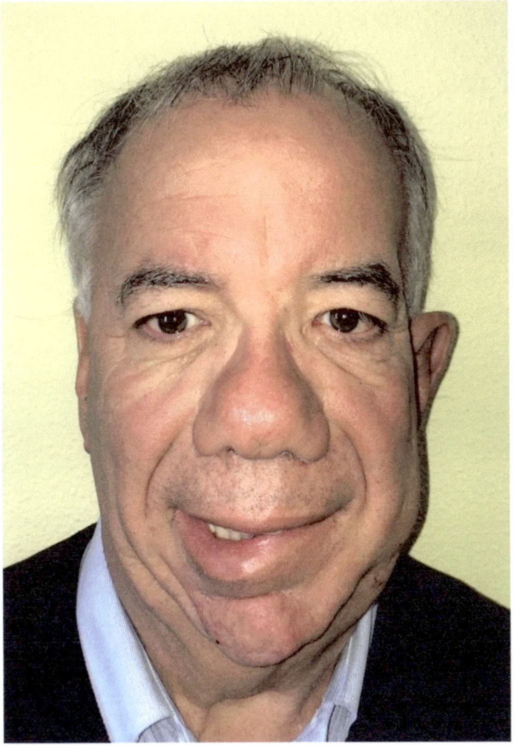

reconstruction: in this case one or two ribs and a myocutaneous free-flap based on the latissimus dorsi and the thoracodorsal vessels may be harvested together with nerve [24]. Although rib has demonstrated to be effective for mandibular reconstruction even in case of postoperative radiotherapy if coupled with a vascularized latissimus dorsi flap, other options to be taken into consideration is the vascularized scapular border [25]. That is surely more difficult to be utilized as a part of a chimeric reconstruction.

In spite of the neural choice of reconstruction, physiotherapy is advocated to better functional result. Physical therapy is even more necessary if the masseteric nerve is utilized as motor source instead of the facial nerve trunk.

Other adjunctive procedures as fascia lata suspensions, upper lid lipofilling, and cross-face nerve grafting may be added simultaneously or later to enhance functional and esthetic outcome.

14.3.3.2 Recent Paralysis Treatment

When paralysis does not solve spontaneously or an immediate reconstruction of the facial nerve has not been provided during surgery, facial reanimation must take place. Depending on the presence of viable mimetic muscles, we deal with two different situations: recent paralysis, requiring a new neural input, and long-standing ones, where extinguished muscles must be substituted [26].

The time limit between the two groups is generally 18–24 months after the onset of palsy, when the absence of neural input leads to an irreversible fibrotic metaplasia of mimetic muscles. If a subclinical neural stimulation is still present, the time limit may extend; if a previous palsy happened, the limit may shorten. An accurate electromyographic evaluation ascertains muscle status in each specific area and muscle group of the face: front, upper, and lower eyelids, zygomatic muscles, upper lip levator muscles, orbicularis oris muscle, depressor of the lower lip muscles, platisma. Viable muscles produce fibrillations at EMG, while fibrotic ones no.

Timing to decide when to give up waiting for a spontaneous recovery of the nerve must be clear: if after 8 months there is no evidence of

Fig. 14.2 Good symmetry of the face of the patient and good ability to smile 12 months after surgery and radiotherapy ended

of the facial nerve may be reconstructed. During surgery, the facial nerve trunk and its branches are easily identified dissecting tissues by spreading the tips of the scissors parallel to facial nerve branches at the periphery of the parotid margins. The facial nerve trunk is identified in a traditional manner at the exit from the stylomastoid foramen. At the end of oncological resection the microsurgical reconstruction takes place, utilizing 10/0 or 11/0 sutures for the neurorrhaphies. By this way the loss of axons is reduced, because of almost perfect matching of all anastomotic sites.

In case the trunk of the facial nerve is not available for neurorrhaphy because of its invasion by the tumor, the masseteric nerve may be used as motor source with very good results. If an extended parotidectomy is performed, including also the skin or the mandibular bone, the lateral thoracic wall allows to add other tissue components from the same site to make a composite movements, facial reanimation must take place because the possibilities to register a good facial nerve functional recovery droop down to null! If after 8 months some movements are present, waiting is mandatory up to 18 months. At that time, microsurgery and ancillary procedures may be taken into consideration if deficits are evident.

If a recent paralysis is diagnosed, a new neural input must be given by anastomosing a new neural source to the extracranial facial nerve. EMG has also the aim to map exactly the status of potential neural sources to be used.

Neural sources are divided into quantitative and qualitative (Table 14.2). A quantitative source gives a powerful neural input, it may convert its original function into the new one by a phenomena called cerebral adaptation, but almost never converts its function into the perfect one. A typical example is the masseteric nerve changing its function from biting to smiling: immediately after the onset of first smiling movements, generally 3–5 months after the reanimation procedure, the patient must clench the teeth to produce a smile. Cerebral adaptation generally takes in few months, leading to smiling without the need to clenching the teeth. After few other months, patients do not have to think about giving a specific stimulus because it all happens automatically. Cerebral adaptation process is facilitated by exercising with a dedicated physiotherapist.

Laughing because of a funny emotion is a completely different matter, almost impossible to obtain by utilizing the masseteric nerve as motor source. A little empathic smile, involuntarily produced while talking to someone, is an even more difficult goal to reach. In fact that is given by a much lighter stimulus, and only facial nerve branches for the zygomatic muscles are involved in those situations. All those findings are easily found recording patient face while watching a funny movie or during a relaxed meet up [6].

The only nerve sources able to give the correct natural stimulus are facial nerve branches: the zygomatic muscle branches for smiling, the orbicularis oculi branches for blinking, etc. We consider those as the qualitative sources. As restitutio ad integrum is nowadays a mirage, the two main functional goals of facial reanimation are blinking and smiling recovery. The first one to give health to the cornea, the second one because it is the main communicative facial movement. So, only reconstructing precisely the branches for the orbicularis oculi and for the zygomatic muscles ensures this goals. Exaggerating this concept, even the homolateral facial nerve trunk is partially incorrect, because its stimulus will not be selective as that given by the single branches of the facial nerve. As an example, blinking stimulus is given by specific axons normally concentrated into the branches for the orbicularis oculi: if the trunk of the facial nerve is used as the proximal motor nerve of the neurorrhaphy, the axons for blinking will spread all over the distal facial nerve branches, with low possibilities to produce blinking. Instead, if a branch for the orbicularis oculi is anastomosed to a severed branch with the same function, the axons leading to blinking will reach their target! Considering a stronger stimulus like smiling, driven by much more branches in the midface, the lack of selectivity of the trunk is partially hidden because a high number of axons will reach the zygomatic muscles anyhow, producing a natural smile at the right time. Though so, other muscles will involuntarily be activated contemporarily, producing a synkinetic movements in the whole face. So, the trunk of the facial nerve

Table 14.2 Neural sources

Quantitative	Qualitative
Masseteric n. (optimal for movement restitution—easy for anastomosing)	Homolateral facial n. trunk (powerful—correct stimulus but leading to several synkinesis)
Deep temporalis n. (optimal for movement—difficult for anastomosing)	Homolateral facial n. branches (ideal—seldom available)
Hypoglossus n. (optimal for muscle tone at rest—poor for movement reinstitution)	Contralateral facial n. branches (ideal—via cross-face nerve grafting—lacking of power)
Spinal n. (optimal for muscle tone at rest—poor for movement reinstitution)	
Others	

provides the correct stimulus only partially because not enogh selective.

Given that the correct stimulus to facial movements is guaranteed only by facial nerve branches, contralateral ones must be taken into consideration if the homolateral are not available. In this case, a long nerve grafting might by-pass the gap with a cross-face positioning. The donor branch must ideally contain a minimum of 900 axons [27, 28] and should be cut at the anterior margin of the parotid gland in order to avoid an evident deficit in the donor side. If two cross-face grafts are planned, one significant facial nerve branch must be left intact between the two, to avoid a facial nerve deficit in the donor site. The classical nerve graft is the suralis because of its length, constant anatomy, and low morbidity. It is set reverse to avoid wasting axonal ingrowth through its few lateral branches. After several months (generally between 6 and 12), the axonal ingrowth through the nerve graft reaches its distal end. If a distal neurorrhaphy has been done at the time of grafting, a scar might partially obstacle axonal growth through it. Results are much more guaranteed if a two times procedure is choosen, accomplishing the distal neurorrhaphy only after complete axonal ingrowth. That is easily checked by the Tinel's sign: a little nip over the distal end of the graft evokes tingling at the anastomotic site.

Unfortunately, in spite of a two-times procedure, the quantity of axons arriving via the cross-face nerve craft is generally insufficient to produce the full movement. Because of that, mixing quantitative stimuli to qualitative ones ensures the best facial reanimation (Table 14.2).

Characteristics of quantitative motor sources help much to decide the better surgical strategies. Particularly the masseteric nerve has proven to be best for movement replacement and lesser to recover a good tone at rest [29, 30]. The opposite is true for the hypoglossus nerve.

Triple innervation (Scheme 14.2, Figs. 14.3, 14.4, 14.5, 14.6, 14.7 and 14.8) provided by masseteric, hypoglossus, and contralateral facial nerve is nowadays the most complete reinnervation technique proposed till now [31]: it utilizes two quantitative stimuli given by the masseteric

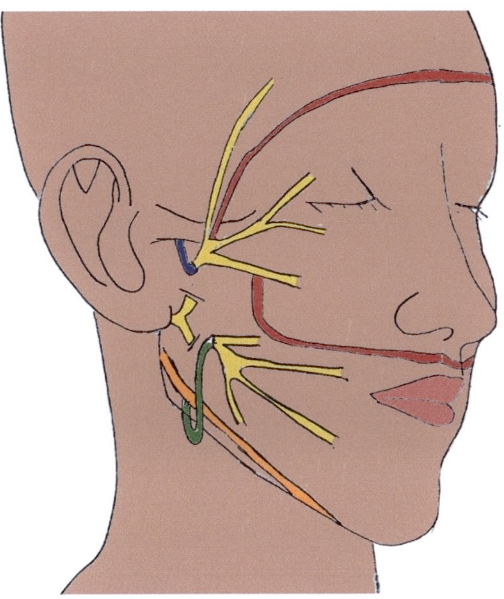

Scheme 14.2 Triple innervation technique. The masseteric nerve (blue) provides stimulus mainly to eyelid closure and smiling. Thirty percent of the hypoglossus nerve (orange) is utilized to guarantee a healthy tone to the mimetic musculature of the lower third of the face. Two cross-face suralis nerve grafts (red) convey the qualitative stimuli of the contralateral facial nerve for blinking and emotional smiling

nerve and part of the hypoglossus nerve, plus qualitative stimuli coming from two contralateral facial nerve branches [32, 33]—one branch to recover blinking and one for smiling. Generally, static procedures are added to better the symmetry: a fascia lata graft from the nasolabial sulcus to the infraorbital margin corrects the middle third soft tissue ptosis and a small lateral tarsorrhaphy adjusts lagophthalmos. Adding 2 ml lipofilling to the upper lid gives immediate corneal relief and better final blinking restitution.

Lower lip paralysis is particularly evident during talking and smiling. That is partially reduced by a reconstituted good muscle tone and an artificial contralateral depressor labii inhibition (by botulinum toxin injection or marginal mandibulae severing). The hypoglossus side-to-end neurorrhaphy ensures good recovery of the muscle tone. Severing completely the hypoglossus nerve leads to unacceptable speech, chewing, and swallowing deficits. Instead, utilizing only 30% of its fibers allows to obtain a good tone at rest of the

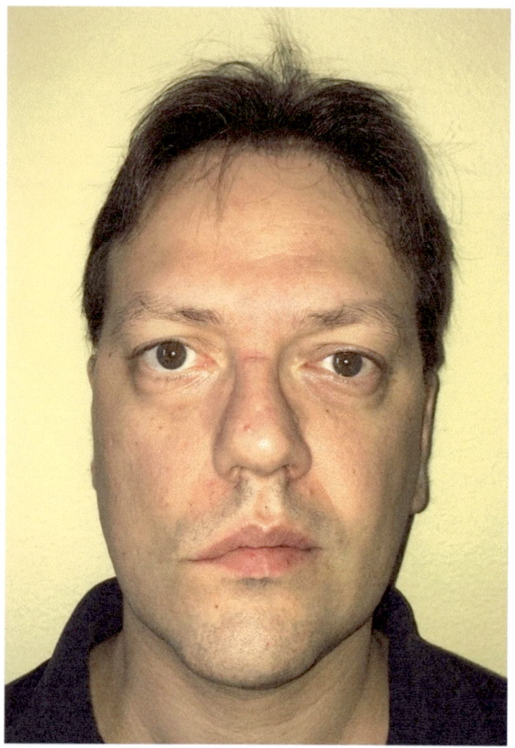

Fig. 14.3 Patient affected by a recent facial paralysis. Appearance of the face at rest prior to triple innervation. During surgery, a fascia lata graft is added to enhance symmetry at rest, and 2 ml lipofilling of the upper lid is accomplished to improve blinking

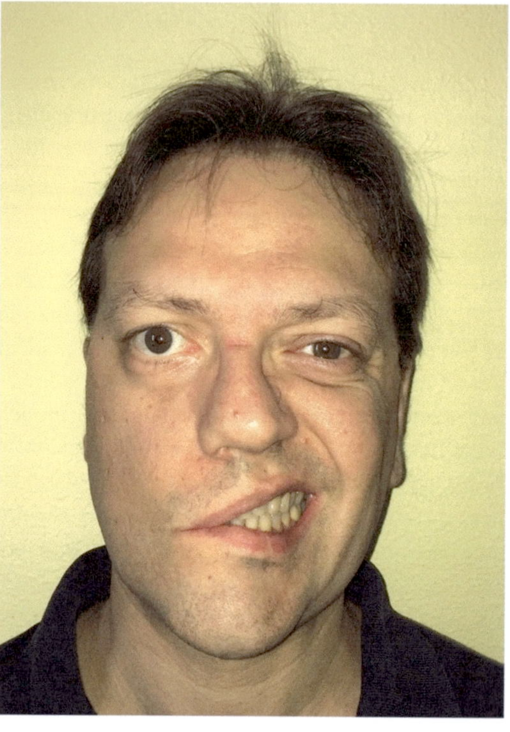

Fig. 14.4 Appearance of the face during smiling prior to triple innervation

lower third of the face without any advisable functional drawback.

According to the two-times concept, distal ends of the two cross-face grafts are accomplished 8–12 months after the main surgery. During the second operation, little deficits might be corrected by ancillary procedures.

Once there was the credo that two different neural sources would have thwarted cerebral adaptation, making it difficult to utilize them. As soon as double innervation has been utilized [34, 35], the opposite has proven to be true, leading to much better results. Triple innervation is the natural evolution of this concept and the number of neural sources could be extended in the future.

If a total parotidectomy has been done without any attempt to reconstruct the facial nerve simultaneously, but mimetic muscle fibrillations are detected at EMG, facial nerve branching

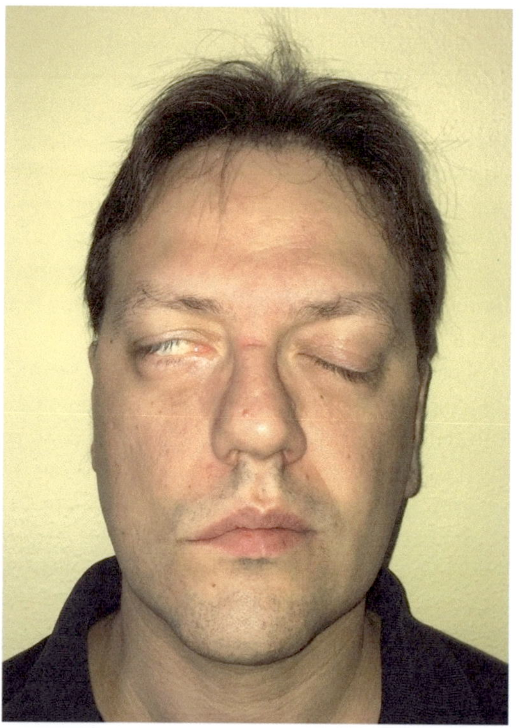

Fig. 14.5 Patient affected by a recent facial paralysis. Appearance of the face and eyelid closure prior to triple innervation

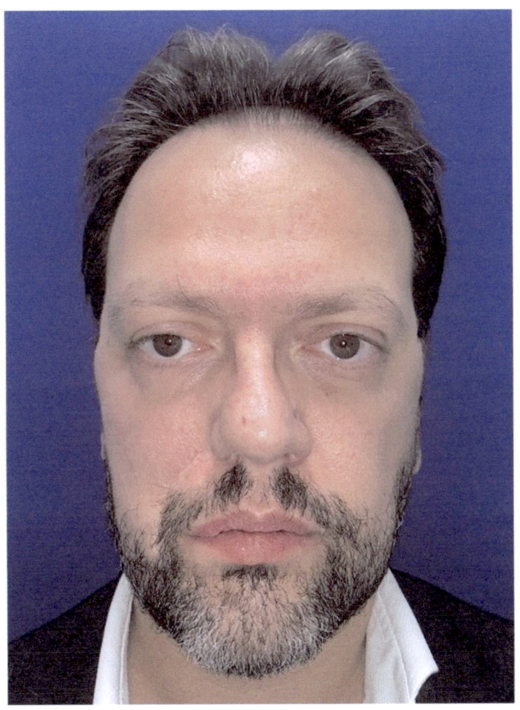

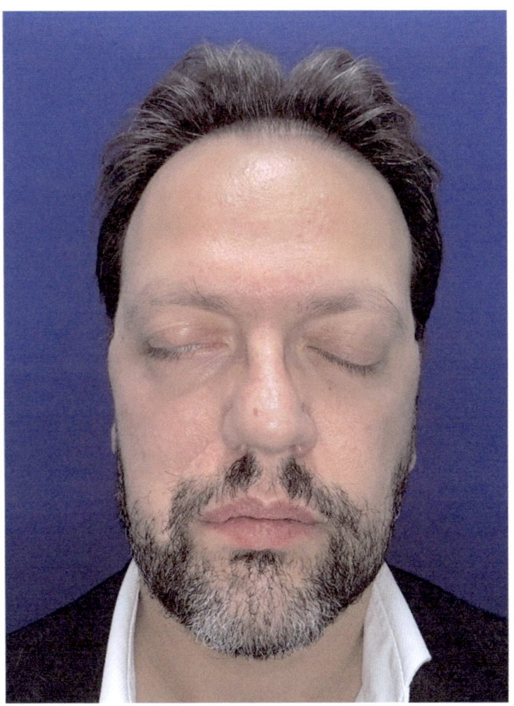

Fig. 14.6 Appearance of the patient at rest, 8 months after surgery

Fig. 14.8 Eyelids closure, 8 months after surgery

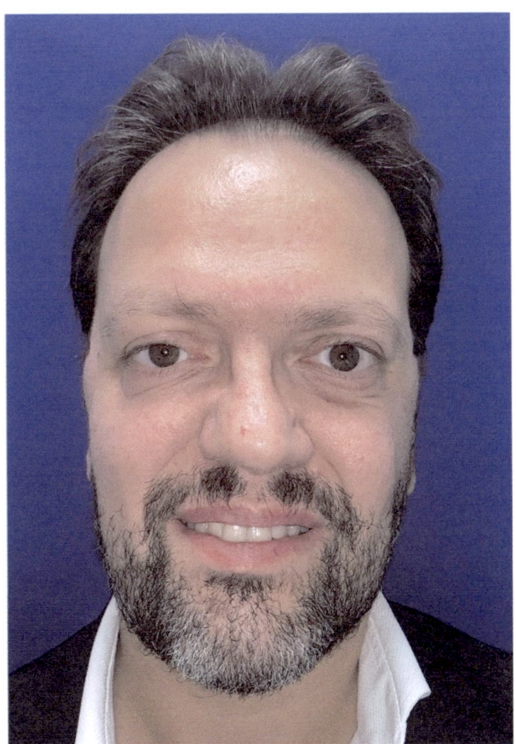

Fig. 14.7 Smiling, 8 months after surgery

reconstruction by a thoracodorsal nerve grafting might be accomplished. At the same time, an early re-opening of the oncologic field might be risky for residual tumor unaware spreading. Moreover, a quick and high-grade fibrosis of muscles and soft tissue could have taken place if postoperative radiotherapy has been delivered to the patient.

In those cases, it might be chosen to obtain a very guaranteed static rehabilitation with a lesser dynamic expectation. The temporalis muscle tendon is identified and rotated medially through the nasolabial sulcus by cutting the coronoid process with a piezoelectric device [36]. A small graft of fascia lata helps distributing better the suspension to all the sulcus. By doing so, the parotid region is left completely untouched. The temporalis muscle, partially devascularized by previous external carotid artery cut and radiotherapy, is left in place without any adjunctive reduction of its vascular flow. The quantity of smiling recovery is less than what is obtainable with thoracodorsal nerve grafting but static symmetry is much guaranteed and oncological safety justifies this technical solution. Corneal protection is obtained by lateral tarsorrhaphy and upper lid lipofilling, described in the following section.

14.3.3.3 Long-Standing Paralysis

After a medium period of 18–24 months, the mimetic musculature is irreversibly changed into fibrotic-fatty tissue and a new neural stimulus would be waisted without any possibility to obtain a visible result [37]. So, facial muscle function has to be substituted, having the realistic goal of focusing on eyelids blinking and smiling as for recent facial paralysis reanimation. Soft tissue ptosis must be addressed at the same time. Before deciding the technique to be proposed to the patient, an accurate anamnesis and a thorough examination of the possible neural sources must be accomplished by EMG. If, for example, the homolateral trigeminus is impaired, a one-time gracilis free-flap may not be proposed because the masseteric nerve is not viable, nor a temporalis muscle flap will produce any movement. If a contralateral neurinoma of the VIII cn is present but does not cause any facial nerve deficit, it is improvident to use the contralateral facial nerve source by a cross-face nerve grafting because it could be impaired in the near future.

Several techniques are devised to replace eyelids closure, missing actually to correct the main functional problem, that is, the lack of eyelid lubrication. That is caused by the loss of blinking, sometimes associated to a reduction of lacrimal gland production because of the damage of its innervation due to facial nerve severing. Blinking takes place 10–19 times a minute [38], and it is the natural way to distribute the lacrimal secretion from the gland to the puncta, protecting the cornea. Spontaneous eyelid closure is seldom utilized to improve the cornea status, mainly to antagonize a situation of great sufferance of it, surely with incomparable lesser frequency than blinking. So, blinking is much more important to be replaced than voluntary eyelids closure and techniques ignoring that, as temporalis flap rotation, fail to correct the main functional problem [39].

Blinking is accomplished by a spontaneous relaxation of the upper lid levator, immediately followed by the contraction of the orbicularis oculi. That process takes few milliseconds. As the first muscle is innervated by the healthy III cn, during facial paralysis only the orbicular oculi contraction is inhibited because depending on the VII cn. The transposition of a platisma graft into the upper lid and its direct neurotization several months after a cross-face grafting procedure has the aim to restore orbicularis oculi function but fails in half of the cases to obtain the goal. That gives reason of its rare use [40].

The most common surgical solution utilized to eyelids closure is the simple procedure of insetting of a plate into the upper lid [41]. This surgical procedure fails to correct blinking because the weight applied, generally 1.4 g, is calculated to let the levator open up the eyelids during vision, allowing at the same time to close the eyelids during voluntary relaxation of the levator muscle. This action takes up to several seconds. In order to guarantee the vision, levator muscle remains full contracted to counteract the weight of the plate, de facto never relaxing spontaneously. By doing that, both muscular actions of blinking are inhibited: levator relaxation by its continuous contraction and orbicularis oculi by facial nerve impairment. The extension of this concept is that a lighter upper lid weight, insufficient to obtain eyelids closure, leads to a lesser contraction of the levator muscle. That allows to increase upper lid lowering during blinking, adding efficiency to it. Gold lid plate has several disadvantages and has been unpleasant esthetically because much visible throughout the skin, in addition to being frequently dislocated and extruded. Most of all, patients often refer discomfort related to the presence of the plate. Utilizing a titanium plate, heavier and consequently smaller, reduces those drawbacks but does not clear them completely.

The best option is to make a 2 ml/1.6 g lipofilling of upper lid: the initial weight decreases much during the first 2 months because of spontaneous partial self-reabsorption. The exact residual weight is impossible to be established, but what is important is that patients refer much comfort related to the procedure and increase of blinking is evident. Fifteen percent of patients still feel discomfort after the first procedure, and a second lipofilling may be repeated easily under local anesthesia. If the quantity of fat injected leads to an unacceptable upper lid ptosis during day-vision, some fat may be taken out under local anesthesia: that is a very rare event.

Lengthening of upper lid levator muscle acts in a similar way to lipofilling, increasing its relaxation action during blinking, but requires a higher surgical skill [42].

Often lids rehabilitation requires correction of lagophthalmos, by a small lateral tarsorrhaphy and sometimes a canthopexy. Several other options may improve the morphological and functional results.

Correction of the lower two-thirds of the face ptosis is fundamental and may be obtained by fascia lata grafting, deep face lifting, and temporalis tendon suspensions [43]. Fascia lata has the big advantage that may be coupled with free-flap surgery, contemporarily increasing static symmetry, and recovering smiling function. Other quicker static techniques carry on several complications: suture threads suspension cut through soft tissues, losing their function in a short period. On the other side, alloplastic strips are easily felt by patients, became often visible throughout the skin, until they get extruded. Finally, reabsorbable threads lose quickly their positive action.

Smiling recovery may be obtained by masticatory muscles transposition and free-flap surgery. The first one is nowadays concentrated into temporalis flap use with several variants. The most common being temporalis lengthening myoplasty in two different variants [44, 45]. The temporalis muscle is innervated by the V cn so, unless it was damaged together with the VII cn, it is available for reanimation surgery. Strongest points of the procedure are a quick and easy operation, without any microsurgical step, which makes it suitable by all reconstructive surgeons. On the contrary, trigeminus innervation, as extensively debated for recent facial reanimation, almost nerve activates because of emotions. The quantity of smiling is often null to little, surely much less than what registered with free-flap transposition. Instead, suspension given to soft tissues by the temporalis tendon is the best among

static remedies. That explains why the visual impression of smiling replacement is much higher than real: a more symmetric start leads to a higher corner of the mouth position at the end of smiling. So, in spite of a little movement, the smile looks lesser asymmetric and the final result is fairly good. An efficient variant of the temporalis flap harvesting with less extensive surgery is by catching the lower tendon through the incision of the nasolabial sulcus, avoiding muscular body exposure. A little graft of fascia lata is necessary to better distribute its insertion to sulcus. Taking account of pros and odds makes this flap a good choice for older people who desire an immediate result, one surgery, with little surgical discomfort.

A more complete result can be obtained using a muscular free-flap. That might be accomplished in one-time surgery or in two operations. Two-step surgery is the most utilized technique: a cross-face nerve graft is anastomized on the healthy semi-face to a branch of the facial nerve for the zygomatic muscles. After 6–12 months, when the Tinel's sign is positive, the muscular free-flap is transposed and its motor nerve anastomized to the distal end of the suralis graft. By utilizing this procedure, the most qualitative neural source is utilized, assuring a very spontaneous smiling. On the contrary, accomplishing two neurorrhaphies and utilizing such a long graft, gives variability to final obtainable contraction of the flap. Most popular muscular free-flaps are latissimus dorsi, gracilis, and pectoralis minor: none of them proving to be better than the other [46, 47].

One of the most utilized one-step procedure is the latissimus dorsi transposition [48, 49]: that flap allows also to make a two-bellies smiling reanimation for those rare cases having a full-dental smile [50]. The advantages are obvious: less hospitalization, reduced psychological effort and shorter recovery time for the patient. On the contrary, the quantity of axons reaching the flap may be reduced because tracing the thoracodorsal nerve up to 15 cm in order to reach the contralateral side of the face for anastomosing requires severing of collateral branches. Incoming axons may be wasted through those branches. Another very common technique is the transposition of a gracilis free-flap innervated by the masseteric nerve. Because of the anatomy of the proper motor nerve of the gracilis without collateral branches and the powerful axonal sprouting of the masseteric nerve, the contraction of the flap is much more consistent [51, 52], although it lacks of emotionality. In order to overcome this problem, mixing the quantitative stimulus of the masseteric with the qualitative stimulus driven by a cross-face nerve graft led to the conception of double innervated gracilis free-flap (Scheme 14.3, Figs. 14.9, 14.10, 14.11, and 14.12) [53, 54]. The procedure may be accomplished in one time, but grafting the suralis nerve 6–12 months prior to the main surgery leads to better percentages of emotional smiling recovery.

Static suspensions must always be added to smiling reanimation surgery [55]. That may be easily accomplished by setting under the free-flap a fascia lata graft, anchoring it cranially to the infraorbital rim and caudally to the same stitches utilized for the free-flap at the nasolabial sulcus.

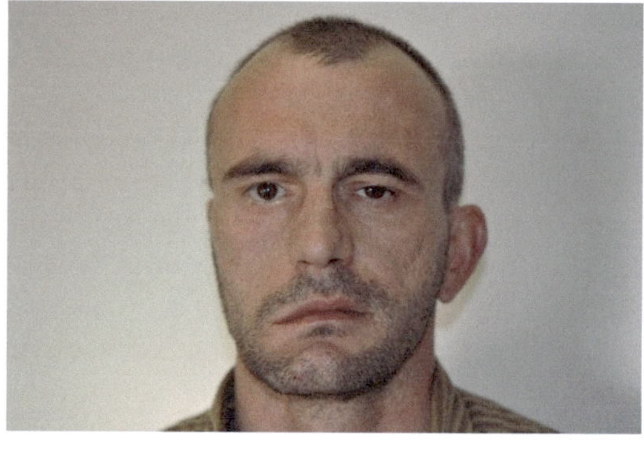

Fig. 14.9 Patient affected by a 5-year-long paralysis. Preoperative appearance of the face at rest

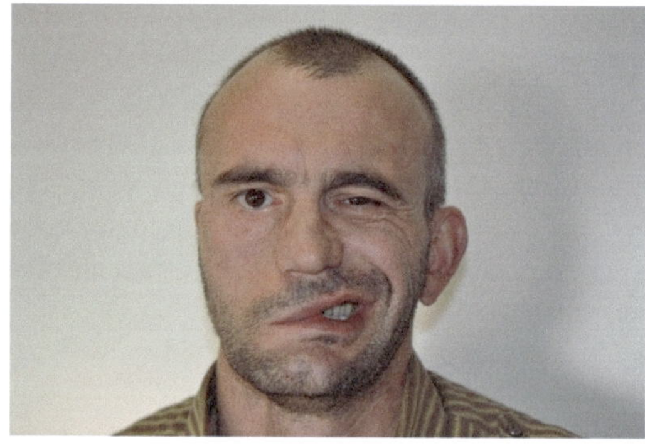

Fig. 14.10 Preoperative appearance of the face of the same patient during smiling

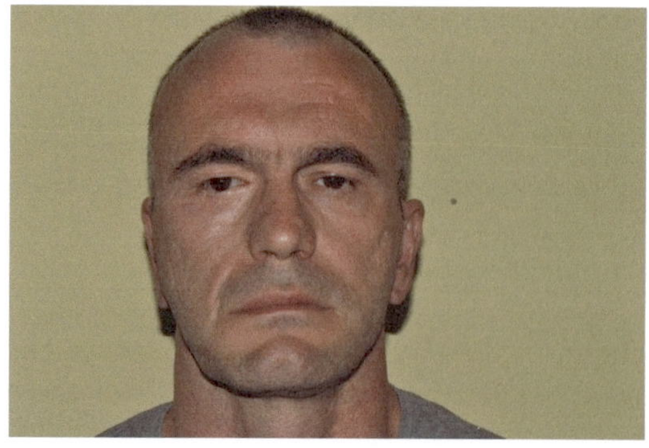

Fig. 14.11 Static symmetry of the face one year after surgery

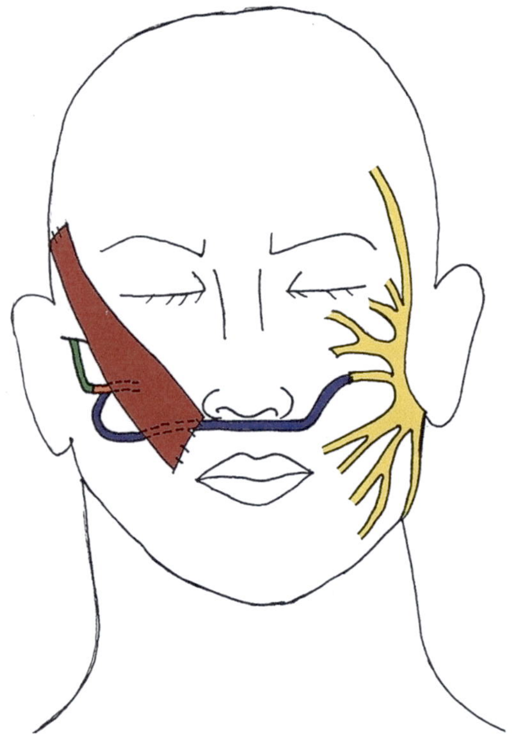

Scheme 14.3 Gracilis free-flap with double innervation. The power of contraction is provided by the masseteric nerve (green), while smiling according to emotions depends on the contralateral facial nerve stimulus, via a cross-face nerve graft (blue)

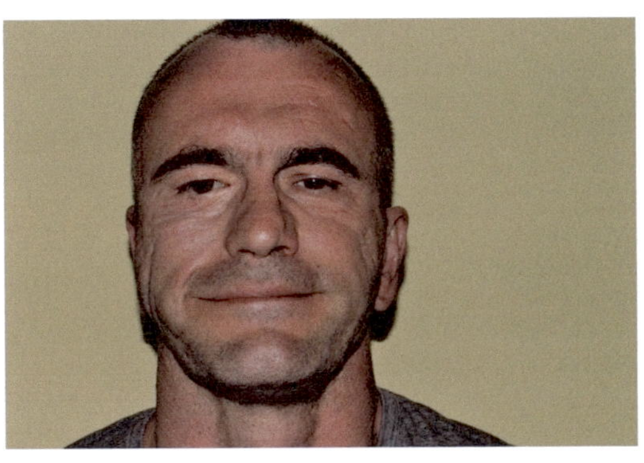

Fig. 14.12 Symmetric smile one year after surgery

Other reanimation targets as eyebrows elevation or lower lip movements are very difficult to be obtained and realistic goals are symmetrization of static and camouflage of the deficient movement. The front paralysis may be addressed by suspending the eyebrows in several ways and reducing contralateral movement by botulinum toxin injection.

Atrophy of the lower lip may be hidden by lipofilling, but it is impossible to reproduce its complex movement during talking with current techniques, the best being contralateral lower lip depressor treatment by botulinum toxin [56]. By doing that, asymmetry of the lower lip during talking and smiling is hidden. The contralateral marginalis mandibulae branch may be severed under local anaesthesia to obtain a long-term similar result.

Several other secondary surgeries help much to improve results, the main ones being nasalabial sulcus revision, free-flap debunking, and repositioning [57].

Bilateral facial palsy is fortunately rare, mainly related to extended brain disease or neurosurgery complications. Another etiology relates to Moebius syndrome, a particular malformation including several cranial nerves impairments. In those cases, the donor nerves to reanimate the face are reduced, and the contralateral facial nerve is not available. That leads necessarily to lower facial reanimation expectation, with less natural appearance of the movements. Eyelid reanimation follows the path of monolateral facial palsy, while smiling surgery may choose among one of the two: bilateral temporalis flap

rotation or double gracilis free-flap transplantation [58]. Both solutions have pros and odds, the microsurgical option being the most utilized worldwide.

14.4 Paresis - Synkinesis - Mimetic Muscle Contracture

Facial paresis differs from paralysis because of the presence of a reduced movement. This particular clinical condition may be congenital or may be caused by an incomplete recovery from various types of facial paralysis (it accounts for 30% of Bell's palsy cases) [59, 60]. Flaccid paresis (FP) differ from non-flaccid ones (NFP) because the last ones are accompanied by hypertone/contracture of mimetic muscles at rest because of an augmented facial nerve stimulus. Synkinetic movements are often present in those cases, due to an erroneous path of reinnervation of mimetic muscles. Substantially some of the axons directed toward a specific muscle compartment grow into a different facial nerve branch from the original one. The result is an involuntary unpleasant synkinetic movement during the voluntary one: for example, eyelids closure while smiling and vice versa.

Treatment of FP requires often a static correction by fascia lata suspension plus an increased neural stimulus: that might be provided by adding end-to-side the masseteric nerve axons with or without contralateral facial nerve ones via a cross-face nerve graft. If the paresis is high graded, free-flap surgery might be more indicated.

Possible treatments of NFP are physiotherapy, botulinum toxin injections, and microsurgery. Physiotherapy is efficient in low-severity cases, reducing contractions by specific massages (but the effect is temporary) and teaching how to lower the evidence of synkinesis by avoiding wide movements. The same has to be done on the healthy side to symmetrize facial mimicry. Specific exercise have the aim to increase muscle force, trying to camouflage the paresis; that is the less efficient part of the treatment.

Botulinum toxin injections are particularly efficient to reduce hypertone at rest. Their use is particularly delicate because an excessive dosage might cause a temporary paralysis, while an under-dosage does not reach the desired effect. EMG and ecographic guidance helps the precision of treatment. Little results may be reached also on synkinesis, but it must be remembered that the toxin inhibits the neuromuscular junction. So, in order to reduce synkinesis, the toxin also reduces the desired movement. As an example, synkinetic smiling during eyelids closure might be reduced at the price of lowering it also during a correct stimulus. Surgical proposal to reduce synkinesis is typically related to selective neurectomies and myectomies [61, 62]. Those are particularly efficient to increase smiling when applied to block the depressor angulis oris (DAO) and upper platisma activation during smiling. Because of those two muscle contraction counteracts of the zygomatic muscle complex, their inhibition allows to reach a much more complete smile.

If paresis, synkinesis, and hypertone at rest are contemporarily present, the pathological neural stimulus must be substituted by a healthy mix of quantitative and qualitative stimuli (Fig. 14.3) [63]. The masseteric nerve is anastomized end-to-end to the facial nerve branch for the paretic musculature in order to provide the correct muscle tone at rest together with a powerful movement when required. A cross-face sural nerve graft is added by an end-to-side neurorrhaphy (an end-to-end is accomplished on the healthy side to guarantee a full axonal ingrowth) to obtain a natural stimulus. By doing so, the synkinetic movement is elided because of a new axonal pathway. As an example, a typical eyelid closure-smiling synkinesis might be considered: when the stimulus is given to the orbicularis oculi, contemporary smiling does not take place anymore because the axons for the zygomatic muscles do not belong to the pathological facial nerve but to the masseteric nerve and the cross-face nerve graft. Moreover, muscles contracture is solved because of the healty masseteric nerve input, wich also leads to powerful movement.

Bibliography

1. House JW, Brackmann DE. Facial nerve grading system. Otolaryngol Head Neck Surg. 1985;93:146–7.

2. Ross BG, Fradet G, Nedzelski JM. Development of a sensitive clinical facial grading system. Otolaryngol Head Neck Surg. 1996;114:380–6.
3. Sforza C, Ulaj E, Gibelli DM, Allevi F, Pucciarelli V, Tarabbia F, Ciprandi D, Dell'Aversana Orabona G, Dolci C, Biglioli F. Three-dimensional superimposition for patients with facial palsy: an innovative method for assessing the success of facial reanimation procedures. Br J Oral Maxillofac Surg. 2018;56(1):3–7.
4. Banks CA, Bhama PK, Park J, Hadlock CR, Hadlock TA. Clinician-graded electronic facial paralysis assessment: the eFACE. Plast Reconstr Surg. 2015;136(2):223e–30e.
5. Banks CA, Jowett N, Azizzadeh B, Beurskens C, Bhama P, Borschel G, Coombs C, Coulson S, Croxon G, Diels J, Fattah A, Frey M, Gavilan J, Henstrom D, Hohman M, Kim J, Marres H, Redett R, Snyder-Warwick A, Hadlock T. Worldwide testing of the eFACE Facial Nerve Clinician-Graded Scale. Plast Reconstr Surg. 2017;139(2):491e–8e.
6. Biglioli F, Colombo V, Tarabbia F, Autelitano L, Rabbiosi D, Colletti G, Giovanditto F, Battista V, Frigerio A. Recovery of emotional smiling function in free-flap facial reanimation. J Oral Maxillofac Surg. 2012;70(10):2413–8.
7. Dalla Toffola E, Tinelli C, Lozza A, Bejor M, Pavese C, Degli Agosti I, Petrucci L. Choosing the best rehabilitation treatment for Bell's palsy. Eur J Phys Rehabil Med. 2012;48(4):635–42.
8. Pavese C, Cecini M, Lozza A, Biglioli F, Lisi C, Bejor M, Dalla TE. Rehabilitation and functional recovery after masseteric-facial nerve anastomosis. Eur J Phys Rehabil Med. 2016;52(3):379–88.
9. Cooper L, Lui M, Nduka C. Botulinum toxin treatment for facial palsy: a systematic review. J Plast Reconstr Aesthet Surg. 2017;70(6):833–41.
10. Vaughan ED, Richardson D. Facial nerve reconstruction following ablative parotid surgery. Br J Oral Maxillofac Surg. 1993;31:274–80.
11. Reddy PG, Arden RL, Mathog RH. Facial nerve rehabilitation after radical parotidectomy. Laryngoscope. 1999;109(6):894–9.
12. Meyer RA. Nerve harvesting procedures. Atlas Oral Maxillofac Surg Clin North Am. 2001;9(2):77e91.
13. Humphrey CD, Kriet JD. Nerve repair and cable grafting for facial paralysis. Facial Plast Surg. 2008;24(2):170–6.
14. Hyodo I, Ozawa T, Hasegawa Y, Ogawa T, Terada A, Torii S. Management of a total parotidectomy defect with a gastrocnemius muscle transfer and vascularized sural nerve grafting. Ann Plast Surg. 2007;58(6):677–82.
15. Biglioli F, Colombo V, Rabbiosi D, Colletti G, Frigerio A. Facial nerve reconstruction using a thoracodorsal nerve graft after radical parotidectomy. Plast Reconstr Surg. 2012;129(5):852e–3e.
16. Brown PD, Eshleman JS, Foote RL, Strome SE. An analysis of facial nerve function in irradiated and unirradiated facial nerve grafts. Int J Radiat Oncol Biol Phys. 2000;48(3):737–43.

17. Haller JR, Shelton C. Medial antebrachial cutaneous nerve: a new donor graft for repair of facial nerve defects at the skull base. Laryngoscope. 1997;107(8):1048–52.
18. Schultes G, Gaggl A, Kärcher H. Reconstruction of accessory nerve defects with vascularized long thoracic vs. non-vascularized thoracodorsal nerve. J Reconstr Microsurg. 1999;15(4):265–70.
19. Iida T, Nakagawa M, Asano T, Fukushima C, Tachi K. Free vascularized lateral femoral cutaneous nerve graft with anterolateral thigh flap for reconstruction of facial nerve defects. J Reconstr Microsurg. 2006;22(5):343–8.
20. Takushima A, Harii K, Asato H, Ueda K, Yamada A. Neurovascular free-muscle transfer for the treatment of established facial paralysis following ablative surgery in the parotid region. Plast Reconstr Surg. 2004;113(6):1563–72.
21. Lu L, Ding Y, Lin Y, Xu Z, Li Z, Qu J, et al. Greater auricular nerve graft for repair of facial nerve defects. J Clin Otorhinolaryngol Head Neck Surg. 2010;24(7):293–7.
22. Theeuwes HP, Gosselink MP, Bruynzeel H, Kleinrensink GJ, Walbeehm ET. Anatomical study of the length of the neural pedicle after the bifurcation of the thoracodorsal nerve: implications for innervated free partial latissimus dorsi flaps. Plast Reconstr Surg. 2011;127(1):210–4.
23. Biglioli F, Tarabbia F, Allevi F, Colombo V, Giovanditto F, Latiff M, Lozza A, Previtera A, Cupello S, Rabbiosi D. Immediate facial reanimation in oncological parotid surgery with neurorrhaphy of the masseteric-thoracodorsal-facial nerve branch. Br J Oral Maxillofac Surg. 2016;54(5):520–5.
24. Biglioli F, Pedrazzoli M, Rabbiosi D, Colletti G, Colombo V, Frigerio A, Autelitano L. Reconstruction of complex defects of the parotid region using a lateral thoracic wall donor site. J Craniomaxillofac Surg. 2013;41(3):265–9.
25. Fairbanks GA, Hallock GG. Facial reconstruction using a combined flap of the subscapular axis simultaneously including separate medial and lateral scapular vascularized bone grafts. Ann Plast Surg. 2002;49(1):104–8.
26. Biglioli F. Facial reanimations: part I--recent paralyses. Br J Oral Maxillofac Surg. 2015;53(10):901–6.
27. Terzis JK, Karypidis D. Therapeutic strategies in post-facial paralysis synkinesis in adult patients. Plast Reconstr Surg. 2012;129(6):925e–39e.
28. Hembd A, Nagarkar PA, Saba S, Wan D, Kutz JW, Isaacson B, Gupta S, White CL III, Rohrich RJ, Rozen SM. Facial nerve axonal analysis and anatomical localization in donor nerve: optimizing axonal load for cross-facial nerve grafting in facial reanimation. Plast Reconstr Surg. 2017;139(1):177–83.
29. Biglioli F, Frigerio A, Colombo V, Colletti G, Rabbiosi D, Mortini P, Dalla Toffola E, Lozza A, Brusati R. Masseteric-facial nerve anastomosis for early facial reanimation. J Craniomaxillofac Surg. 2012;40(2):149–55.
30. Sforza C, Tarabbia F, Mapelli A, Colombo V, Sidequersky FV, Rabbiosi D, Annoni I, Biglioli F. Facial reanimation with masseteric to facial nerve transfer: a three-dimensional longitudinal quantitative evaluation. J Plast Reconstr Aesthet Surg. 2014;67(10):1378–86.
31. Biglioli F, Allevi F, Rabbiosi D, Cupello S, Battista VMA, Saibene AM, Colletti G. Triple innervation for re-animation of recent facial paralysis. J Craniomaxillofac Surg. 2018;46(5):851–7.
32. Gibelli D, Tarabbia F, Restelli S, Allevi F, Dolci C, Dell'Aversana Orabona G, Cappella A, Codari M, Sforza C, Biglioli F. Three-dimensional assessment of restored smiling mobility after reanimation of unilateral facial palsy by triple innervation technique. Int J Oral Maxillofac Surg. 2020;49:536.
33. Sforza C, Tarabbia F, Mapelli A, Colombo V, Sidequersky FV, Rabbiosi D, Annoni I, Biglioli F. Facial reanimation with masseteric to facial nerve transfer: a three-dimensional longitudinal quantitative evaluation. J Plast Reconstr Aesthet Surg. 2014;67(10):1378–86.
34. Watanabe Y, Akizuki T, Ozawa T, Yoshimura K, Agawa K, Ota T. Dual innervation method using one-stage reconstruction with free latissimus dorsi muscle transfer for re-animation of established facial paralysis: simultaneous reinnervation of the ipsilateral masseter motor nerve and the contralateral facial nerve to improve the quality of smile and emotional facial expressions. J Plast Reconstr Aesthet Surg. 2009;62(12):1589–97.
35. Tomita K, Hosokawa K, Yano K. Reanimation of reversible facial paralysis by the double innervation technique using an intraneural-dissected sural nerve graft. J Plast Reconstr Aesthet Surg. 2010;63:e535–9.
36. Boahene KD. Principles and biomechanics of muscle tendon unit transfer: application in temporalis muscle tendon transposition for smile improvement in facial paralysis. Laryngoscope. 2013;123(2):350–5.
37. Biglioli F. Facial reanimations: part II--long-standing paralyses. Br J Oral Maxillofac Surg. 2015;53(10):907–12.
38. Sforza C, Rango M, Galante D, Bresolin N, Ferrario VF. Spontaneous blinking in healthy persons: an opto-electronic study of eyelid motion. Ophthalmic Physiol Opt. 2008;28(4):345–53.
39. Gillies HD, Millard DR. The principles and art of plastic surgery. Boston: Little, Brown; 1957. p. 21.
40. Biglioli F, Zago M, Allevi F, Ciprandi D, Dell'Aversana Orabona G, Pucciarelli V, Rabbiosi D, Pacifici I, Tarabbia F, Sforza C. Reanimation of the paralyzed lids by cross-face nerve graft and platysma transfer. J Craniomaxillofac Surg. 2018;46(3):521–6.
41. May M. Gold weight and wirespring implants as alternatives to tarsorrhaphy. Arch Otolaryngol Head Neck Surg. 1987;113:656–60.
42. Tessier P, delbet JP, Pastoriza J, et al. Paralized eyelids. Ann Chir Plast. 1969;14:215–23.
43. Biglioli F, Frigerio A, Autelitano L, Colletti G, Rabbiosi D, Brusati R. Deep-planes lift associ-

ated with free flap surgery for facial reanimation. J Craniomaxillofac Surg. 2011;39(7):475–81.

44. Labbé D. Lengthening of temporalis myoplasty and reanimation of lips. Ann Chir Plast Esthet. 1997;42(1):44–7.

45. Labbé D. Lengthening of temporalis myoplasty V.2. and lip reanimation. Ann Chir Plast Esthet. 2009;54(6):571–6.

46. Vedung S, Hakelius L, Stålberg E. Cross-face nerve grafting followed by free muscle transplantation in young patients with long-standing facial paralysis. Reanimation of the cheek and the angle of the mouth. Scand J Plast Reconstr Surg. 1984;18(2):201–8.

47. Frey M, Michaelidou M, Tzou CH, Hold A, Pona I, Placheta E. Proven and innovative operative techniques for reanimation of the paralyzed face. Handchir Mikrochir Plast Chir. 2010;42(2):81–9.

48. Harii K, Asato H, Yoshimura K, Sugawara Y, Nakatsuka T, Ueda K. One-stage transfer of the latissimus dorsi muscle for reanimation of a paralyzed face: a new alternative. Plast Reconstr Surg. 1998;102(4):941–51.

49. Biglioli F, Frigerio A, Rabbiosi D, Brusati R. Single-stage facial reanimation in the surgical treatment of unilateral established facial paralysis. Plast Reconstr Surg. 2009;124(1):124–33.

50. Allevi F, Motta G, Colombo V, Biglioli F. Double-bellied latissimus dorsi free flap to correct full dental smile palsy. BMJ Case Rep. 2015;2015.

51. Harii K, Ohmori K, Torii S. Free gracilis muscle transplantation with microneurovascular anastomoses for the treatment of facial paralysis. Plast Reconstr Surg. 1976;57:133.

52. Manktelow RT, Zuker RM. Muscle transplantation by fascicular territory. Plast Reconstr Surg. 1984;73:751.

53. Biglioli F, Colombo V, Tarabbia F, Pedrazzoli M, Battista V, Giovanditto F, Dalla Toffola E, Lozza A, Frigerio A. Double innervation in free-flap surgery for long-standing facial paralysis. J Plast Reconstr Aesthet Surg. 2012;65(10):1343–9.

54. Sforza C, Frigerio A, Mapelli A, Tarabbia F, Annoni I, Colombo V, Latiff M, Pimenta Ferreira CL, Rabbiosi D, Sidequersky FV, Zago M, Biglioli F. Double-powered free gracilis muscle transfer for smile reanimation: a longitudinal optoelectronic study. J Plast Reconstr Aesthet Surg. 2015;68(7):930–9.

55. Kiefer J, Braig D, Thiele JR, Bannasch H, Stark GB, Eisenhardt SU. Comparison of symmetry after smile reconstruction for flaccid facial paralysis with combined fascia lata grafts and functional gracilis transfer for static suspension or gracilis transfer alone. Microsurgery. 2018;38(6):634–42.

56. Biglioli F, Allevi F, Battista VM, Colombo V, Pedrazzoli M, Rabbiosi D. Lipofilling of the atrophied lip in facial palsy patients. Minerva Stomatol. 2014;63(3):69–75.

57. Takushima A, Harii K, Asato H, Momosawa A. Revisional operations improve results of neurovascular free muscle transfer for treatment of facial paralysis. Plast Reconstr Surg. 2005;116(2):371–80.

58. Zuker RM, Goldberg CS, Manktelow RT. Facial animation in children with Möbius syndrome after segmental gracilis muscle transplant. Plast Reconstr Surg. 2000;106(1):1–8.

59. Terzis JK, Anesti K. Developmental facial paralysis: a review. J Plast Reconstr Aesthet Surg. 2011;64(10):1318–33.

60. Biglioli F, Kutanovaite O, Rabbiosi D, Colletti G, Mohammed MAS, Saibene AM, Cupello S, Privitera A, Battista VMA, Lozza A, Allevi F. Surgical treatment of synkinesis between smiling and eyelid closure. J Craniomaxillofac Surg. 2017;45(12):1996–2001.

61. Azizzadeh B, Irvine LE, Diels J, Slattery WH, Massry GG, Larian B, Riedler KL, Peng GL. Modified selective neurectomy for the treatment of post-facial paralysis synkinesis. Plast Reconstr Surg. 2019;143(5):1483–96.

62. Labbé D, Bénichou L, Iodice A, Giot JP. Depressor anguli oris sign (DAO) in facial paresis. How to search it and release the smile (technical note). Ann Chir Plast Esthet. 2012;57(3):281–5.

63. Biglioli F, Soliman M, El-Shazly M, Saadeldeen W, Abda EA, Allevi F, Rabbiosi D, Tarabbia F, Lozza A, Cupello S, Privitera A, Dell'Aversana Orabona G, Califano L. Use of the masseteric nerve to treat segmental midface paresis. Br J Oral Maxillofac Surg. 2018;56(8):719–26.

Marcus Couey, Ashish Patel, and R. Bryan Bell

15.1 Introduction

Robotic-assisted surgery (RAS) became a reality in 1985, when the PUMA 560 robotic arm was first used for precision needle placement for neurosurgical biopsies. Around that time, under a Small Business Innovation Research contract from the National Aeronautics and Space Administration (NASA), Computer Motion, Inc. began developing the AESOP endoscope robotic arm, which was cleared for use by the Food and Drug Administration (FDA) in 1994. The AESOP platform was then taken a step further by adding two robotic arms capable of carrying out surgical procedures under the control of a surgeon operator. This system, known as the ZEUS Robotic Surgical System, received FDA approval in 2001 [1].

Concurrent to the development of the ZEUS system, Intuitive Surgical, Inc. was developing a competing robotic technology. Early systems were named Lenny (short for Leonardo) and Mona, the latter being used in the first robotic-assisted general surgical procedure, a cholecystectomy in 1997. Intuitive named Mona's successor da Vinci, and this more-capable robotic system was granted FDA approval for general

surgery procedures in 2000 [2]. Since then, the da Vinci has been embraced by numerous surgical specialties, including urology, gynecologic oncology, general surgery, cardiothoracic surgery and head and neck surgery. Since its approval in 2009 for resection of T1 and T2 oropharyngeal tumors, use of da Vinci robotic systems for transoral robotic surgery (TORS) was rapidly adopted throughout Head and Neck Surgery programs in the USA [3].

15.2 Advantages of Robotic Surgery

Robotic surgery offers a number of technical advantages over conventional surgery. Possibly the most unique benefit of RAS over other methods is high-definition three-dimensional optics that provide outstanding clarity and magnification. Another important advantage is the reduction of physiologic hand tremor. The ability to preserve depth perception with 3D optics, as with the da Vinci system, offers a substantial benefit over endoscopic techniques. The benefit of high-definition visualization, combined with the reduction of hand tremor, may be particularly advantageous for microsurgical procedures.

As with endoscopic techniques, RAS allows for minimally invasive surgical approaches. However, the dexterity of robotic instrumentation, such as the da Vinci EndoWrist® instruments

M. Couey · A. Patel · R. B. Bell (✉)
Head and Neck Cancer Program, Providence Cancer
Institute, Portland, OR, USA
e-mail: Marcus.Couey@providence.org;
Ashish.Patel@providence.org;
Richard.Bell@providence.org

© Springer Nature Switzerland AG 2021
J. Acero (ed.), *Innovations and New Developments in Craniomaxillofacial Reconstruction*,
https://doi.org/10.1007/978-3-030-74322-2_15

which provides 7 degrees of freedom (the same as the human wrist) and 90° of articulation, allows for movements that are not possible with conventional endoscopic surgery. This versatility of movement has facilitated minimally invasive approaches to common head and neck procedures such as thyroidectomy, parathyroidectomy, and sleep apnea surgery [4]. Further, robotic instrumentation is capable of and is particularly appealing from a reconstructive surgery perspective.

15.3 Limitations of Robotic Surgery

A commonly cited disadvantage of robotic surgery is the upfront costs of the robotic system and maintenance, as well as the cost per case. The impact of this may be offset in instances where improved outcomes or safety can be demonstrated. Further, in the case of TORS with or without flap reconstruction, there is evidence that RAS may reduce costs compared with traditional open surgery, and even compared with definitive chemoradiation in select cases [5–7].

Another limitation of some robotic systems is the lack of haptic feedback. This may be especially relevant to microsurgery, where excess forces could cause vessel tearing or breakage of microsuture. While this has been cited as a drawback to RAS, several groups have argued that visual feedback can compensate for lack of haptic feedback and that visual feedback is in fact more important than tactile feedback in traditional microsurgery [8]. Nonetheless, robotic systems can generate excessive forces and the lack of tactile feedback can lead to bending of needles, particularly when handled by two robotic arms at the same time [9]. At least four new robotic systems have actually incorporated haptic feedback in various forms, including the Flex (Medrobotics Inc., Raynham, MA), Senhance Surgical Robotic System (TransEnterix, Morrisville, NC), Versius Robotic System (Cambridge Medical Robotics, CMR Surgical, Cambridge, UK), and the Yomi dental implant robot (Neocis, Miami, FL) [10, 11].

Other potential disadvantages include the steep learning curve and interruptions in work flow, including the additional time required for robotic setup and converting between RAS and conventional surgery at different points in the procedure [12].

15.4 Applications of Robotic-Assisted Surgery in Head and Neck Reconstruction

15.4.1 Oropharyngeal Reconstruction

Traditionally, surgical access to oropharyngeal cancers required highly invasive approaches such as a lip split with mandibulotomy or transcervical pharyngotomy. While these approaches carry substantial morbidity [13, 14], reconstruction of the resultant defect is fairly straightforward, given the wide exposure that is obtained [15]. Transoral resection offers an alternative approach that is substantially less invasive; however, access to the oropharynx is limited with conventional instrumentation. RAS has largely solved the problem of transoral surgical access to the oropharynx. While TORS utilization has expanded rapidly in the USA [3], adoption in Europe has been relatively slow, likely due to widespread and decade-long history of transoral laser microsurgery for oropharyngeal and laryngeal cancers in the region [16]. However, as advances in technology that allow for deeper, more versatile robotic access such as the da Vinci SP (Intuitive Surgical Inc., Sunnyvale, CA; Fig. 15.1) and Flex (Medrobotics Inc., Raynham, MA; Fig. 15.2) become available, the shift toward RAS in head and neck surgery has potential for further expansion. Both of these systems employ a single port mechanism with a drivable robotic camera, eliminating the need for straight-line transoral access.

For oropharyngeal cancer cases requiring reconstruction after TORS, robotic instrumentation affords the same advantages concerning access, visualization, and dexterity as it does for the oncologic resection, which has particular utility for regional or free flap inset.

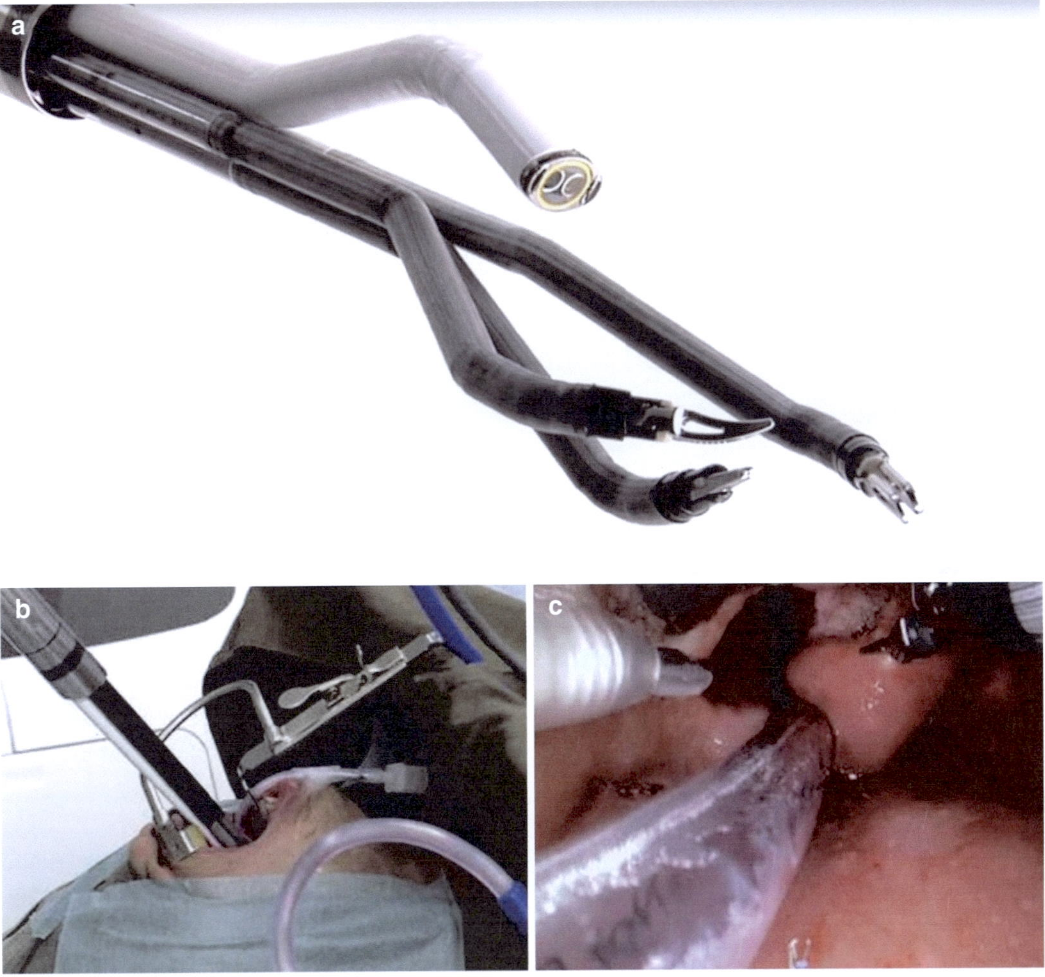

Fig. 15.1 (**a**) da Vinci SP system with three arms and fully wristed camera deployed. *Courtesy of Intuitive Surgical.* (**b, c**) SP system in use for transoral robotic surgery [17]

- Indications

  de Almeida et al. proposed an algorithm to determine which defects require reconstruction after TORS [18]. They suggested that defects lacking adverse features such as exposed carotid artery, pharyngocervical fistula, or a >50% soft palate defect could be left to heal by secondary intention or managed with primary closure or local flaps. For defects with any of these adverse features, they recommended reconstruction with regional or free flaps. In our institution, post-TORS defects without these adverse features are generally managed with secondary healing; however, RAS has proven useful for flap inset in cases requiring vascular coverage or closure of pharyngocervical fistula. Reconstruction of soft palate defects involving more than 50% of the antero-posterior dimension are best treated with robot-assisted flap reconstruction to prevent nasal emission speech and nasal regurgitation of food.

Use of RAS for immediate reconstruction after TORS oropharyngectomy seems a natural application of the technology, as in this scenario the robot, instrumentation and support staff are already present in the OR for the ablative procedure. Numerous case series have demonstrated the feasibility of robot-assisted flap inset in the oropharynx and

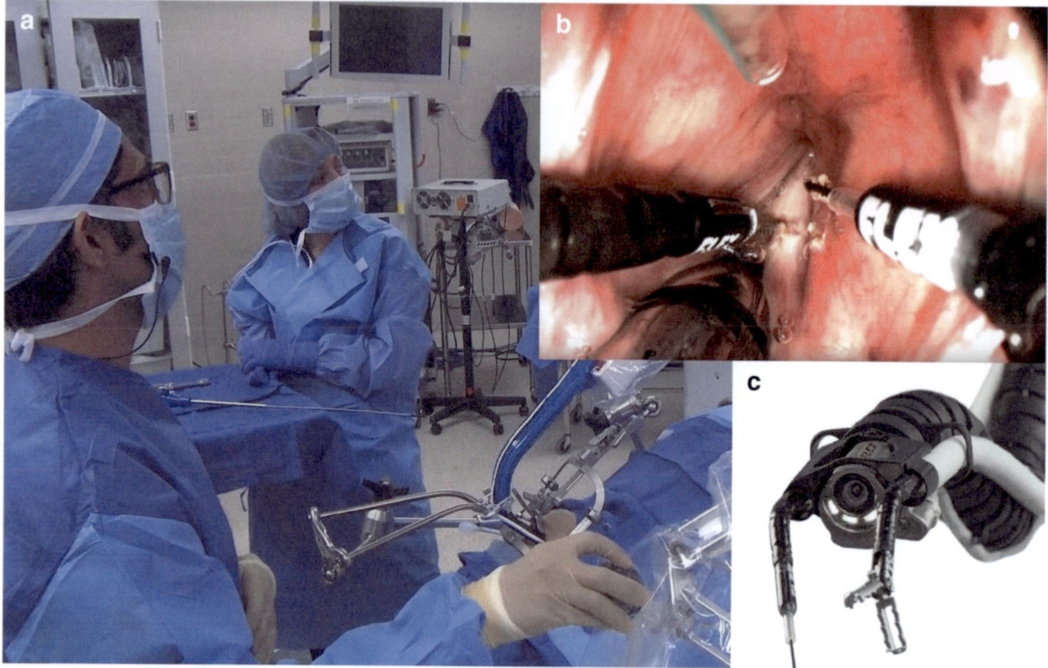

Fig. 15.2 (**a**) Surgeon positioning the Flex robotic system for transoral robotic surgery. (**b**) Flex system in use for vocal cord resection. (**c**) Flex robotic system with central camera and two instrument arms displayed. *Courtesy of Medrobotics Corporation*

hypopharynx [19, 20]. Additionally, several authors have described RAS for raising local and regional flaps including superior constrictor musculomucosal flaps and facial artery musculomucosal flaps [21, 22].

– Technique: Flap Inset

In some cases, particularly when there is a pharyngocervical communication post-TORS and concomitant neck dissection, there may be access for inserting a flap through the pharyngeal defect distally and through a standard oral cavity approach proximally. However, many cases may benefit from use of the surgical robot. A particular example is for coverage of the carotid artery. In this case, a pharyngotomy is still required for passage of the vascular pedicle, but this opening can be minimized by robotic suturing from within the pharynx, which may reduce the risk of leakage of pharyngeal contents. Transcervical inset of a flap to close a small pharyngotomy or fistula oftentimes requires expanding the defect for sufficient access. Creating a watertight suture line can be difficult at the level of

the lingual gutter or superior hypopharynx as these areas are difficult to visualize via standard transcervical or transoral approaches.

The setup for RAS flap inset is the same as for TORS resection (Fig. 15.3). Using a Feyh-Kastenbauer, Dingman, or Crowe–Davis retractor, the robot is positioned at a 45° angle toward the head of the patient. Two needle driver instruments are loaded onto the robot, and a 0 or 30° scope is loaded, depending on the angle of view necessary. The operator then uses the robotic arms to suture the flap to the oropharyngeal defect, and the assistant can cut sutures when appropriate under direct visualization. It is important to properly orient the flap and pass the pedicle into the neck prior to docking the robot. Once engaged, the field of view is magnified, and re-positioning the entire flap may be challenging.

– Functional Outcomes

There are currently no data we are aware of that compare outcomes of robot-assisted free flap reconstruction with conventional free flap reconstruction, and such a comparison would

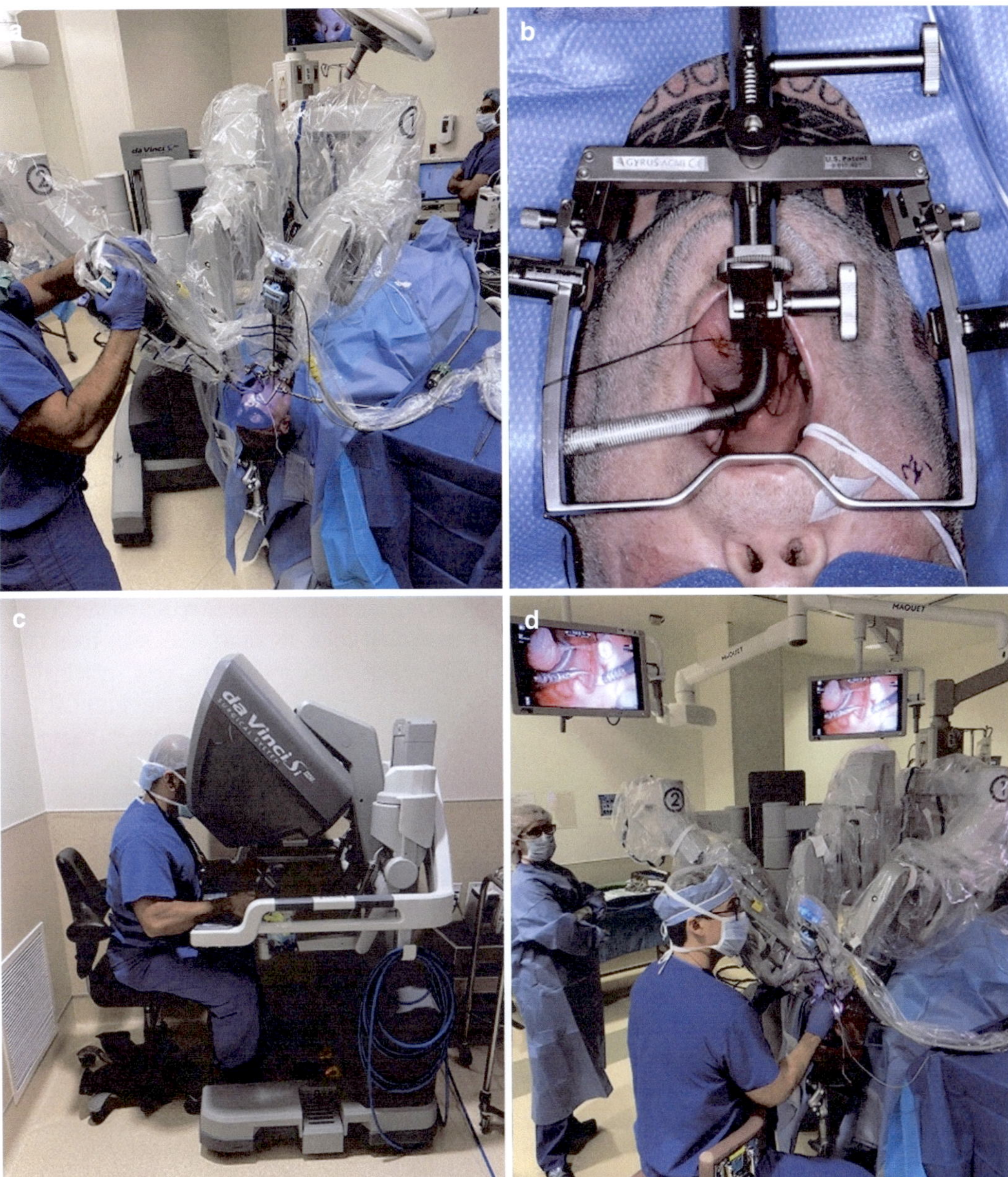

Fig. 15.3 (**a**) Positioning the robotic arms of the da Vinci Si system. (**b**) FK-WO retractor in position for view of the oropharynx. (**c**) Surgeon console in use. (**d**) Assistant at the head retracting and suctioning as needed

be unlikely to show objective differences in outcomes as these are simply differences in instrumentation to perform the same procedure. However, outcome data for free flap reconstruction after TORS, with or without robotic-assisted inset, is available, as are some comparisons with conventional mandibulotomy and free flap reconstruction.

A retrospective study by Al-khudari et al. reported the rate of G-tube dependence in patients who underwent TORS oropharyngectomy. Nine of their patients underwent robot-assisted free flap reconstruction owing to large defect size or need for great vessel coverage. Six (80%) of these patients required a G-tube, and four (44%) remained G-tube-dependent at

1 year. There was no comparator arm of flap reconstruction of conventional mandibulotomy or lateral pharyngotomy approaches; however, other reports of open flap reconstruction of oropharyngeal defects have shown long-term G-tube dependence rates of 9–65% [15, 23–25].

One group ostensibly reported superior swallowing and speech outcomes for robot-assisted flap inset vs. a standard technique in patients receiving radial forearm free flaps for oropharyngeal reconstruction [26]. However, the "conventional surgery" comparison group underwent lip split and mandibulotomy, which oddly seemed to be for reconstructive access rather than ablation, and this represents a tremendous confounder to their analysis. Further, only one patient in each arm actually had a tumor originating in the oropharynx; all other patients had oral cavity primaries, which in our practice do not require lip split or mandibulotomy and are reconstructed using conventional free flap inset.

Biron et al. performed a case–control study of radial forearm free flap reconstruction following either TORS or open mandibulotomy approach for oropharyngeal cancer [5]. They found significantly decreased hospital stay and decreased estimated total cost in the TORS group, and no significant difference in operating time. There were fewer adverse events overall in the TORS group, though the study was not powered to compare rates with those of open surgery. They concluded that free flap reconstruction may potentially decrease costs associated with resection of advanced oropharyngeal tumors and provides better cosmesis and a less invasive approach.

The overarching theme in the available literature regarding robot-assisted oropharyngeal flap inset is that robotic instrumentation to maneuver within the tight confines of the oropharynx is well-established in oncologic surgery, and this utility can be extended to reconstructive procedures (Figs. 15.4 and 15.5).

15.4.2 Robot-Assisted Flap Harvest

Muscle flaps and adipofascial flaps are well-established in the reconstruction of craniomaxillofacial defects [27–29]. As these flaps do not require a skin paddle, RAS may facilitate minimally invasive approaches to the harvest, with the goal of minimizing the associated scar. Two recent studies demonstrated the feasibility of robot-assisted flap harvest, each procedure using only three small incisions. Selber et al. used the da Vinci robot to harvest eight latissimus dorsi muscle flaps, two of which were free flaps used for scalp reconstruction [30]. Pedersen et al. then demonstrated intraperitoneal robot-assisted harvest of ten rectus abdominus muscle flaps, four of which were free flaps used for extremity reconstruction [31]. All flaps were completely viable following harvest, and none required conversion to open technique. Ibrahim et al. later found that RAS rectus abdominus harvest resulted in reduced postoperative pain, shorter hospital stay, and accelerated functional recovery compared with an open approach, though these findings were anecdotal and not quantified [32].

In addition to reducing the extent of scar through minimally invasive approaches, some RAS systems have the capability to assess flap perfusion and assist in identifying vessels. The Firefly® feature of newer da Vinci systems uses near-infrared fluorescence that can assess tissue perfusion using intravenous indocyanine green (ICG) (Fig. 15.6). The applications of this ICG fluorescence for reconstructive flap surgery and surgical treatment of lymphedema have been widely reported [33], and this may further expand the utility of RAS reconstructive surgery.

15.4.3 Robot-Assisted Microsurgery

Robot-assisted surgery has been explored for the completion of pedicle dissection and microvascular anastomosis. Potential advantages of RAS for microsurgery include reduction of physiologic tremor, motion scaling, and high-definition 3D magnification. Numerous preclinical and clinical studies have demonstrated the feasibility of RAS microsurgery including vascular anastomosis [34–36].

The advantages of scalability of movement and high-definition optics may find particular applicability in the field of supermicrosurgery. Lymphovenous anastomosis is increasingly used in the treatment of severe lymphedema of the extremities, and this technique has recently been applied for the treatment of facial lymphedema [37, 38]. However, performing surgery at submillimeter scale requires extraordinary precision. Robotic systems have the capability of translating large movements into very small movements

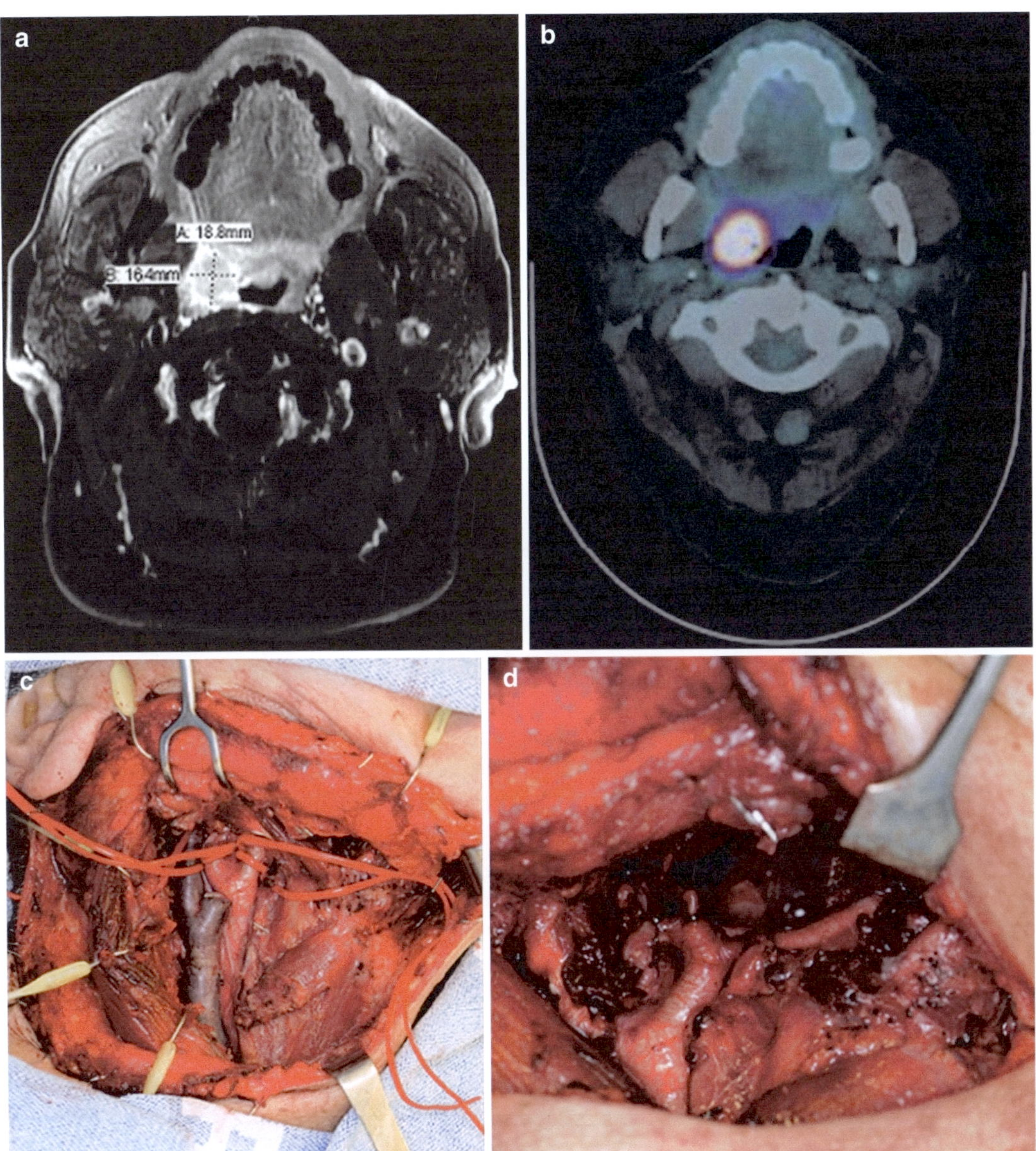

Fig. 15.4 (**a**) Preoperative MRI showing a right-sided squamous cell carcinoma of the right tonsillar fossa. (**b**) Hypermetabolic activity of the oropharyngeal tumor on PET/CT. (**c**) Intraoperative view following neck dissection and isolation of the great vessels. (**d**) Transcervical pharyngotomy. (**e**) Free flap design and inset for complex oropharyngeal reconstruction. (**f**) Postoperative appearance after complete healing

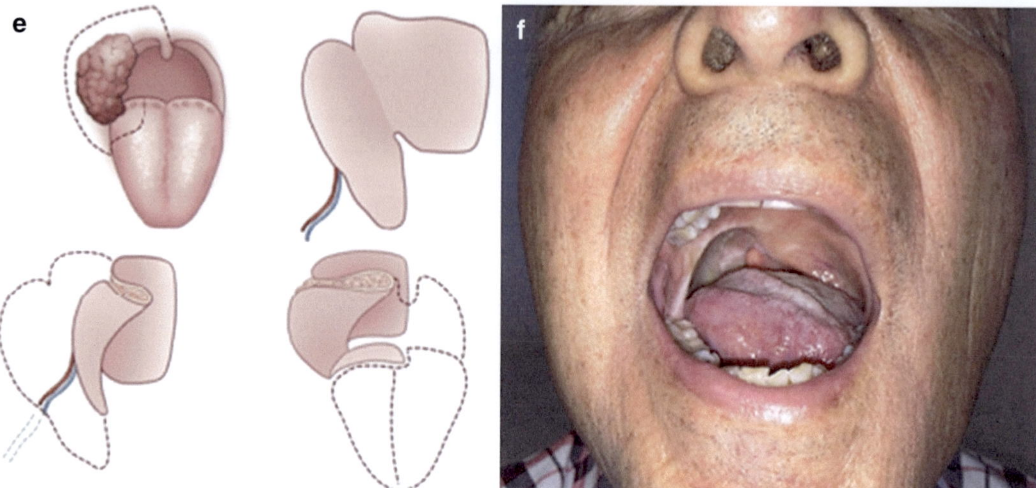

Fig. 15.4 (continued)

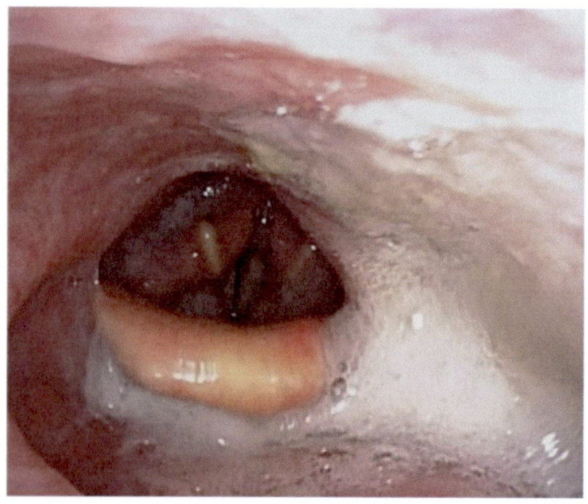

Fig. 15.5 Flexible laryngoscopy showing healed radial forearm free flap for reconstruction of a large defect following TORS radical tonsillectomy

as well as filtering physiological tremor, potentially improving surgical precision beyond the limits of human manual dexterity.

15.4.4 Transoral Robotic Cleft Surgery

Recently, Nadjmi used the da Vinci robot to perform modified Furlow palatoplasty on 10 patients with cleft palate. They found that RAS provided enhanced dexterity and precision, with excellent visibility and relatively easy soft tissue handling and intraoral suturing. They found that surgery was significantly longer with the robotic system and that introduction of a third robotic arm was not possible due to space constraints intraorally [39]. Two preclinical studies have since corroborated the feasibility and potential advantages of RAS cleft palate surgery [40, 41].

15.4.5 Craniofacial Reconstruction

In 2008, the ROBODOC® became the first (and currently the only) robotic surgical system cleared by the FDA for orthopedic surgery. This programmable, fully automated robotic system uses technology akin to CAD/CAM manufacturing processes to perform the bone-milling and implant placement portions of total hip arthroplasty based on preoperative computed tomography imaging. Clinical trials using the ROBODOC showed improved implant fit and alignment of robotically placed hip prostheses compared with the conventional technique [42].

Applications of similar technology for craniomaxillofacial surgery have recently been investigated in preclinical studies. Using a commercial industrial robot, Sun et al. tested the feasibility of a fully automated process for creating the osteotomies for a mandibular sagittal split, first using 3D printed mandibular models, and then in

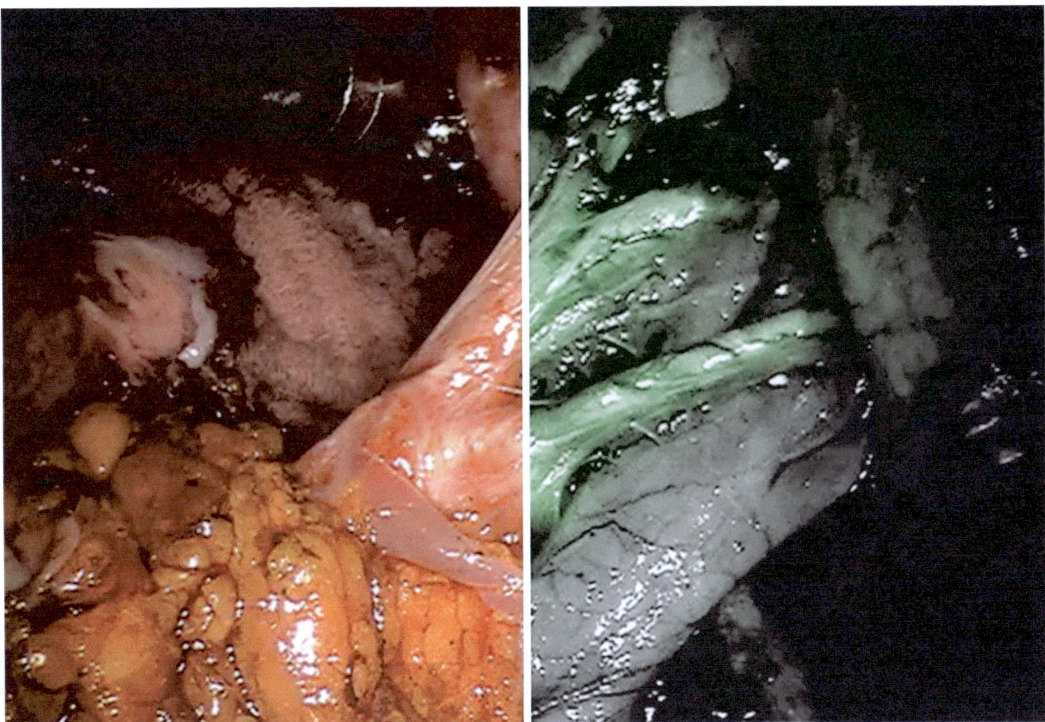

Fig. 15.6 da Vinci Firefly® near-infrared fluorescence activated around the renal hilum. *Courtesy of Intuitive Surgical*

animal experiments [43]. They found that the process was possible; however, there was roughly 1.5 and 2.75 mm error in the phantom and animal experiments, respectively. The larger error in the animal experiments was partially attributed to soft tissue interference.

Two similar studies by Kong et al. and Zhu et al. evaluated RAS for fibular reconstruction of the mandible [44, 45]. Their workflow included preoperative CT, virtual surgical planning, intra-operative navigation, and automated robotic positioning of the fibular segment into the mandibular defect. With the fibula held in position by the robot, the surgeon then proceeded with fixation to complete the reconstruction. Both studies found a mean deviation of roughly 1.5 mm from the preoperative plan in phantom models and animal surgery.

The success of the ROBODOC system in orthopedic surgery is proof-of-concept for the use of automated robotics in osseous surgery. With advancement of this technology and the development of dedicated instrumentation for craniomax-

illofacial surgery, there great potential in the fields of orthognathic surgery, pediatric craniofacial surgery, and craniomaxillofacial trauma surgery.

15.4.6 Dental Reconstruction

In 2017, Neocis received FDA 510(k) approval for its Yomi dental implant robot, the first and only application of robotics in dentistry and dental implant surgery. Unlike surgical robots used in head and neck soft tissue resection and reconstruction, the Yomi incorporates computer aided surgical simulation (CASS) into its software platform, allowing surgeons to digitally plan and simulate dental implant placement using patient-specific computed tomography (CT) data. Though this is common in implant dentistry, Yomi's robotic hardware uses this data to assist the surgeon in positioning the implant drill and burr over the desired osteotomy site in the oral cavity. Once the desired coordinates match the planned position and angles, the robot arm is locked in the x and y axes, allowing the surgeon to drill only to the desired and predetermined depth of the osteotomy.

As with other robotic platforms, the major advantage lies in removing human error including inaccurate and imprecise osteotomy creation. It is unclear whether robot-assisted dental implant surgery will have major indication advantages over readily available guided implant surgery using CASS and 3D printed guides, or real-time dynamic navigation. Data is currently limited on whether or not this approach is advantageous in the scope of dental reconstruction and rehabilitation, and no long-term data on implant success rates, restorability, or adverse outcomes are available at this time. According to a January 2020 press release by Neocis, 1000 dental implants were placed under robotic guidance in 2019 [46].

15.5 Conclusions

Over the last decade, transoral robotic surgery (TORS) has become a fixture in the therapeutic arsenal of many head and neck surgery programs within the USA [3]. TORS allows for minimally invasive access to the upper aerodigestive tract, particularly for tumors of the oropharynx, for which surgical resection would otherwise require considerably more invasive approaches. However, the capabilities of robot-assisted surgery for head and neck reconstruction are just beginning to be realized. Robotic surgery has the potential to improve upon current surgical techniques, potentially improving reconstructive precision and allowing for the advancement of minimally invasive approaches that would otherwise not be possible. Further, the development of instrumentation and end effectors specific to microsurgery may expand the field beyond what is currently possible with conventional techniques. With the recent arrival of new and unique robotic systems into clinical practice, the applications of RAS for head and neck reconstruction are sure to expand and have marked impact on the field in the years to come.

References

1. Shah J, Vyas A, Vyas D. The history of robotics in surgical specialties. Am J Robot Surg. 2014;1(1):12–20.
2. George EI, Brand TC, LaPorta A, Marescaux J, Satava RM. Origins of robotic surgery: from skepticism to standard of care. JSLS. 2018;22(4):e2018.00039.
3. Baliga S, Kabarriti R, Jiang J, Mehta V, Guha C, Kalnicki S, et al. Utilization of Transoral Robotic Surgery (TORS) in patients with oropharyngeal squamous cell carcinoma and its impact on survival and use of chemotherapy. Oral Oncol. 2018;86:75–80.
4. Garas G, Arora A. Robotic head and neck surgery: history, technical evolution and the future. ORL. 2018;80(3–4):117–24.
5. Biron VL, O'Connell DA, Barber B, Clark JM, Andrews C, Jeffery CC, et al. Transoral robotic surgery with radial forearm free flap reconstruction: case control analysis. J Otolaryngol Head Neck Surg. 2017;46(1):20.
6. Richmon JD, Quon H, Gourin CG. The effect of transoral robotic surgery on short-term outcomes and cost of care after oropharyngeal cancer surgery. Laryngoscope. 2014;124(1):165–71.
7. Tam K, Orosco RK, Dimitrios Colevas A, Bedi N, Starmer HM, Beadle BM, et al. Cost comparison of treatment for oropharyngeal carcinoma. Laryngoscope. 2019;129(7):1604–9.
8. Katz RD, Rosson GD, Taylor JA, Singh NK. Robotics in microsurgery: use of a surgical robot to perform a free flap in a pig. Microsurgery. 2005;25(7):566–9.
9. Nectoux E, Taleb C, Liverneaux P. Nerve repair in telemicrosurgery: an experimental study. J Reconstr Microsurg. 2009;25(04):261–5.
10. Wottawa CR, Genovese B, Nowroozi BN, Hart SD, Bisley JW, Grundfest WS, et al. Evaluating tactile feedback in robotic surgery for potential clinical application using an animal model. Surg Endosc. 2016;30(8):3198–209.
11. Tamaki A, Rocco JW, Ozer E. The future of robotic surgery in otolaryngology–head and neck surgery. Oral Oncol. 2020;101:104510.
12. Chalmers R, Schlabe J, Yeung E, Kerawala C, Cascarini L, Paleri V. Robot-assisted reconstruction in head and neck surgical oncology: the evolving role of the reconstructive microsurgeon. ORL. 2018;80(3–4):178–85.
13. Dubner S, Spiro RH. Median mandibulotomy: a critical assessment. Head Neck. 1991;13(5):389–93.
14. Parsons JT, Mendenhall WM, Stringer SP, Amdur RJ, Hinerman RW, Villaret DB, et al. Squamous cell carcinoma of the oropharynx: surgery, radiation therapy, or both. Cancer. 2002;94(11):2967–80.
15. Sims JR, Moore EJ. Primary surgical management with radial forearm free flap reconstruction in T4 oropharyngeal cancer: Complications and functional outcomes. Am J Otolaryngol. 2018;39(2):116–21.

16. Lörincz BB, Jowett N, Knecht R. Decision management in transoral robotic surgery: Indications, individual patient selection, and role in the multidisciplinary treatment for head and neck cancer from a European perspective. Head Neck. 2016;38(S1):E2190–6.

17. Chan JY, Wong EW, Tsang RK, Holsinger FC, Tong MC, Chiu PW, et al. Early results of a safety and feasibility clinical trial of a novel single-port flexible robot for transoral robotic surgery. Eur Arch Otorhinolaryngol. 2017;274(11):3993–6.

18. de Almeida JR, Park RCW, Villanueva NL, Miles BA, Teng MS, Genden EM. Reconstructive algorithm and classification system for transoral oropharyngeal defects. Head Neck. 2014;36(7):934–41.

19. Ghanem TA. Transoral robotic-assisted microvascular reconstruction of the oropharynx. Laryngoscope. 2011;121(3):580–2.

20. Hans S, Jouffroy T, Veivers D, Hoffman C, Girod A, Badoual C, et al. Transoral robotic-assisted free flap reconstruction after radiation therapy in hypopharyngeal carcinoma: report of two cases. Eur Arch Otorhinolaryngol. 2013;270(8):2359–64.

21. Genden EM, Kotz T, Tong CC, Smith C, Sikora AG, Teng MS, et al. Transoral robotic resection and reconstruction for head and neck cancer. Laryngoscope. 2011;121(8):1668–74.

22. Bonawitz SC, Duvvuri U. Robotic-assisted FAMM flap for soft palate reconstruction. Laryngoscope. 2013;123(4):870–4.

23. Zafereo ME, Weber RS, Lewin JS, Roberts DB, Hanasono MM. Complications and functional outcomes following complex oropharyngeal reconstruction. Head Neck. 2010;32(8):1003–11.

24. Kostrzewa JP, Lancaster WP, Iseli TA, Desmond RA, Carroll WR, Rosenthal EL. Outcomes of salvage surgery with free flap reconstruction for recurrent oral and oropharyngeal cancer. Laryngoscope. 2010;120(2):267–72.

25. Patel SN, Cohen MA, Givi B, Dixon BJ, Gilbert RW, Gullane PJ, et al. Salvage surgery for locally recurrent oropharyngeal cancer. Head Neck. 2016;38(S1):E658–64.

26. Tsai Y-C, Liu S-A, Lai C-S, Chen Y-W, Lu C-T, Yen J-H, et al. Functional outcomes and complications of Robot-assisted free flap oropharyngeal reconstruction. Ann Plast Surg. 2017;78(3):S76–82.

27. Revenaugh PC, Haffey TM, Seth R, Fritz MA. Anterolateral thigh adipofascial flap in mucosal reconstruction. JAMA Facial Plast Surg. 2014;16(6):395–9.

28. Wolff K-D. Indications for the vastus lateralis flap in oral and maxillofacial surgery. Br J Oral Maxillofac Surg. 1998;36(5):358–64.

29. Hierner R, van Loon J, Goffin J, Van Calenbergh F. Free latissimus dorsi flap transfer for subtotal scalp and cranium defect reconstruction: report of 7 cases. Microsurgery. 2007;27(5):425–8.

30. Selber JC, Baumann DP, Holsinger CF. Robotic harvest of the latissimus dorsi muscle: laboratory and clinical experience. J Reconstr Microsurg. 2012;28(07):457–64.

31. Pedersen J, Song DH, Selber JC. Robotic, intraperitoneal harvest of the rectus abdominis muscle. Plast Reconstr Surg. 2014;134(5):1057–63.

32. Ibrahim AE, Sarhane KA, Pederson JC, Selber JC. Robotic harvest of the rectus abdominis muscle: principles and clinical applications. In: Seminars in plastic surgery. New York: Thieme Medical Publishers; 2014. p. 026–31.

33. Burnier P, Niddam J, Bosc R, Hersant B, Meningaud J-P. Indocyanine green applications in plastic surgery: a review of the literature. J Plast Reconstr Aesthet Surg. 2017;70(6):814–27.

34. Lee J-Y, Mattar T, Parisi TJ, Carlsen BT, Bishop AT, Shin AY. Learning curve of robotic-assisted microvascular anastomosis in the rat. J Reconstr Microsurg. 2012;28(7):451–6.

35. Boyd B, Umansky J, Samson M, Boyd D, Stahl K. Robotic harvest of internal mammary vessels in breast reconstruction. J Reconstr Microsurg. 2006;22(4):261–6.

36. van der Hulst R, Sawor J, Bouvy N. Microvascular anastomosis: is there a role for robotic surgery? J Plast Reconstr Aesthetic Surg. 2007;60(1):101–2.

37. Mihara M, Uchida G, Hara H, Hayashi Y, Moriguchi H, Narushima M, et al. Lymphaticovenous anastomosis for facial lymphoedema after multiple courses of therapy for head-and-neck cancer. J Plast Reconstr Aesthet Surg. 2011;64(9):1221–5.

38. Ayestaray B, Bekara F, Andreoletti J-B. π-Shaped lymphaticovenular anastomosis for head and neck lymphoedema: a preliminary study. J Plast Reconstr Aesthet Surg. 2013;66(2):201–6.

39. Nadjmi N. Transoral robotic cleft palate surgery. Cleft Palate Craniofac J. 2016;53(3):326–31.

40. Khan K, Dobbs T, Swan MC, Weinstein GS, Goodacre TE. Trans-oral robotic cleft surgery (TORCS) for palate and posterior pharyngeal wall reconstruction: a feasibility study. J Plast Reconstr Aesthet Surg. 2016;69(1):97–100.

41. Podolsky DJ, Fisher DM, Riff KWW, Looi T, Drake JM, Forrest CR. Infant robotic cleft palate surgery: a feasibility assessment using a realistic cleft palate simulator. Plast Reconstr Surg. 2017;139(2):455e–65e.

42. Bargar WL, Parise CA, Hankins A, Marlen NA, Campanelli V, Netravali NA. Fourteen year follow-up of randomized clinical trials of active robotic-assisted total hip arthroplasty. J Arthroplasty. 2018;33(3):810–4.

43. Sun M, Chai Y, Chai G, Zheng X. Fully automatic robot-assisted surgery for mandibular angle split osteotomy. J Craniofac Surg. 2020;31:336–9.

44. Kong X, Duan X, Wang Y. An integrated system for planning, navigation and robotic assistance for man-

dible reconstruction surgery. Intell Serv Robotics. 2016;9(2):113–21.

45. Zhu J-H, Deng J, Liu X-J, Wang J, Guo Y-X, Guo C-B. Prospects of robot-assisted mandibular reconstruction with fibula flap: comparison with a computer-assisted navigation system and freehand technique. J Reconstr Microsurg. 2016;32(09):661–9.

46. Neocis. The first surgical robot designed for dental implant surgery, Yomi®, surpasses 1000 implants. 2020. https://www.neocis.com/news-category/press-release/

Reconstructive Options in the Vessel-Depleted Neck: Past, Present and Future Strategies

Andreas M. Fichter and Klaus-Dietrich Wolff

16.1 Introduction: Definition and Development of the Vessel-Depleted Neck

The routinely performed neck dissection has improved the disease-free survival in oral cancer patients [1]. However, during this intervention, arterial and venous blood vessels are ligated and are lost as potential recipient vessels for microsurgical procedures. While after tumour resection and selective neck dissection potential recipient vessels in the ipsilateral neck can be missing in 39% of cases [2], practically no suitable vessels remain after radical or modified radical neck dissection [3].

Adjuvant (chemo)radiation has also improved disease-free survival in head and neck cancer patients [4], but is also associated with adverse side effects, particularly to the cervical tissue. Severe fibrosis, scarring and loss of tissue planes are unpleasant accompanying symptoms in the neck region and may lead to complications like wound healing disturbances and osteoradionecrosis that may require additional surgery [5–7]. Radiation therapy also evokes endothelial changes like intimal fibrosis which can lead to atherosclerosis and activate the coagulation cascade [8–10]. The resulting increased risk of thrombosis [10, 11] is held responsible for a significantly higher complication and failure rate after free flap transfer in irradiated patients [10]. Tumour recurrence and surgery- or radiation-related complications like fistulae, extensive wound healing disorders and osteoradionecrosis but also the patients' wishes to improve quality of life may require additional surgical steps [12]. Due to fibrosis and excessive scarring, tissue layers can be hard to discern and accidental vascular injury can lead to a high risk of potential life-threatening bleeding in the pre-treated neck [3, 13]. With each additional intervention, the risk for therapy-related complications rises and patients end up in a vicious circle that will leave 7% of them completely devoid of potential cervical recipient vessel [14]. This medical condition is referred to as vessel-depleted (VDN) or frozen neck (Fig. 16.1) [14, 15]. Frequently, microvascular transplants of undamaged tissue quality are the last chance to provide functional reconstructions in areas of disrupted anatomy. However, in the absence of adequate recipient vessels, microvascular transfer can only be achieved through detours—or not at all. Therefore, knowledge of past, present and future therapeutic strategies is important to achieve stable situations even in the most extreme cases.

A. M. Fichter (✉) · K.-D. Wolff
Department of Oral and Maxillofacial Surgery, Klinikum rechts der Isar, Technical University Munich, Munich, Germany
e-mail: andreas.fichter@tum.de; klaus-dietrich.wolff@tum.de

© Springer Nature Switzerland AG 2021
J. Acero (ed.), *Innovations and New Developments in Craniomaxillofacial Reconstruction*,
https://doi.org/10.1007/978-3-030-74322-2_16

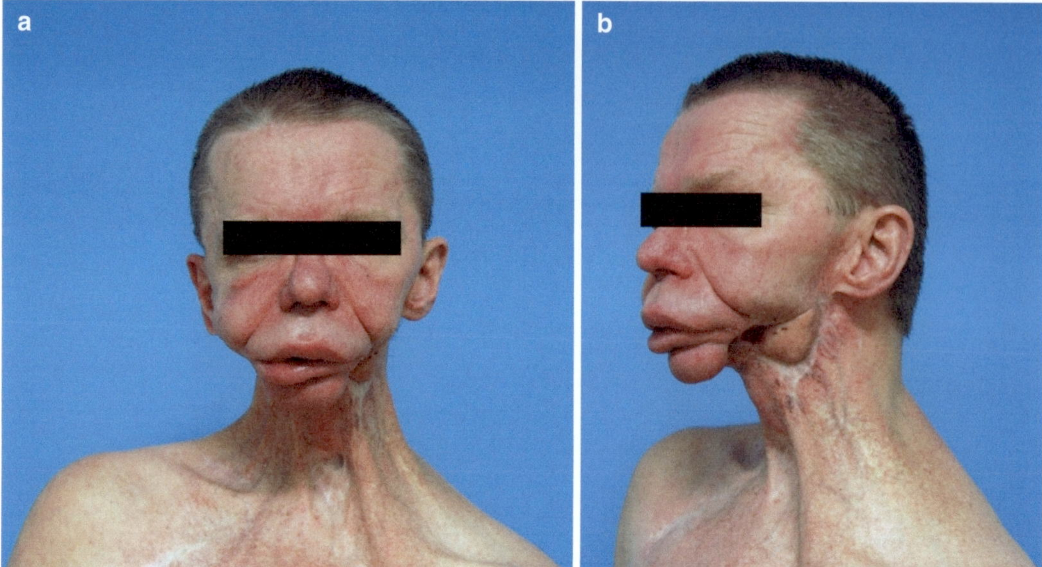

Fig. 16.1 Clinical image of patient with vessel-depleted neck. Patient suffering from vessel-depleted neck after radiation therapy and multiple surgeries for oral cancer and therapy-related complications. (**a**) En face view, (**b**) profile view

16.2 Therapy Options in the Vessel-Depleted Neck

Due to the complexity of the deformity, treatment of patients with vessel-depleted neck is highly individual. For most reconstructive problems in this patient collective, microvascular transfer is the most reliable option, but this option may not be possible in the absence of adequate recipient vessels. In many cases, the use of flaps with long pedicles, the choice of more distant recipient vessels or the interposition of vein grafts will help to facilitate successful free flap transfer. When all microvascular endeavours fail, it might make sense to go down a rung or two on the reconstructive ladder or switch to a more conservative treatment concept, accepting a long healing process and inferior functional outcome.

16.2.1 Microvascular Options in the Absence of Local Recipient Vessels

In highly pre-treated necks, the standard vascular network used for microsurgical reconstructions

defined by branches of the external carotid artery and the jugular vein is inaccessible. Surgical exposure of recipient vessels in a field of radiation-induced skin damage, scar contraction and disrupted anatomy is a highly demanding challenge with a risk of uncontrollable bleeding, consecutive wound healing disorders and aggravation of functional impairment. Nevertheless, microvascular reconstructions still outplay most alternative options with regard to success rate and functional outcome, and all options to achieve microvascular tissue transfer should be exploited. In the following section, we aim to discuss the most favoured options for vessel anastomosis and transplant selection in the VDN.

16.2.1.1 The Ideal Recipient Vessels

The vessels most commonly used in head and neck reconstruction are branches of the ipsilateral external carotid artery and internal jugular vein or the external jugular vein [15, 16]. Following repetitive surgery and radiation therapy, this standard vascular network for microsurgical anastomoses is often inaccessible. In the field of radiation (Fig. 16.2), surgical exposure of recipient vessels is highly demanding due to skin

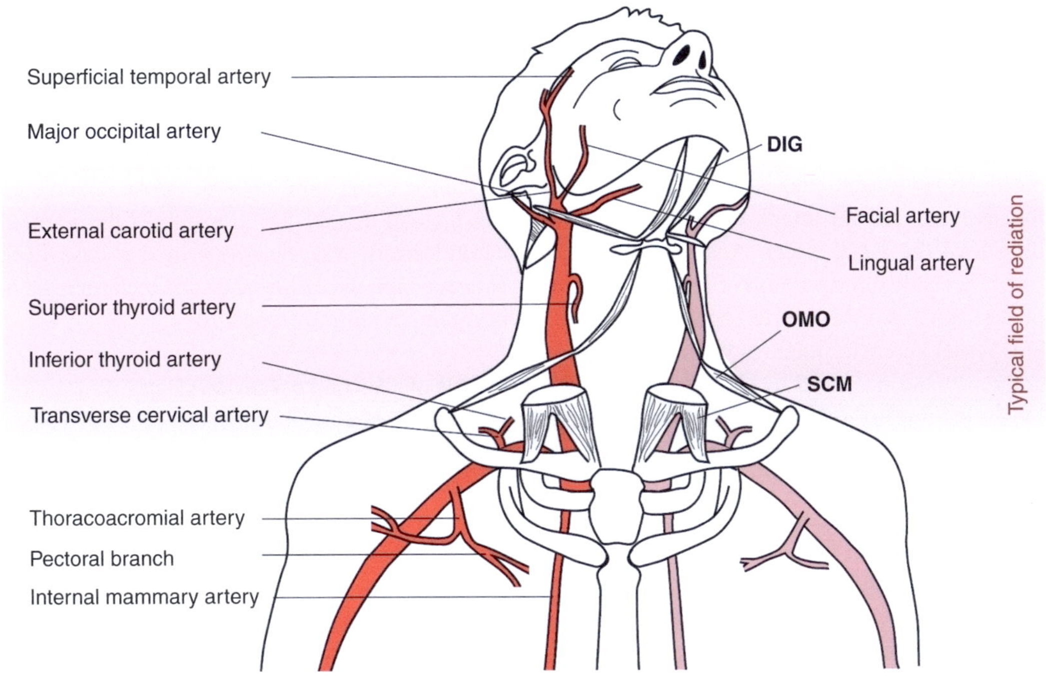

Fig. 16.2 Anatomy of potential donor arteries in the head and neck area. The most common arteries used for microvascular reconstructions are branches of the external carotid artery like the superior thyroid, facial and occasionally the lingual artery. If these vessels are missing, the transverse cervical, thoracoacromial or internal mammary artery can be used. Important muscles of the neck are shown hatched: *SCM* sternocleidomastoid muscle, transected, *OMO* omohyoid muscle, *DIG* anterior belly of the digastric muscle

damage, scar contraction and a disrupted anatomy [3]. Disturbed wound healing, aggravation of functional impairment and, most importantly, vascular damage can occur when accessing the neck. The carotid artery often lies quite superficially and is scarred to the skin, evoking a potential risk of uncontrollable, potentially life-threatening bleeding. Therefore, alternative solutions for reliable microvascular anastomosis are vital for successful reconstruction. The ideal alternative vessels should fulfil three qualifications: (1) the vessels need to be of reliable anatomical appearance, length and calibre as there is little or no room for alternatives in cases of failure, (2) surgical exposure of the recipient vessels should not cause any further damage to the pre-treated neck and (3) the vessels should lie in a non-irradiated part of the body [12].

16.2.1.2 Alternative Recipient Vessels

The most commonly used arteries for reconstructions in the VDN are (in order of frequency): the internal mammary artery (28%), the transverse cervical artery (15.9%), the superficial temporal artery (14.9%), arteries from the contralateral neck (14.5%), the thoracoacromial artery (10.7%), the supraclavicular artery (10.4%) and the external carotid artery above the facial artery (2.4%) [12]. The dorsal scapular artery, the internal carotid artery, the inferior thyroid artery, the arterial pedicle of a previous microvascular flap anastomosis and the use of a wrist-carrier (radial artery) are described in case reports [12]. In the following text, the most common and most important alternative vessels are discussed, and an algorithm for finding adequate vessels is provided at the end of the chapter.

Vessels in Proximity to the Defect Area

External Carotid Artery
Even if all major branches of the external carotid artery are lacking, the cranial portion of the ***external carotid artery*** (above the facial artery)

still provides a high calibre and high blood flow. The vessel lies within the field of radiation and vessels access can be very demanding and risky in the frozen neck. The accessible part of the artery is located underneath the posterior belly of the digastric muscle and is found by following the external carotid artery upwards above the branch of the facial artery. Anastomosis can at times be challenging because of the high location of the vessel and the interference by the mandible. Vessel geometry requires bending the vessel anteriorly and may lead to kinking after anastomosis, but this is rarely a problem due to the high flow of the artery. Despite numerous ipsi- and contralateral collaterals, this procedure should only be performed at one side of the neck to avoid trophic impairment of the facial skin and potential necrosis of the tongue.

The Contralateral Neck

If the ipsilateral neck is depleted of suitable vessels located in proximity to the defect area, the major external carotid branches of the contralateral neck are an option, offering the same advantages of the ipsilateral major external carotid branches like good calibre and blood flow. Depending on the type of defect and intended reconstruction, the contralateral neck often lies in proximity to the defect area, i.e. in multi-segmented mandible reconstructions. In these cases, access to the contralateral neck is required anyway, making the contralateral neck vessels attractive for microvascular reconstruction. However, radiation changes usually affect the contralateral neck as well and after bilateral neck dissection, this pool of alternative vessels may be depleted as well [14, 15]. If flaps with long pedicles or interpositional vein grafts are required to bridge the distance between recipient vessel and defect area, the risk of flap failure is increased due to venous thrombosis or compression of the pedicle by the scarred integument when crossing the mid-line [17–21].

Common Carotid Artery and Internal Carotid Artery

End-to-side anastomoses to the *common* and even *internal carotid artery* have been described, using balloon shunts to bridge the proximal internal carotid artery and the common carotid artery in an effort to minimize cerebral ischaemia time during anastomosis [22]. Preoperative internal carotid artery balloon test occlusion is mandatory to reduce the risk of cerebral stroke. Even successful end-to-side flap transfer to the internal carotid artery was described in one case [22]. However, the risks disqualify this technique from becoming a routine procedure.

Pedicle of a Second or Previous Flap

The pedicle of a previous flap can be used as blood supply for a new flap, as long as it is not obliterated and still provides enough blood flow. Although trophic impairment of the previous flap is unlikely due to rapid autonomization [23, 24], there have been reports of flap loss after transecting the supplying artery even years after the first surgery, in particular in jejunal flaps [25–27]. Preparation of the pedicle of a previous flap is usually demanding due to heavy scarring and radiation-induced changes. This is especially true for the veins.

If more than one flap is raised during the same operation, the number of required recipient vessels can be reduced by connecting the second flap to the pedicle of the first flap (end-to-side or using a side branch) [15]. Alternatively, two flaps can be connected in a serial way, meaning that one flap is daisy-chained to the distal artery of a 'flow-through' flap [28, 29]. However, both techniques still rely on the presence of a local recipient artery. Serial anastomosis implies that ischaemia of the first flap will result in the loss of both flaps.

'Pedicle-sharing' should therefore always be performed knowing that, if everything goes wrong, the patient will not only lose one but two flaps and might end up with severe functional impairment.

Small, Less Common Local Vessels

Complex reconstructions in the central midface can sometimes be achieved using small, less common arteries like the *facial artery with an intraoral approach*, the *angular* and the *major occipital artery* [20]. Vessel preparation and anastomosis require special supermicrosurgical instruments and high magnification [20]. Due to their small calibre and blood volume, these vessels are primarily suited for low-volume reconstructions [20].

Distant Vessels

If no suitable vessels in proximity to the defect area can be located, more distant areas have to be considered. Vessels in these areas are usually located outside the direct field of radiation and previous surgeries, making access to the vessels easier and less risky. The distance between recipient vessel and defect area, however, has to be bridged using either flaps with a long pedicle or interpositional vein grafts, potentially increasing the risk for flap failure [16–21]. For the vessels to reach the defect area, a risky neck access or at least tunnelling of the irradiated integument of the neck is still required in most cases.

If all branches of the external carotid artery are lacking, the superficial temporal [30] and branches of the subclavian artery [14, 15] can be recommended for microvascular reconstructions.

Superficial Temporal Artery

For upper midface reconstruction, the *superficial temporal artery* can be an easily accessible vessel as long as it remained unaffected of previous irradiation. The superficial temporal artery arises from the external carotid artery and runs preauricularly towards the scalp (Fig. 16.2), between the temporal and temporoparietal fascia. It can be detected by palpation or Doppler probe. The artery has a calibre of 1.8–2.7 mm, while the comitant vein has a slightly larger calibre of 2.1–3.3 mm but is very fragile, hard to dissect and lacks in 15% of cases [30]. Vessel geometry is unfavourable for caudally directed vessel connections and may lead to kinking [30]. The temporal artery is also known to be susceptible to vasospasm. Since the achievable pedicle length is limited, the indication spectrum is usually limited to defects of the scalp and upper two thirds of the face [16]. Despite these potential pitfalls, the temporal vessels have been successfully used for intraoral reconstructions in the VDN [31]. Even multi-segmented mandible reconstructions become possible using just a preauricular access,

making these vessels an attractive alternative if a risky cervical access is preferred to be avoided in the irradiated patient [30].

The Subclavian/Brachiocephalical System

Branches of the subclavian artery, such as the thyrocervical trunk with its transverse cervical artery and inferior thyroid artery or the supraclavicular artery, constitute advanced alternatives. The *transverse cervical artery (= A. transversa colli)* and accompanying vein are missing in 6% and 12% of cases, respectively [15]. Despite their location in the field of irradiation and scarred tissue, Urken considered the transverse cervical vessels as 'the best-recipient vessels' for head and neck reconstruction because the axis of the vascular pedicle lies in a longitudinal direction to the head and neck and provides ideal flow and blood pressure characteristics [32]. Critical evaluation of the defect location is necessary as areas above the mandible often require interposition vein grafts due to limited pedicle length. Pedicle length can be increased by dissecting the vessels laterally, but this comes at the cost of calibre. Furthermore, if dissection is carried out beneath the clavicle or far deep into the supraclavicular fat pad, thoracic duct injuries can occur.

The *internal mammary (= internal thoracic) artery* is the most frequently used alternative vessel in the VDN (28%) and the only alternative that follows all three principles for ideal recipient vessels mentioned above [12]. The artery derives from the subclavian artery, whereas the accompanying vein drains into the brachiocephalic vein [16]. Parasternally, both vessels run caudally on the underside of the sternum and the upper six ribs. Due to their location, vessel access is demanding [16] and usually requires the osteotomy of one or two ribs to mobilize the vessels [33]. Anastomosis is complicated by the patient's respiration [33]. Pneumothorax, thoracic duct injury, neuralgia, herniation and chest wall deformities have been described as serious risks during vessel access [3, 16]. Furthermore, the cardiac status of the patient has to be considered as bypass surgery with an internal mammary graft is a contraindication for vessel dissection. Apart from losing a potential donor vessel for coronary bypass surgery, the tedious venous preparation [33], short vessel length and long, subcutaneous run of the pedicle risking compression are additional drawbacks of this approach. Moreover, in most cases, interpositional grafts are required. For these reasons, the internal mammary vessels should be considered a final resort if no other suitable vessels can be located.

The *inferior thyroid artery* deriving from the thyrocervical trunk is usually of inferior calibre and only plays a subordinated relevance in head and neck reconstructions. The same applies for the *supraclavicular artery* which is a descendent from the transverse cervical artery and represents the pedicle of the supraclavicular island flap.

Thoracoacromial System

Further caudally, the *thoracoacromial artery* derives from the axillary artery and divides into four separate branches: the pectoral, clavicular, deltoid and acromial branch [16]. The accompanying veins drain into the external jugular or subclavian vein [16] and are inexistent in 12% of the cases [15]. The thoracoacromial system has been successfully used to provide blood supply for microvascular flaps [34].

While the thoracoacromial artery with a calibre of 1.2–2.4 mm usually matches the calibre of the donor vessel, the calibre of the individual branches often lies below 1 mm [34]. If either the pectoral branch or the thoracoacromial artery itself are used as recipient vessels, the blood supply to the pectoralis major flap is cut, which means closing the door on an important back up procedure ('safety net') reserved for desperate cases when all microvascular procedures have failed. Another major restriction is the frequent need of an interposition graft due to the caudal location of this vascular network [14].

Venous Options

According to the current literature, the veins most commonly used for microvascular anastomosis in the VDN in the absence of branches of the internal jugular vein are the cephalic vein (25.9%), the internal mammary vein (24.4%), the superficial temporal vein (15.4%), the supracla-

vicular vein (9.3%), the transverse cervical vein (8.3%), the thoracoacromial vein (4.9%) and the external (2.2%) or internal jugular vein (1.2%) [12]. In most cases, the most obvious option for venous drainage is to use the accompanying vein of the arterial branch as practiced for the internal mammary, thoracoacromial, transverse cervical and superficial temporal veins. However, these veins are often inconsistent.

End-to-Side Anastomosis to the Internal Jugular Vein

The venous phase of a preoperative CT scan is helpful to assess the patency of the *internal jugular vein*, which can be obliterated following surgery and/or radiation therapy due to thromboses and is completely missing after radical neck dissection. Provided adequate outflow, an end-to-side anastomosis to the internal jugular vein should be considered. However, careful microsurgical planning of location and size of the incision in the internal jugular vein is mandatory to avoid kinking or collapse of the donor vein due to an unfavourable entry angle.

Transposition of the Cephalic Vein

If cervical veins are absent or venous drainage is poor, the *cephalic vein* usually provides a reliable outflow. The cephalic vein runs from the dorsal part of the thumb along the radial flexor tendons towards the elbow, and along the biceps brachii muscle into the clavipectoral triangle between the major pectoral and deltoid muscle, and it drains into the axillary vein [14]. This long vein can be dissected either solely for venous transposition or with a pedicle vessel of a semi-free radial forearm flap [28, 35]. Its numerous advantages have been described extensively and include a consistent anatomy in a non-irradiated graft area, as well as a sufficient calibre. Moreover, the pedicle drains into a high-flow and low-pressure system that bears little risk for stasis and thrombosis [14–16, 35, 36]. Attention has to be paid in terms of kinking and compression of the vein, especially where it crosses the clavicle. Nevertheless, the cephalic vein is a safe and feasible option for venous drainage in the VDN and is considered a 'lifeboat for head and neck free-flap reconstruction' [37]. The cephalic vein is also essential for the Corlett loop [38] (see next section).

Interpositional Vein Grafts, Loops and Shunts

If the pedicle length is too short to bridge the gap between recipient vessel and defect area, vein grafts can be interposed between donor and recipient vessel [17]. The most commonly used *interpositional vein grafts* are the saphenous vein and the cephalic vein [16, 39].

Temporary *arterio-venous loops or shunts* are an alternative bridging technique. A long vein graft is harvested, and each end is sutured to the artery and vein of a free flap, respectively. In the next step, this 'loop' is pulled through a subcutaneous tunnel to the recipient vessels where the loop is transected and the newly generated artery and vein are sutured to their respective recipient vessel. The *Corlett loop* [38] is a different approach to facilitate a vessel connection by interposing the cephalic vein between the contralateral external carotid artery (end-to-side or via a side branch) in a first step. In a second step, the vein is transected distally and the free end is sutured to the flap's artery. The distal segment of the vein, draining into the axillary vein, is sutured to the flap's vein.

The additional harvesting procedure and associated donor site morbidity as well as the fact that twice as many anastomoses have to be conducted leads to an extended operation time. The higher number of anastomoses and often required subcutaneous tunnel under an irradiated integument are also associated with a fourfold higher risk of thrombosis and flap failure when using vein grafts [16–19, 21]. Therefore, other options like the use of flaps with longer pedicles or alternative vascular networks should first be considered before deciding to use vein grafts.

Vessel-Sparing and Vessel-Sharing Techniques

Patients with a history of previous surgery and radiation therapy are likely to require future free flap reconstructions due to complications (infections, radiation ulcer, fistula, etc.) or recurrent cancer. Progressive vessel-depletion following each therapeutic intervention evokes a vicious circle that in turn leads to therapy-related complications, requiring additional interventions. To slow down this spiral, vessel-sparing and vessel-sharing techniques during neck dissection and microvascular interventions can help to reduce trophic impairment to the facial and cervical skin and preserve potential future recipient vessels. *End-to-side anastomosis* to large calibre vessels (i.e. internal jugular vein) is often more challenging then end-to-end anastomoses, but has similar success rates.

As described above, if more than one flap is raised, the *pedicle of a first flap* can be used to connect a second flap to spare local recipient vessels. This can be achieved either by using a side branch of the proximal artery or the distal end of the artery of the first flap as recipient vessel. If the flaps are connected in a serial fashion, the first flap becomes a 'flow-through' flap. The concept of *flow-through flaps* can also be applied to spare recipient vessels if only a single flap is raised by interposing the flap between the two ends of a transected recipient artery. Soutar et al. [40] established a blood flow between the external carotid artery and the distal facial artery by interposing a radial forearm flap. Apart from the radial forearm flap, numerous flow-through flaps have been described [22], mostly for the treatment of ischaemic foot. *Venous flow-through flaps*, based on a single flow-through vein, are yet another option in regions with limited arterial vascular supply [41]. Safak and Akyurek [29] describe successful reconstruction of a patient with severe burns in the neck and chest area using a cephalic vein-based venous flap from the anteromedial upper arm. The main disadvantage of venous flaps is the high failure rate of up to 40%, especially when used for intraoral reconstructions [42, 43]. If no arterial vessels with sufficient arterial outflow can be located, *reverse-flow arteries* might be an alternative. Due to countless collaterals, the distal facial artery provides 76% of the systemic blood pressure and was successfully used as recipient vessel for perforator flaps [23]. Calibre (1.3 mm) and close proximity to the defect area are ideal for short-pedicled perforator flaps. However, in the irradiated patient, paramandibular scarring will impede identification and preservation of the distal vessel stump. Moreover, calibre and flow of the distal facial artery may be too low for larger reconstructions.

16.2.1.3 Algorithm for Locating Recipient Vessels

Based on our experience, the following algorithm for locating adequate recipient vessels in the VDN can be recommended (Fig. 16.3). Although few or no potential recipient vessel will meet all recommended criteria, choice of vessels should always be carried out for each individual patient with the criteria for ideal recipient vessels in mind: (1) reliable anatomical appearance, length and calibre, (2) prevention of further damage to the pre-treated neck and (3) location outside the field of radiation [12].

16.2.1.4 Considerations for Flap Choice

A plethora of different flaps described today usually offers a number of different possibilities for defect coverage with comparable aesthetic and functional outcome. If a flap with a long pedicle is raised, the contralateral neck side or distant ipsilateral recipient vessels can be reached without the need for interpositional vein grafts [2, 16].

The most common flaps used in the VDN are the anterolateral-thigh (ALT) flap (25.8%), the radial forearm flaps (23.7%), flaps from the trunk (DIEP, TRAM, FRAM) (9.4%), the supraclavicular island flap (9.1%) and the free fibula flap (8.2%) [12]. The main concern when harvesting a flap in this patient collective is the unconditional need for success. Apart from defect configuration and required amount and composition of tissue,

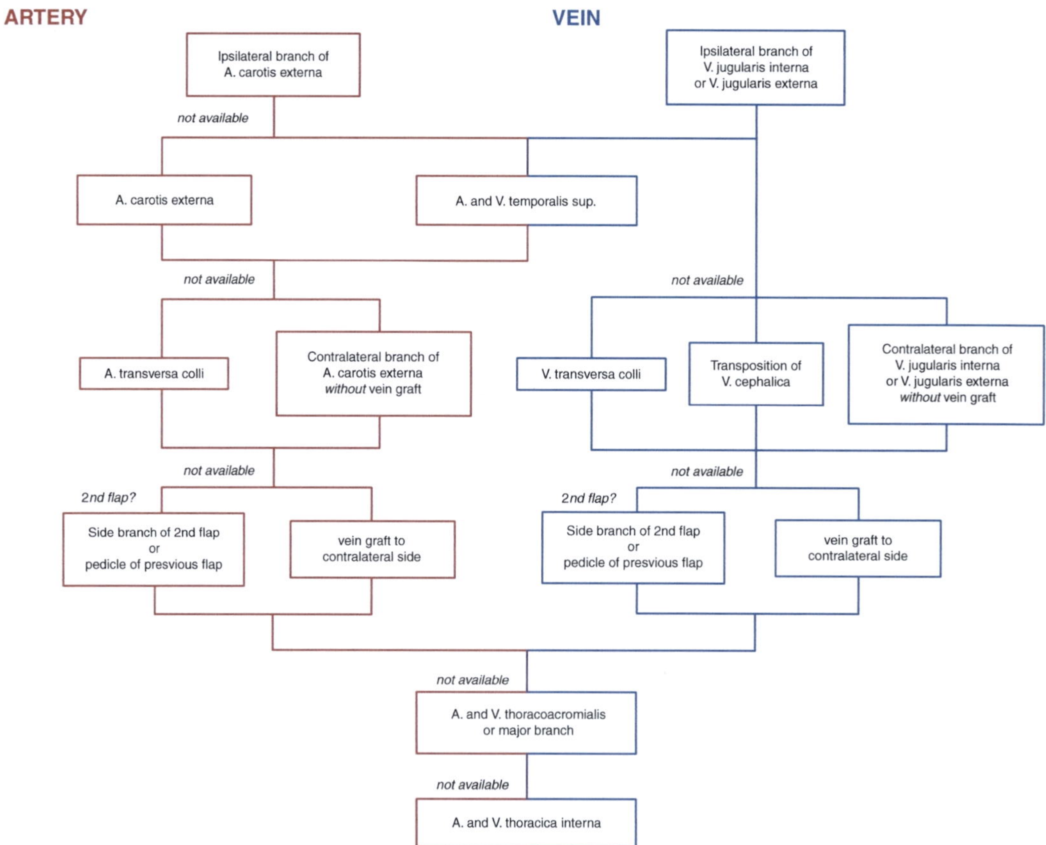

Fig. 16.3 Algorithm for locating alternative vessels for microvascular reconstruction in the vessel-depleted neck. Modified and extended based on Hanasono et al. [8]

criteria for flap choice should therefore include reliability of the flap, personal experience and skills of the surgeon and required pedicle length. Reliable transplants of predictable surgical routine are of first choice, whereas functional and aesthetical aspects play an inferior role compared to primary surgery. Detailed description of all possible flaps is beyond the scope of this chapter, but due to its extreme pedicle length, the reverse-flow thoracoacromial artery-based scapula flap is worth mentioning here. For the interested reader, a comprehensive overview of the most commonly used free flaps in the VDN is provided by Frohwitter et al. [12].

Reverse-Flow Thoracodorsal, Artery-Based Scapula Flap

Jacobson et al. [14] describe a technique to prolong the pedicle length of an existing osteomyocutaneos flap model (scapula flap) to facilitate reconstructions without the need for interpositional vein grafts. The thoracodorsal artery is raised together with the distal portion of the subscapular artery and its descending circumflex scapular artery. In contrast to the conventional scapula flap based on the circumflex scapular artery, in this model, the thoracodorsal artery is used as arterial donor vessel with a reverse flow: The blood flows reversely through the thoracodorsal artery to the subscapular artery, which is ligated, and enters the flap through the circumflex scapular artery. This way, very long pedicle lengths can be achieved. For venous anastomosis, vein grafts are often required [16]. Alternatively, transposition of the cephalic vein should be considered. However, harvesting the thoracodorsal artery means losing a potential 'safety net' flap for neck and lower face reconstructions: the (pedicled) latissimus dorsi flap [14].

16.2.2 Microvascular Options Without Anastomosis in the Head and Neck Region

16.2.2.1 The Principle of Ischaemic Preconditioning

Especially in the irradiated wound bed, transfer of well-vascularized is imperative to avoid wound healing disorders, fistulae and surgical re-interventions. Even towards the end of the middle ages, long before the invention of the operating microscope, techniques for transferring vascularized tissues were known and are based on a stepwise tissue transfer, temporarily preserving the original blood supply. A prerequisite for these procedure to work is rapid *autonomization* of the transferred tissue in the wound bed [24, 44, 45], which means that the transferred tissue has to revascularize in the wound bed and become independent from its original blood supply. Hypoxia constitutes a strong promoter of angio- and vasculogenesis [46], and revascularization follows a hypoxia-gradient directed from well-perfused towards less-perfused tissues [47]. Unfortunately, ischaemia-induced necrosis often develops more rapidly than angiogenesis promoted by hypoxia [48]. In compromised wound beds (i.e. irradiated neck), the hypoxia-gradient might even be reversed, promoting a spread of the vascular network from the flap to the surrounding tissues instead of the other way around. In this scenario, the flap would likely remain dependent on its original blood supply. Using the principal of *ischaemic conditioning*, however, the hypoxia gradient can be redirected towards the flap by reducing flap oxygenation levels below the levels of the surrounding tissues, potentially risking hypoxic injury to the transferred tissue.

16.2.2.2 Tubed Flaps

Almost 500 years ago, the Italian plastic surgeon Gaspare Tagliacozzi [49] described a technique to transfer compound tissues without anastomosis for nasal reconstruction using a tubed upper arm flap. The upper arm was fixed for several weeks to the head using a custom-made hooded leather west, until revascularization of the transferred tissue had occurred from the surrounding tissues and the pedicle could be transected. Today, tubed flaps are of historical relevance [50] but might be considered for small-volume reconstructions in desolate cases of VDN. Due to trophic impairment following radiation therapy, revascularization of transferred tissue may take longer in an irradiated wound bed, but does seem to occur eventually [24, 51]. Tubed flaps also build the intellectual base for the carrier flap, which allows transfer of microvascular flaps without local vessel connections.

16.2.2.3 The Carrier Flap Technique

The carrier flap is the link between historic methods for tissue transfer and modern microvascular techniques. Like with its historical predecessor, the tubed flap, tissue transfer can be achieved without anastomosis in proximity to the defect. The radial artery is used as a wrist carrier as temporary blood supply for one or more microvascular free flaps. The flap(s) can then be used to reconstruct defects in the head and neck area without local vessel access. As with the tubed flap, the patient's arm is fixed to the head for several weeks until revascularization in the recipient wound bed has occurred and the wrist carrier can be ligated. Wolff et al. [24, 51] describe complex soft and hard tissue reconstructions using serial (flow-through) double flaps consisting of an ALT and a free fibula flap for mandible and lower face reconstructions in a patient with VDN. After 18 days, the wrist carrier could be safely ligated. Due to the high operative expense, risk of rupture of the pedicle, inconvenient dressing changes, high donor site morbidity and mandatory immobilization of the shoulder, which can lead to shoulder stiffness, the carrier flap is considered a reserve procedure [20].

16.2.2.4 Extracorporeal Perfusion of Microvascular Free Flaps

We know from animal experiments and organ preservation studies that living tissues can be vitally stored for several days using extracorporeal perfusion [52–57]. While perfusion-based organ preservation has since become a routine clinical procedure, extracorporeal perfusion of free flaps has only recently been demonstrated in the clinical setting to bridge the time to anastomosis in an effort to salvage extremity replants [58] or critically perfused free flaps [59, 60].

Instead of using a wrist carrier as blood supply, free flap perfusion can be maintained temporarily using an extracorporeal perfusion device until revascularization from surrounding tissues has occurred [61], theoretically paving the way to free flap transfer *without* any kind of anastomosis. Following the above-mentioned principle of *ischaemic conditioning*, even in irradiated wound beds, rapid revascularization of voluminous composite free flaps was observed and free flaps survived after cutting off the original blood supply 2–3 weeks after transfer [24, 51, 61, 62]. Based on this observation it seems feasible to apply a temporary extracorporeal flap perfusion in patients suffering from vessel-depleted neck, pre-irradiation, severe atherosclerosis or other conditions associated with a high perioperative risk during free tissue transfer. Preliminary animal experiments have shown promising results [41], and only recently, the first clinical cases with successful flap transfer using an extracorporeal perfusion system for reconstructions of the lower face in patients with VDN have been reported [61–63]. The necessity for continuous monitoring of an immobilized and sedated patient on the ICU, continuous (24 h) surveillance of the extracorporeal membrane oxygenation by a trained physician, high blood loss due to the fact that the venous return is often not reinfused for risk of systemic infection, significant tendency for local oedema formation, partial or total flap necrosis and infection of the perfusate are common risks associated with this procedure in its current form [7, 61, 63].

To make the clinical application more feasible, we have since switched to a simplified, blood-saving, intermittent one-way perfusion using a modified commercial extracorporeal membrane oxygenation system for paediatric lung perfusion [63]. With this setup, successful transfer of primarily thinned ALT flaps to the irradiated neck was performed. Monitoring of both patient and perfusion system was reduced, and patients were able to ambulate on the ward between perfusion cycles. However, decreasing the complexity of the system also led to a higher risk of wound infection and partial or complete epithelial loss and even subtotal flap loss [63]. When using extracorporeal flap perfusion, a delicate balance between a hypoxia-promoted revascularization within a tolerable time frame on the one hand, and a perfusion high enough for crucial parts of the transplanted tissues to survive on the other hand has to be found, respecting the varying ischaemia tolerance of different tissues. It should therefore not surprise that extracorporeal flap perfusion is usually associated with inferior results in comparison with conventional microsurgical techniques, especially in its early stage of development.

Extracorporeal free flap perfusion is an innovative, but still challenging procedure. In comparison with conventional microsurgical tissue transfer, no vascular preparation and microanastomoses have to be performed and operation time is drastically reduced. As of today, however, this technique is still highly experimental, and results are still inferior to conventional microsurgical techniques. Therefore, extracorporeal flap perfusion should be considered a reserve procedure and should only be performed in select cases in specialized centres.

16.2.3 Down the Reconstructive Ladder

Transfer of compound and bulky, well-vascularized tissue is a prerequisite for functional recovery and long-term success in patients with VDN, which is why microvascular reconstructions are still the first choice in this patient collective. However, if all microvascular endeavours fail or if the patient's general health status prohibits lengthy operations, one has to consider stepping down one or two rungs on the reconstructive ladder, gradually accepting inferior functional outcome.

16.2.3.1 Pedicled Myocutaneous Flaps

Pedicled regional muscle flaps, like the *pectoralis major* and *pedicled latissimus dorsi* or the *pedicled trapezius flap*, can also provide healthy, vascularized tissues from non-irradiated regions of the body [64]. Pedicled flaps can be quickly raised and require no microvascular anastomoses, making them ideal for patients in bad general health. Representative of this group of flaps, the pectoralis major flap as an important 'safety net' flap for difficult cases, is discussed in more detail.

The *pedicled myocutaneous pectoral muscle* flap was first described in 1979 [65] and served as a 'working horse' flap in reconstructive head and neck surgery for decades [66]. The major pectoral muscle consists of a clavicular and a sternal part, perfused by branches of the thoracoacromial and lateral thoracic artery, respectively [66]. The flap with its large skin island and sufficient volume is considered very reliable and versatile and is often used for contouring the neck, covering the large cervical vessels and covering intraoral and through-and-through defects as a solid alternative after free flap loss [66]. It can also be combined with a rib graft but this is not recommended in the irradiated neck [13]. The fixed position and restricted pedicle length and rotational axis limits the applicability of this flap to the neck and lower face [67]. Trophic impairment of the skin island is commonly observed, resulting in a considerably high complication rate, especially after radiation therapy [67, 68]. Especially the coverage of exposed osteoradionecrotic bone and the combination with reconstruction plates seem to be problematic [64, 69]. The combination with a reconstruction plate cannot be recommended [64] and functional and aesthetic outcome is usually inferior in comparison with microvascular reconstructions [70, 71], which is of special importance in female patients due to a distortion of the breast [68].

16.2.3.2 Locoregional Fasciocutaneous Flaps

Local random pattern flaps and free skin grafts are not recommended in the irradiated integument because of a high risk of failure [13]. However, a number of locoregional, primarily axial pattern fasciocutaneous flaps exist that still play a role for reconstructions in the previously operated, irradiated neck even in the age of microsurgery [72, 73]. The most commonly used representatives of this group are the *deltopectoral flap* [73], the fasciocutaneous *temporal muscle flap* and the *supraclavicular island flap*.

The *deltopectoral or 'Bakamijan' flap*, a thin, pliable fasciocutaneous flap based on perforators from the internal thoracic artery, perfectly matches the colour and texture of the cervical skin [73]. The donor site is located at the anterior aspect of the shoulder and upper chest wall and thus usually lies outside the field of radiation in an aesthetically favourable location [64]. The flap is suited for reconstructions of the lower face, oral mucosa, cheek and neck and can be combined with the major pectoral flap for complex reconstructions like through-and-through defects [73]. Functional deficits in the donor region are minimal, but primary closure is not possible and requires skin grafting [73]. Today, the deltopectoral flap has lost its status as a 'working horse' flap but remains a valuable option as a salvage technique after free flap loss in the VDN [74].

The *supraclavicular island flap* has recently relived a revival in popularity [12]. Based on the supraclavicular artery, a branch from the transverse cervical artery, skin islands from the supraclavicular and shoulder region of up to 25×10 cm can be harvested with the option to primarily close the donor site [72]. The flap is used for reconstructions of the lower third of the face, the oral cavity and the pharynx [64, 75] and has also proven a valuable alternative in the VDN [76]. However, the low pedicle length (1–7 cm) and anatomical variability of the supraclavicular artery limit the application spectrum. The supraclavicular artery can be missing after level V neck dissection and preoperative radiological imaging of the vessels in cases of radical neck dissection, and radiochemotherapy is frustrating [77]. With complication rates of up to 38% [76, 78], the supraclavicular island flap can therefore not be recommended after level V neck dissection [64]. Nevertheless, the flap offers extraordinarily well-fitting tissue for head and neck reconstruction with regard to texture and skin quality and may be used as a free or pedicled flap.

The *myocutaneous platysma flap* with complication rates of around 40% after neoadjuvant chemo- or radiation therapy is considered unreliable [79–81]. Other locoregional flaps occasionally used in previously operated and irradiated patients are the *temporal muscle flap*, the *tongue flap*, the *cheek flap*, the *lateral neck flap*, the *submental island flap* and the *facial artery musculomucosal (FAMM) flap* [64, 72, 82–84].

The main disadvantage of all locoregional flaps is their lack of bulk, making them unsuited for complex, multi-layered defect coverage. Bone defects cannot be bridged with fasciocutaneous flaps alone and a combination with reconstruction plates is prone to fail due to the lack of a soft tissue. A combination with pedicled muscle flaps may provide enough soft tissue coverage in these cases.

16.2.3.3 Alternative and Additional Surgical Techniques

Tissue expansion using subcutaneous expanders with increasing volumes to expand the local skin provides healthy, well-vascularized tissue and has been used by some authors to treat radiation ulcer [13]. Although at least two operative steps are required for implementation and explanation and reconstruction, operation time and donor morbidity can be drastically reduced in comparison with free flap surgery [13]. Due to anatomical limitations for tissue expansion in the head and neck area and due to a lack of bulk of the expanded tissue, the field of application of this method in the VDN is limited. However, combination with other techniques, i.e. locoregional flaps from the shoulder/chest wall might be an option in select cases.

Reaching the bottom of the reconstructive ladder, when all reconstructive endeavours have failed, stabile wound conditions can be achieved by way of secondary wound healing given enough time and accepting considerable functional and aesthetic impairment. The process of secondary wound healing can be dramatically accelerated using *vacuum-assisted closure (VAC) therapy*. The principle of this therapy is to distribute a suction effect evenly onto the wound surface using a porous sponge to provoke wound granulation and contraction and insure continuous wound drainage [85]. VAC therapy is contraindicated in proximity to large blood vessels (cave: irradiated vessels!) and malign tumour wounds, and the decision to use this technique in the irradiated neck should therefore be made with great caution and consideration.

In cases of therapy-resistant through-and-through fistulae or osteoradionecrosis of the lower jaw, removal of parts of the jaw resulting in *soft tissue collapse* can be a method of last resort to achieve soft-tissue coverage. In most cases, stability of the lower face and posterior airway space are maintained due to severe paramandibular scarring, and patients are often able to breathe without tracheostoma. However, swallowing and speech are usually drastically impaired, and patients end up with a bird-like profile due to the missing mandible, known as the Gump Deformity.

Despite immense progress in the field of *tissue engineering* in the past decades, this technique is still experimental and the transfer of large, vascularized tissues to a compromised wound bed is not yet possible and would also require the presence of local recipient vessels [39, 86].

16.3 Treatment Algorithm

Despite the progressive development in medical research, an *evidence-based* algorithm for reconstructive techniques in patients with VDN cannot be provided. The presented flowchart (Fig. 16.4) is based on our personal experience and the review of the literature and can serve as a general guideline. The complexity of reconstructive problems in the VDN demands highly individual solutions that are prone to surgical revision. Often, expectations of both patient and surgeon must be lowered in advance with regard to functional and aesthetic outcome. As mentioned previously in this chapter, although access to local recipient vessels in irradiated areas is demanding

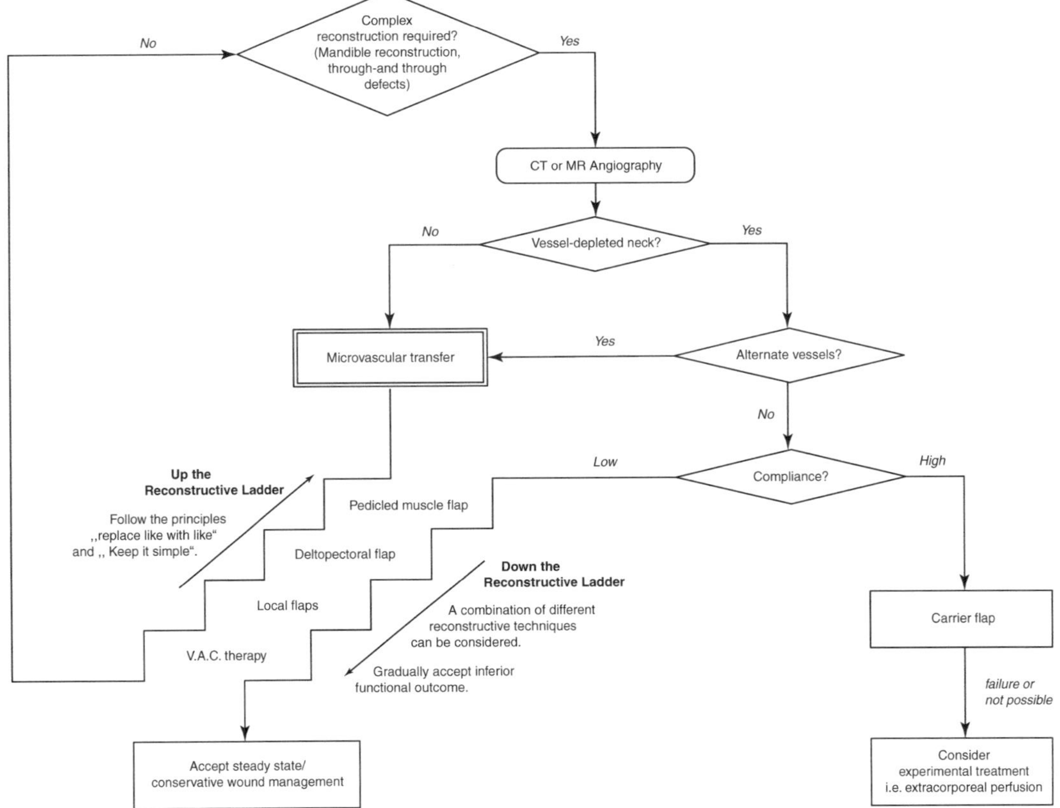

Fig. 16.4 Algorithm for the treatment of complex defects in the vessel-depleted neck. Treatment of the vessel-depleted neck is highly individual, and the depicted algorithm should only be interpreted as a rough guideline to help in the decision-making process

and risky, microvascular reconstructions are still the method of choice for the treatment of complex defects, as this technique provides healthy, well-vascularized tissue with enough bulk. If adequate local recipient vessels can be located or distant recipient vessels reached with a long pedicle, free flaps still have a higher success rate than most other techniques in the VDN. If microvascular transfer is not feasible, the carrier flap technique might be considered as an alternative method to deliver high amounts of soft and hard tissue without relying on local blood supply. However, a high amount of compliance from the patient is required. If all microvascular techniques fail, the reconstructive ladder can be descended rung by rung, gradually accepting inferior functional outcome. As a means of last resort, experimental treatment options like extracorporeal free flap perfusion may offer acceptable outcomes in select patients but should only be performed in specialized centres.

16.4 Conclusion

This chapter comprises a magnitude of options for challenging surgical solutions. However, the final decision of the reconstructive option is highly individual and based on the patient's condition and the individual skills of the surgeon. With complication rates of 34.5%, reconstruction in this patient collective demands highly individual solutions that are prone to surgical revision. Due to the complexity of the deformity and due to the fact that present concepts like free flaps may not be suitable, the knowledge of past concepts is just as important as continuous ongoing scientific effort in finding new ways for treating this deformity.

Bibliography

1. Fasunla AJ, et al. A meta-analysis of the randomized controlled trials on elective neck dissection versus therapeutic neck dissection in oral cavity cancers with clinically node-negative neck. Oral Oncol. 2011;47(5):320–4.
2. Head C, et al. Microvascular reconstruction after previous neck dissection. Arch Otolaryngol Head Neck Surg. 2002;128(3):328–31.
3. Sturtz G, Heidekruger PI, Ninkovic M. The internal thoracic vessels as alternative recipient vessels for microsurgical reconstruction in the head and neck area in patients with a vessel-depleted neck. Handchir Mikrochir Plast Chir. 2012;44(2):75–9.
4. Cooper JS, et al. Postoperative concurrent radiotherapy and chemotherapy for high-risk squamous-cell carcinoma of the head and neck. N Engl J Med. 2004;350(19):1937–44.
5. Shih HS, et al. An alternative option to overcome difficult venous return in head and neck free flap reconstruction. J Plast Reconstr Aesthet Surg. 2013;66(9):1243–7.
6. Koerdt S, et al. Radiotherapy for oral cancer decreases the cutaneous expression of host defence peptides. J Craniomaxillofac Surg. 2016;44(7):882–9.
7. Koerdt S, et al. An immunohistochemical study on the role of oxidative and nitrosative stress in irradiated skin. Cells Tissues Organs. 2017;203(1):12–9.
8. Kiener JL, Hoffman WY, Mathes SJ. Influence of radiotherapy on microvascular reconstruction in the head and neck region. Am J Surg. 1991;162(4):404–7.
9. Momeni A, et al. The effect of preoperative radiotherapy on complication rate after microsurgical head and neck reconstruction. J Plast Reconstr Aesthet Surg. 2011;64(11):1454–9.
10. Tall J, et al. Vascular complications after radiotherapy in head and neck free flap reconstruction: clinical outcome related to vascular biology. Ann Plast Surg. 2015;75(3):309–15.
11. Rudolph R, Arganese T, Woodward M. The ultrastructure and etiology of chronic radiotherapy damage in human skin. Ann Plast Surg. 1982;9(4):282–92.
12. Frohwitter G, et al. Microvascular reconstruction in the vessel depleted neck - a systematic review. J Craniomaxillofac Surg. 2018;46(9):1652–8.
13. Fujioka M. Surgical reconstruction of radiation injuries. Adv Wound Care (New Rochelle). 2014;3(1):25–37.
14. Jacobson AS, et al. Vessel-depleted neck: techniques for achieving microvascular reconstruction. Head Neck. 2008;30(2):201–7.
15. Hanasono MM, Barnea Y, Skoracki RJ. Microvascular surgery in the previously operated and irradiated neck. Microsurgery. 2009;29(1):1–7.
16. Wong KK, Higgins KM, Enepekides DJ. Microvascular reconstruction in the vessel-depleted neck. Curr Opin Otolaryngol Head Neck Surg. 2010;18(4):223–6.
17. Miller MJ, et al. Interposition vein grafting in head and neck reconstructive microsurgery. J Reconstr Microsurg. 1993;9(3):245–51; discussion 251–2.
18. Bozikov K, Arnez ZM. Factors predicting free flap complications in head and neck reconstruction. J Plast Reconstr Aesthet Surg. 2006;59(7):737–42.

19. Salgarello M, et al. The Pruitt-Inahara carotid shunt as an assisting tool to anastomose the arterial free flap pedicle to the internal carotid artery in the vessel-depleted neck. Microsurgery. 2011;31(3):234–6.
20. Gießler GA. [Der mikrochirurgische Gefäßanschluss am bestrahlten und gefäßverarmten Hals]. Face. 2013;1:6–9.
21. Maricevich M, et al. Interposition vein grafting in head and neck free flap reconstruction. Plast Reconstr Surg. 2018;142(4):1025–34.
22. Bullocks J, et al. Flow-through flaps: a review of current knowledge and a novel classification system. Microsurgery. 2006;26(6):439–49.
23. Holzle F, et al. Reverse flow facial artery as recipient vessel for perforator flaps. Microsurgery. 2009;29(6):437–42.
24. Wolff KD, et al. Rapid autonomisation of a combined fibular- and anterolateral thigh flap transferred by a wrist carrier to an irradiated and vessel depleted neck. J Surg Oncol. 2009;99(2):123–6.
25. Machens HG, et al. Persistence of pedicle blood flow up to 10 years after free musculocutaneous tissue transfer. Plast Reconstr Surg. 1998;101(3):719–26.
26. Moolenburgh SE, van Huizum MA, Hofer SO. DIEP-flap failure after pedicle division three years following transfer. Br J Plast Surg. 2005;58(7):1000–3.
27. Heitland AS, et al. Early and long-term evaluation of perfusion changes in free DIEP-flaps for breast reconstruction via IC-view and duplex ultrasound: autonomous or peripheral perfusion? J Reconstr Microsurg. 2009;25(2):139–45.
28. Nakayama Y, Soeda S, Iino T. A radial forearm flap based on an extended dissection of the cephalic vein. The longest venous pedicle? Case report. Br J Plast Surg. 1986;39(4):454–7.
29. Safak T, Akyurek M. Cephalic vein-pedicled arterialized anteromedial arm venous flap for head and neck reconstruction. Ann Plast Surg. 2001;47(4):446–9.
30. Shimizu F, et al. Superficial temporal vessels as a reserve recipient site for microvascular head and neck reconstruction in vessel-depleted neck. Ann Plast Surg. 2009;62(2):134–8.
31. Sudirman SR, et al. Superficial temporal vessels, both anterograde and retrograde limbs, are viable recipient vessels for recurrent head and neck reconstruction in patients with frozen neck. Head Neck. 2019;41(10):3618–23.
32. Urken ML, et al. Geometry of the vascular pedicle in free tissue transfers to the head and neck. Arch Otolaryngol Head Neck Surg. 1989;115(8):954–60.
33. Ninkovic M, et al. Internal mammary vessels: a reliable recipient system for free flaps in breast reconstruction. Br J Plast Surg. 1995;48(8):533–9.
34. Harris JR, et al. The thoracoacromial/cephalic vascular system for microvascular anastomoses in the vessel-depleted neck. Arch Otolaryngol Head Neck Surg. 2002;128(3):319–23.
35. Quilichini J, et al. Semi-free radial forearm flap for head and neck reconstruction in vessel-depleted

36. Vasilakis V, Patel HD, Chen HC. Head and neck reconstruction using cephalic vein transposition in the vessel-depleted neck. Microsurgery. 2009;29(8):598–602.
37. Horng SY, Chen MT. Reversed cephalic vein: a lifeboat in head and neck free-flap reconstruction. Plast Reconstr Surg. 1993;92(4):752–3.
38. Ethunandan M, Cole R, Flood TR. Corlett loop for microvascular reconstruction in a neck depleted of vessels. Br J Oral Maxillofac Surg. 2007;45(6):493–5.
39. Chang KP, et al. Use of single saphenous interposition vein graft for primary arterial circuit and secondary recipient site in head and neck reconstruction: a case report. Head Neck. 2007;29(4):412–5.
40. Soutar DS, et al. The radial forearm flap: a versatile method for intra-oral reconstruction. Br J Plast Surg. 1983;36(1):1–8.
41. Maeda M, et al. Extracorporeal circulation for tissue transplantation (in the case of venous flaps). Plast Reconstr Surg. 1993;91(1):113–24; discussion 125–6.
42. Kovacs AF. Comparison of two types of arterialized venous forearm flaps for oral reconstruction and proposal of a reliable procedure. J Craniomaxillofac Surg. 1998;26(4):249–54.
43. Klein C. [Experiences with an arterialized venous flap for intraoral defect reconstruction]. Zentralbl Chir. 2000;125(1):51–5.
44. Gundeslioglu AO, et al. Neo-vascularisation of musculocutaneous and muscle flaps after division of the major vascular supply: an experimental study. J Plast Reconstr Aesthet Surg. 2013;66(7):978–86.
45. Wise SR, et al. Free flap survival despite early loss of the vascular pedicle. Head Neck. 2011;33(7):1068–71.
46. Namiki A, et al. Hypoxia induces vascular endothelial growth factor in cultured human endothelial cells. J Biol Chem. 1995;270(52):31189–95.
47. Tomanek RJ, et al. Vascular endothelial growth factor expression coincides with coronary vasculogenesis and angiogenesis. Dev Dyn. 1999;215(1):54–61.
48. Weng R, et al. Mimic hypoxia improves angiogenesis in ischaemic random flaps. J Plast Reconstr Aesthet Surg. 2010;63(12):2152–9.
49. Tagliacozzi G. De Curtorum Chirurgia per Insitionem: Libri Duo. De Curtorum Chirurgia per Insitionem: Libri Duo. Ad Serenissimum Principem d. Vincentium Gonzagam. Venice: Apud Gasparem Bindonum Luniorem; 1597.
50. Dragu A, et al. [Prinzipien der Lappenplastiken: Eine Übersicht]. CHAZ. 2009;9(2):59–66.
51. Wolff KD, Holzle F, Eufinger H. The radial forearm flap as a carrier for the osteocutaneous fibula graft in mandibular reconstruction. Int J Oral Maxillofac Surg. 2003;32(6):614–8.
52. Dragu A, et al. Extracorporeal perfusion of free muscle flaps in a porcine model using a miniaturized perfusion system. Arch Orthop Trauma Surg. 2011;131(6):849–55.

53. Slater NJ, et al. Ex-vivo oxygenated perfusion of free flaps during ischemia time: a feasibility study in a porcine model and preliminary results. J Surg Res. 2016;205(2):292–5.

54. Fichter AM, et al. Development of an extracorporeal perfusion device for small animal free flaps. PLoS One. 2016;11(1):e0147755.

55. Worner M, et al. A low-cost, small volume circuit for autologous blood normothermic perfusion of rabbit organs. Artif Organs. 2014;38(4):352–61.

56. Herold C, et al. A normothermic perfusion bioreactor to preserve viability of rat groin flaps extracorporally. Transplant Proc. 2009;41(10):4382–8.

57. Mayer B. Significance of extracorporally perfused microsurgical free flaps. Laryngorhinootologie. 2002;81(9):640–3.

58. Greaney PJ Jr, et al. Use of an extracorporeal membrane oxygenation circuit as a bridge to salvage a major upper-extremity replant in a critically ill patient. J Reconstr Microsurg. 2010;26(8):517–22.

59. Fichter AM, et al. Free flap rescue using an extracorporeal perfusion device. J Craniomaxillofac Surg. 2016;44(12):1889–95.

60. Taeger CD, et al. Extracorporeal free flap perfusion in case of prolonged ischemia time. Plast Reconstr Surg Glob Open. 2016;4(4):e682.

61. Wolff KD, et al. Free flap transplantation using an extracorporeal perfusion device: first three cases. J Craniomaxillofac Surg. 2016;44(2):148–54.

62. Wolff KD. New aspects in free flap surgery: MINI-perforator flaps and extracorporeal flap perfusion. J Stomatol Oral Maxillofac Surg. 2017;118(4):238–41.

63. Wolff KD, et al. In vivo perfusion of free skin flaps using extracorporeal membrane oxygenation. Under review. 2019.

64. Hayden RE, Nagel TH. The evolving role of free flaps and pedicled flaps in head and neck reconstruction. Curr Opin Otolaryngol Head Neck Surg. 2013;21(4):305–10.

65. Ariyan S. The pectoralis major myocutaneous flap. A versatile flap for reconstruction in the head and neck. Plast Reconstr Surg. 1979;63(1):73–81.

66. Teo KG, Rozen WM, Acosta R. The pectoralis major myocutaneous flap. J Reconstr Microsurg. 2013;29(7):449–56.

67. Sakuraba M, et al. Recent advances in reconstructive surgery: head and neck reconstruction. Int J Clin Oncol. 2013;18(4):561–5.

68. Kruse AL, et al. Evaluation of the pectoralis major flap for reconstructive head and neck surgery. Head Neck Oncol. 2011;3:12.

69. Zbar RI, et al. Pectoralis major myofascial flap: a valuable tool in contemporary head and neck reconstruction. Head Neck. 1997;19(5):412–8.

70. Mucke T, et al. Functional outcome after different oncological interventions in head and neck cancer patients. J Cancer Res Clin Oncol. 2012;138(3):371–6.

71. Corbitt C, et al. Free flap failure in head and neck reconstruction. Head Neck. 2014;36(10):1440–5.

72. Colletti G, et al. Autonomized flaps in secondary head and neck reconstructions. Acta Otorhinolaryngol Ital. 2012;32(5):329–35.

73. Chan RC, Chan JY. Deltopectoral flap in the era of microsurgery. Surg Res Pract. 2014;2014:420892.

74. Krijgh DD, Mureau MA. Reconstructive options in patients with late complications after surgery and radiotherapy for head and neck cancer: remember the deltopectoral flap. Ann Plast Surg. 2013;71(2):181–5.

75. Chiu ES, Liu PH, Friedlander PL. Supraclavicular artery island flap for head and neck oncologic reconstruction: indications, complications, and outcomes. Plast Reconstr Surg. 2009;124(1):115–23.

76. Su T, Pirgousis P, Fernandes R. Versatility of supraclavicular artery island flap in head and neck reconstruction of vessel-depleted and difficult necks. J Oral Maxillofac Surg. 2013;71(3):622–7.

77. Adams AS, et al. The use of multislice CT angiography preoperative study for supraclavicular artery island flap harvesting. Ann Plast Surg. 2012;69(3):312–5.

78. Razdan SN, et al. Safety of the supraclavicular artery island flap in the setting of neck dissection and radiation therapy. J Reconstr Microsurg. 2015;31:378–83.

79. Futrell JW, et al. Platysma myocutaneous flap for intraoral reconstruction. Am J Surg. 1978;136(4):504–7.

80. Verschuur HP, et al. Complications of the myocutaneous platysma flap in intraoral reconstruction. Head Neck. 1998;20(7):623–9.

81. Szudek J, Taylor SM. Systematic review of the platysma myocutaneous flap for head and neck reconstruction. Arch Otolaryngol Head Neck Surg. 2007;133(7):655–61.

82. Ceran C, et al. Tongue flap as a reconstructive option in intraoral defects. J Craniofac Surg. 2013;24(3):972–4.

83. Pepper JP, Baker SR. Local flaps: cheek and lip reconstruction. JAMA Facial Plast Surg. 2013;15(5):374–82.

84. Kummoona R. Reconstruction by lateral cervical flap of perioral and oral cavity: clinical and experimental studies. J Craniofac Surg. 2010;21(3):660–5.

85. Palm HG, et al. Vacuum-assisted closure of head and neck wounds. HNO. 2011;59(8):819–30.

86. John S, et al. Development of a tissue-engineered skin substitute on a base of human amniotic membrane. J Tissue Eng. 2019;10:2041731418825378.

Face Transplantation

17

Bernard Devauchelle, Stéphanie Dakpe,
Emmanuel Morelon, Sophie Cremades,
and Sylvie Testelin

17.1 Introduction

Is it possible to have an objective position when it comes to the indication for vascular composite allotransplantation of the face, the face graft as a reconstructive procedure for extensive disfigurement 15 years after the first was performed [1], and with the experience of more than 40 other officially reported cases?

This was also the conclusion of the XIIIth conference of the International Society of Vascularized Composite Allotransplantation (ISVCA) held in Salzburg in 2017 and reported in the *Journal of Transplantation* [2].

We would have to analyze each clinical case, determine all scientific assessment measures, and apply them all to each situation, knowing that methods and ideas have changed since the beginning and that cultural attitudes and behavior in different countries could vary radically. Moreover, the aesthetic dimension of this type of vascularized composite allotransplantation (VCA) is clearly of great importance, adding subjectivity and a double look of the patient himself and the medical staff.

A recent work in sociology reported on the large differences between the two sides of the channel, probably a consequence of their First World War experiences [3]. A similar report was published by the Chauvet Group (including psychologists, psychiatrists, sociologists, and medical doctors) about the differences in decision-making and analyses depending on teams and continents [4].

This inability to reach a consensus on a face transplantation viewpoint could also be an opportunity to ignite discussions [5] and continue research by the involved face transplant teams. Face transplantation should still be considered an experimental work and not thought of as outbid, as it is all too often referred to in papers [6]. It should involve critical thinking from different perspectives. Some could object that it is a biased inside opinion; nevertheless, many questions are technical. There is currently no team actively and successfully involved in this field of face VCA

B. Devauchelle · S. Dakpe · S. Testelin (✉)
Department of Maxillofacial Surgery, University Hospital Amiens Picardie, Amiens Cedex 1, France

Research Unit UR7516 Chimere, Facing Faces Institute, Amiens, France
e-mail: devauchelle.bernard@chu-amiens.fr;
dakpe.stephanie@chu-amiens.fr;
testelin.sylvie@chu-amiens.fr

E. Morelon
Department of Immunology and Transplantation, University Hospital of Lyon, Lyon, France
e-mail: emmanuel.morelon@chu-lyon.fr

S. Cremades
Department of Psychiatry, University Hospital Amiens Picardie, Amiens Cedex 1, France

Research Unit UR7516 Chimere, Facing Faces Institute, Amiens, France
e-mail: crcmadcs.sophie@chu-amiens.fr

© Springer Nature Switzerland AG 2021
J. Acero (ed.), *Innovations and New Developments in Craniomaxillofacial Reconstruction*,
https://doi.org/10.1007/978-3-030-74322-2_17

who has no close links with immunologists, psychologists and philosophers. Techniques cannot break free from whom mastered them, the patients themselves, and the conditions of the procedures as a whole.

All these aspects should be addressed individually in sections.

17.2 Retrospective Analysis of Vascularized Composite Allotransplantations (VCA) of the Face

Despite the existence of the international registry for VCA [7], it is very difficult, if not impossible, to obtain a detailed report for each face transplant performed in the world. Some scientific journals are not fair and regularly accept reports by some teams and refuse others, even though these publishers are responsible for the validity of results and available data.

The exact number of face transplants is not precisely known. More than 40 are identified, but there are probably more. Their geographic distribution was reported in a paper published in 2018 [8]. It points out the difficulty in following up patients due to the distance between the centers and their home. In the USA, it is sometimes more than 2000 km between them, and we know about the Chinese patient living far away in the mountains, more than a 2-day journey from the Xi'an hospital.

Many teams have performed only one face VCA. They claim to be "inexperienced," either in Europe or the USA. We might wonder about the reason for which they attempted this experiment, yet never performed it again. Only two teams (Boston and Paris) have taken the challenge of managing more than seven cases each.

At least 7 of 40 patients have died: one in the early postoperative period, 6 weeks after the transplant procedure due to infection; one 11 years after the transplant; one Spanish case due to the bad immunologic status (indication after previous malignant tumor exeresis context), one did a new suicide and four because of secondary malignant complications under immuno-suppressive treatments. Three chronic rejections have been reported of whom one could be re-transplanted.

These data could be cautiously compared with those of organ transplantation. The mean success time for cardiac transplantation is about 12 years, with no clear determination of the etiology of death. The same thinking should apply to VCA regarding chronic rejection and treatment adherence, or chronic rejection and death.

In a paper in the *British Medical Bulletin*, Maria Siemionov [9], who had extensive expertise in experimental works on VCA, performed the first face VCA in the USA, then gave an optimistic overview of the face transplant 10 years later (2016) on aesthetic and functional aspects. She reported: *"the functional aspects were surprising, and most patients recovered their daily activities and were satisfied with their new faces."* Breathing and feeding are now possible to do naturally, but speech is rather difficult for many transplanted patients (lip mobility is usually insufficient and some words cannot be clearly pronounced). Eyelid closure, despite a recent paper by Rodriguez [10], is not well recovered, exactly as is known in palliative surgery for cases of facial palsy rehabilitation.

Is it actually possible to analyze and judge the aesthetic result? In indications for trauma cases, the result after face transplantation should be compared with the face before the trauma, certainly, illusory. The aesthetic result will be analyzed in terms of the quality of integration of the transplant into the face (shape and color), the slight visibility of the scars, and symmetry. We could imagine that, for this reason, some face transplants are extended beyond the defect area.

Would it be possible to consider aesthetic results when the patient was transplanted because of von Recklinghausen's disease or disfiguring vascular malformations with disfigurement eventually ending in a monstrous face? In the end, each harmonious face would be broken by an unsightly imposter.

The author's optimism should also be tempered by the request for secondary surgical procedures needed to improve these types of results.

In a paper by Rodriguez in 2016 [11], the author reported a partial distribution of the topography of facial defects and studied their etiologies. At that time, there were 37 cases. Lips and noses were always involved. The extension of the transplant was regularly and progressively performed from the center outward to reach the full face for his last case. Deep reconstruction involved only the nose and maxillary bones, with some extension to the orbit. The tongue was partially included in two cases, and entirely in another. Obviously, for aesthetic reasons, no half-face transplants were involving only one profile.

Indications for previously performed face transplants included 40% due to sequelae from ballistic trauma, usually with severe sequalae from the surgery. Thirty percent were burn cases (thermal or chemical etiologies). The other etiologies were animal wounds, neurofibromatosis, and vascular malformations (Figs. 17.1, 17.2, 17.3, 17.4, and 17.5).

There was a real concern among the teams when the first chronic rejection effects occurred. Of course, it was also question raised when for example in one patient who re-attempted suicide. Perhaps it is the reason why the number of face transplants is now stagnant.

The initial hope, almost enthusiastic, led to a real awareness of the complexity of the procedure whose success depends on, beyond the skillful hands of the surgeon, the unknown power of long-term immunosuppressive treatment and unmastered nerve regeneration. Paradoxically, this period is continuously energized by numerous papers and research works on extending transplantation procedures to other skeletal areas and sensory units!

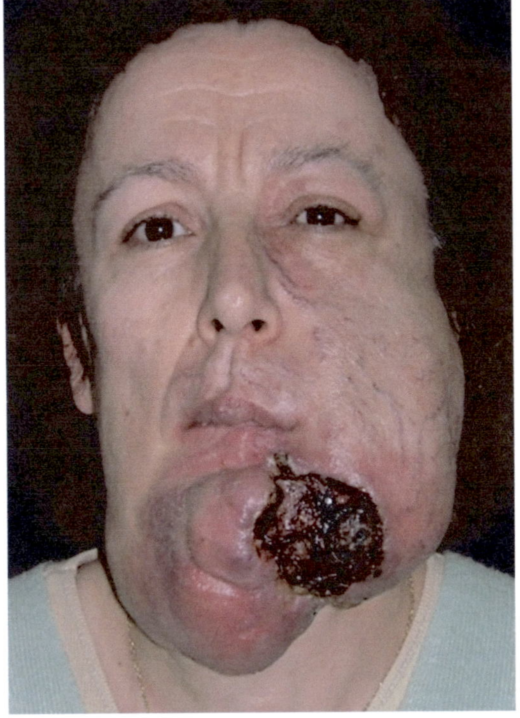

Fig. 17.1 Evolution of the third VCA patient performed in Amiens in 2012 after arteriovenous malformation removal (two times surgery). Initial aspect of the patient with high blood flow arterial malformation 22 years of evolution, highly risk because of daily bleeding, no social life, and many embolization and local surgery

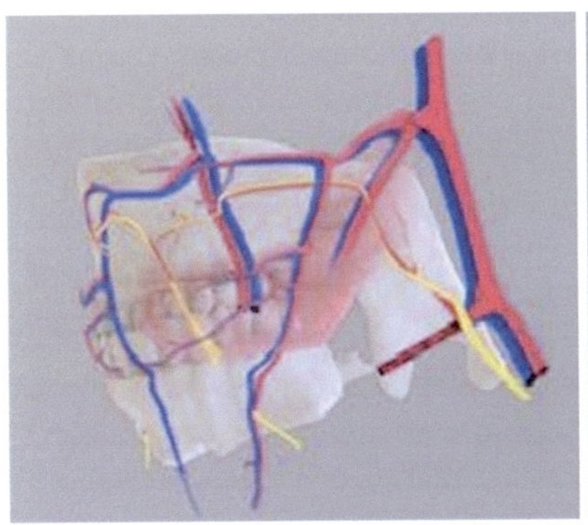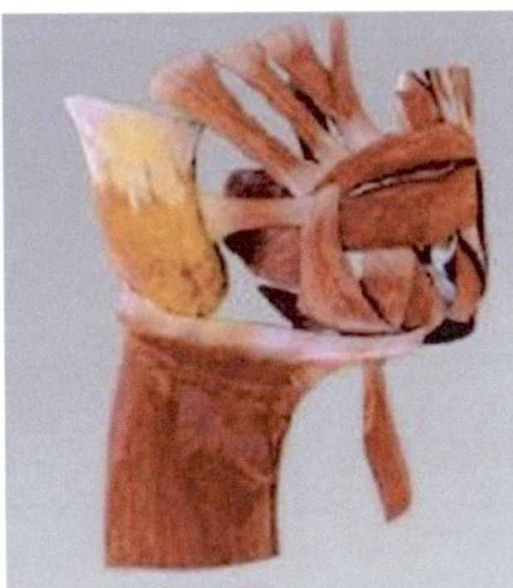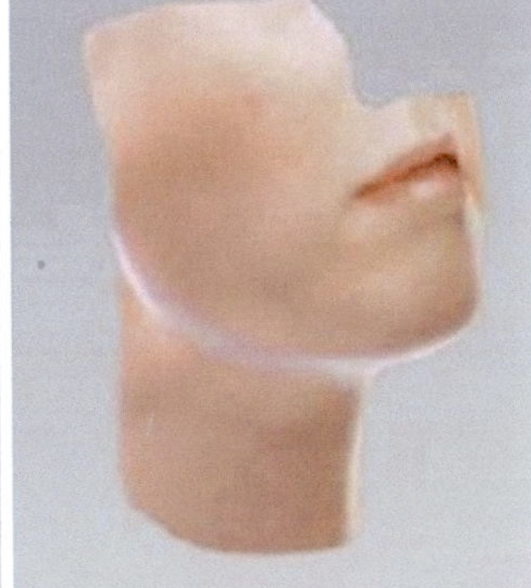

Fig. 17.2 Modelization of the VCA (mandible maxilla, tongue, soft tissue, and skin)

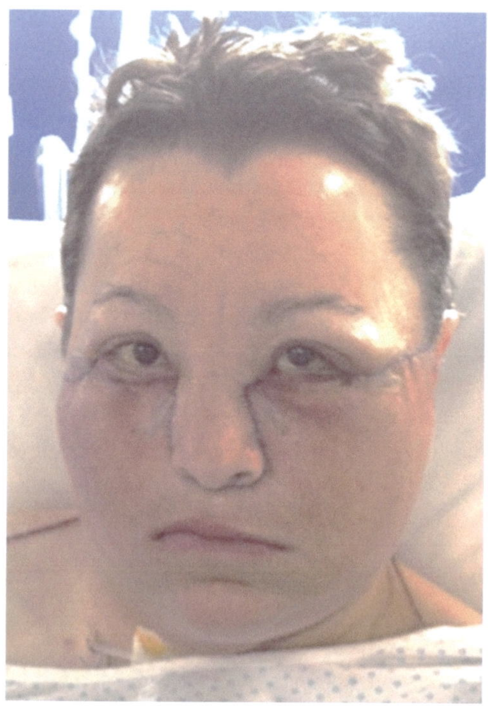

Fig. 17.3 DAY 2 posttransplant

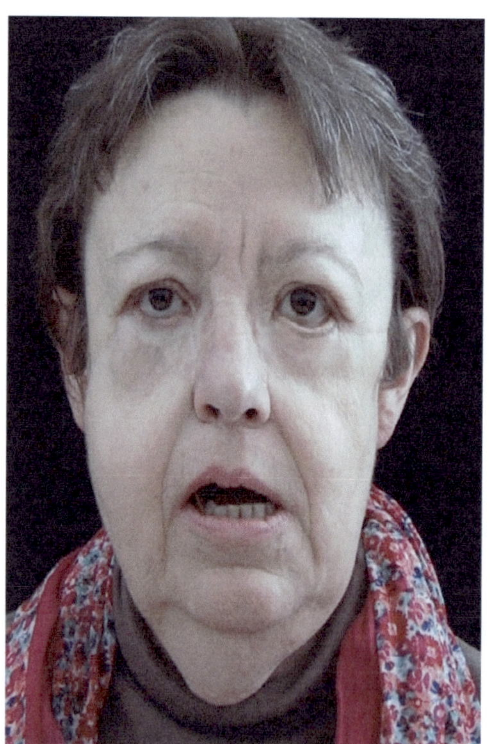

Fig. 17.4 Year 2 posttransplant

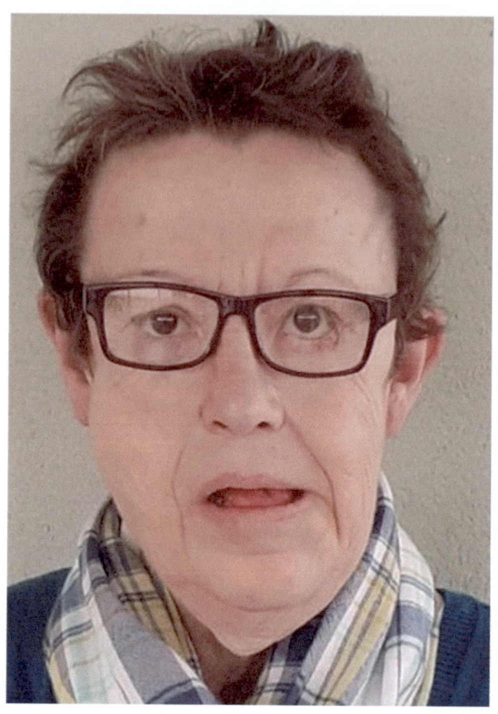

Fig. 17.5 Year 8 posttransplant

17.3 Progressive Extension of Face VCA

At the end of the twentieth century facing a particular treatment deadlock, the willingness to go forward and innovate allowed several reconstructive surgeons to perform a face graft. The example of the hand transplant has existed since 1998, erasing the taboo of skin immunogenicity, which was solved. The hand is part of the history of reconstructive surgery: one more time re-implantation preceded transplantation.

Of course, one could use the same argument regarding the process applied to the face, when a partial face re-transplantation was reported in India after a trauma [12]. Two other clinical cases of partial face transplants had been reported before the first official one in 2005, but were highly controversial from an ethical point of view. Further condemnation was expressed by the scientific community for ear and scalp allotransplantation after a melanoma defect in China and a tongue replacement for cancer surgery in Vienna. Malignancy of the tumors was a clear contraindication for immunosuppressive treatment and for transplantation as well. The two patients died in less than 1 year after surgery.

Independent of the experimental models performed and studied by Siemionow [13], face transplantation was, at that time, thought to be more of a morphologic restitution than functional rehabilitation. Face shape and function are obviously linked. Yet, it was considered more as a concept of covering reconstruction just for skin replacement, as for burn patients although, in despite the remarkable results of the case of Rodriguez [14], the indication for burn cases could only remain in certain conditions. The face allotransplant initially included the surface, then over the years, it was extended to deep tissues including tongue and neck structures for better function and morphological rehabilitation. This was completely natural because of the type of defects themselves: ballistic trauma cases or even electrical burns with complete destruction of the skeletal component of the inferior third of the face as well.

The spatial position of the occlusion plane is actually the key point of functional rehabilitation in terms of mastication. It is easy to understand that the occlusal dimension could only be compromised by the obvious difference between the maxillary bone of the donor and the recipient. The mandibular bone section should be adjustable using the sagittal split surgical procedure. The nasal spine projection verification is a priority to avoid a secondary new osteotomy as reported by Rodriguez, who performed a Le Fort 3 osteotomy 1 year post transplant [15].

On that point, digital technologies could be used to guide spatial positioning, but the problem of the data acquisition from the donor, analysis, and work in such a short time could be incompatible with the requirements of the transplantation. Regarding the extension of the transplant, either spread out or deep, it can be considered that any anatomical element dependent on one branch of the carotid artery or the external artery itself could support a transplant. Thinking in this way, some authors have imagined a transplant that includes the frontal vault and orbital rims. The solution of extending the transplant to the whole bone structure, the skin, all muscles, and all other anatomical elements could allow a risk of real resemblance between the donor and recipient's appearance, which had always been denied before then.

After it was proved that transplantation of the face could properly, though imperfectly, restore sensitivity and motricity, it was very exciting to extend the indication to the other senses. In 2016, the Department of Plastic Surgery in Pittsburg published an interesting anatomical study on a conceptual model of an intraorbital transplant (eye, muscles, and all anatomical elements of the orbit) [6]. A first intranasal endoscopic approach allowed an ethmoidal resection with a sphenoidal osteotomy to access the optical canal. Then, a pteryonal approach was described to perform a retro-dissection of the optical nerve and those of oculomotricity. After retraction of the frontal and temporal brain lobes, the internal carotid and its relation to the chiasma was exposed. Without completely detailing the procedure here, they mention ligating the internal carotid on both sides of the beginning of the ophthalmic artery. The vascular anastomosis could then be done using a double venous shunt with facial vessels. The nerve sutures should be done using a termino-terminal technique.

This anatomical model should raise some questions, especially as it was repeated in an extensive way to the whole orbit, including the lacrimal gland by Siemionov [16], requiring a double arterial revascularization.

At this experimental stage, and because there are only anatomical dissections on the reported paper, only one question comes to mind: Who can claim to restore vision through this "simple" anatomical replacement? Is it not only light perception, but also a completely utopian dream of opening and closing the eyelids and restoring oculomotricity? Some such unthinking nonsense has already been highly mediatized [17].

More wisely, contrary to the ideas above, Rodriguez [18] proved that it is possible to restore a certain degree of eyelid occlusion after transplantation. To succeed, it is very important to understand and see the dissection way of the recipient site, with respect to the tarsal cartilage, the levator muscle of the upper-eyelid, and Mueller's ligament.

There is no organ without function. If the face is an organ, the proof is in its transplantation, where it restores the destroyed shape, it only rehabilitates a part of its function. It is also true for the tongue, the larynx, and the hands.

But the face is also the place for concentration of sensation. Although it was possible to restore taste for our patient without the tongue (the motricity remained poor), a simple nerve suture could not pretend to restore visual function and motor coordination.

17.4 Immunologic Aspects of VCA Acute and Chronic Rejection, Re-transplantation

After the success of the first kidney transplant (the donor was a homozygotic twin) at a time when the HLA system was not yet described (it would be in 1958 by J. Dausset), Joseph Murray stated that no transplant with cutaneous tissue could be tolerated because of skin immunogenicity. The first hand VCA in 1998 completely disconfirmed this principle. Immunosuppressive treatment was usually the same as that used for organ transplants. It is also the same rule for face VCA, with the same secondary effects due to the drugs (e.g., renal insufficiency, diabetes).

In 2016, in the paper entitled "Ten years after face transplantation" [19], M. Siemionov reported the immunologic complications of face VCA. When there were no hyperacute rejection episode, for each face transplant, there were always several acute rejection episodes with clinical signs such as edema, red skin transplant, small cutaneous nodes, or papules. Histologically, lymphoplasmocytic infiltration was noted, either in skin and/or mucosae. In 2007 the Banff classification appeared, describing four grades (I–IV) [20]. The readjustment of the initial treatment, some local uses of tacrolimus, or corticosteroids and possibly phototherapy succeeded in treating these rejection episodes in a few weeks. An acute rejection episode could occur early, after some weeks. These episodes are closely linked to nonadherence to the treatment.

Conversely, immunotherapy could bring with it metabolic, infectious, or tumoral complications. It could also lead to renal insufficiency on different levels for numerous studies, viral (CMV, herpes virus), bacterial, or mycotic infections, often with possible systemic medical treatments. Epstein–Barr virus transmission from the donor to the nonimmunized recipient patient was responsible for the development of a severe B-cell lymphoma.

In 2015, 10 years after the first face transplant, the patient developed partial vascular ischemia of the transplant skin [21]. The context was very specific. Initially, there was the hypothesis of potential chimerism due to stem cell infusion from the donor at the time of the VCA. In fact, nothing like this occurred. She presented the expected rate of rejection episodes. At that time, the benefit of the sentinel flap (transplant of a vascularized flap from the donor used to perform biopsies, avoiding facial scars) was evident because of the reaction on the vascular pedicle, which led to the diagnosis. On the face, several ischemic, then necrotic skin areas appeared and led to new lip reconstruction. In addition, it should be known that the patient had developed uterine epithelioma many years before the face transplant which requested surgical treatment as well as anaplastic cell lung carcinoma around 2015, again benefiting from surgical treatment. We knew for some time about her regular nonadherence to treatment. The question of chronic rejection disease was reported by Kanitakis in a paper in 2016 [22].

It is clearly this chronic rejection disease which also occurred for hand VCA that led to questions about face VCA relevance. In fact, the question addresses the possibility of accepting that, as with heart transplants, composite tissue transplants (non-vital) could be considered for a limited 12-year time period. Another possible alternative could be performing a re-transplantation. For the face, only one re-transplantation appeared to have been done, performed by the Paris team. It is, of course, also very interesting in terms of discussions in surgical and philosophical fields about the problem of time dimension.

17.5 Psychological Background

Before its realization the question was raised of the psychological background of a potential recipient patient for a face transplant because of the idea of living with a part of someone else's face. The unthinkable became a potential reality. Some literature references, often arising from science fiction or humor had already been available on this topic. Strangely, their thinking never dealt with the previous history of disfigurement of patients, a subject that was largely analyzed in the years following the First World War. The one benefit of this question was to encourage philosophical reflection on the tolerance of the other, a situation which is, in our case, forced upon us by immunology.

In November 2012, the American Society of Transplantation, probably due to the unfortunate failure of the first-hand VCA, suggested creating a discussion group on the psychological dimension of hand VCA, which quickly extended to other composite transplants. This group was named the Chauvet Group in reference to the handprints that adorn a French prehistoric cave. In 2014, for the first time in France, a meeting of the Chauvet Group was held and reported in the *Journal of Transplantation* [22]. The ideas concentrated on these points:

- Assessment in terms of self-image, psychological status, trauma history, and ability to adhere to the treatment before transplantation.
- Environment and support from loved ones.
- Postsurgical observation to detect signs of complications, psychological problems, and deterioration of quality of life.
- Support of the medical and surgical teams.
- Discussion on the benefit–risk balance.
- Different aspects and control of the media and communication around the patient.
- Partnership with the ethics committee and compliance with regulations regarding consent and information.
- Requirements for developing objective means of evaluation of the aesthetic and functional results and improvement of quality of life after transplantation.

Even if all these considerations should be clarified, they have already been transferred to face and other types of VCA. The Chauvet Group now meets every 2 years.

Although it is now clearly recognized that the psychological background should be considered in all pre-, per-, and postoperative periods, playing a real role in the selection of the patients, the Chauvet Group pointed out some differences dependent on cultural attitudes and behavior. These differences are not only found between the two sides of the Atlantic but also between the different teams themselves. Surprisingly, tobacco use is considered to be a contraindication for VCA transplantation, not only because of its harmful effects on health status (e.g., microcirculation, lung capacity, increased cancer risk) but more because of the addictive aspect. In a way, a face transplantation can be considered another form of addiction, because of the requirements of a continuing immunosuppressive regimen.

The *Journal of Psychosomatic Research* [23] reported the experience of psychiatrists following the six face transplant cases of the Paris–Mondor team. Between 2000 and 2009, 20 disfigured patients were evaluated. Ten were positively selected after a psychiatric assessment. Seven were transplanted and three were not because of organic impairments. One of the seven patients died from severe sepsis and cardiac failure at 63 days post-transplant, and a second patient died more than 3 years later by suicide.

In the psychological field, the follow-up was carried out by interviews with patients and quantitative assessments (short 36-item health survey form, or the Mini-International Neuro psychiatric Interview [MINI]). Four of six patients suffered from postoperative *delirium tremens* syndrome, certainly due to addiction which was never reported. The patients who were psychologically frail before the transplant showed no improvement, in contrast to the two cases with von Recklinghausen's disease. As a consequence, the authors questioned the indication for VCA for patients with disfigurement due to a suicide attempt.

This retrospective analysis could also explain the relative stagnation of VCA throughout the world.

Finally, without returning to the ethical debates which occurred after the first face VCA, other discussions from different perspectives in related papers (Sociology [24] and Philosophy [25]) have explained differences due to geographic distribution of countries or places where face transplants have or have not been performed.

17.6 Conclusion

Allotransplantation of composite tissue of the face had the great advantage of integrating maxillofacial surgeons into the community of transplant surgeons. In doing so, they discovered new worlds, new cultures, and most of all immunology.

This transplant led them to reconsider anatomy and to explore other dimensions of surgical management. It was an invitation to meet with psychiatrists and to hold debates on philosophy and ethics. From this point of view, facial VCA is not only a technical improvement, but is also a complete form of management of the reconstruction of the disfigured face as a whole.

Because face VCA imparts the surgeon with new responsibilities, it should remain a controlled experimental field. Of course, reflection should focus on technical points, and each facial VCA indication carries with it a duty to be innovative. We should be careful not to fall into the trap of unreasonable indications. The literature has reported on possible sensory recovery which currently is still a utopian dream.

Considering the possibility of performing face transplants in children is more relevant because of the encountering a very severe even rare craniofacial malformation, a disfiguring benign tumor, or a severe vascular facial malformation. Two papers have reported on this subject with comparable conclusions. The first was from the Cleveland team who consider indications premature because of the consequences of immunosuppressive treatment. Similarly, and for numerous reasons, we have the same view, though there are some experimental works on newborn hand transplants. Nonetheless, agenesis of the face does not exist.

On facial transplantation: *"Knowledge is coming, questions remain."*

References

1. Devauchelle B, Badet L, Lengele B, Morelon E, Testelin S, Michallet M, et al. First human face allograft: early report. Lancet. 2016;368(9531):203–9.
2. Weissenbacher A, Cendales L, Morelon E, Petruzzo P, Brandacher G, Friend PJ, Gorantla V, Kaufman C, Krapf J, Scott Levin L, Vrakas G, Schneeberger S. Meeting report of the 13th congress of the international society of vascularized composite allotransplantation. Transplantation. 2018;102(8):1250–2.
3. Le Clainche-Piel M. Ce que charrie la chair. Thèse de doctorat en sociologie présentée le 28 mai 2018 – Ecole des hautes études en sciences sociales.
4. Jowsey-Gregoire SG, Kumnig M, Morelon E, Moreno E, Petruzzo P, Seulin C. The Chauvet 2014 meeting report: psychiatric and psychosocial evaluation and outcomes of upper extremity grafted patients. Transplantation. 2016;100(7):1453–9.
5. Ibid 2.
6. Davidson EH, Wang EW, Yu JY, Fernandez-Miranda JC, Wang DJ, Richards N, Miller M, Schuman JS, Washington KM. Total human eye allotransplantation: developing surgical protocols for donor and recipient procedures. Plast Reconstr Surg. 2016;138:1297–308.
7. Petruzzo P, Dubernard JM. The international registry on hand and composite tissue allotransplantation. Clin Transpl. 2011:247–53.
8. Rifkin WJ, Manjunath A, Kimberly LL, Plana NM, Kantar RS, Leslie Bernstein G, Rodrigo Diaz-Siso J, Rodriguez ED. Long-distance care of face transplant recipients in the United States. J Plast Reconstr Aesthetic Surg. 2018;71:1383–91.
9. Siemionow M. The miracle of face transplantation after 10 years. Br Med Bull. 2016;120:5–14.
10. Grigos MI, Leblanc E, Rifkin WJ, Kantar RS, Greenfield J, Diaz-Siso JR, Rodriguez ED. Total eyelid transplantation in a face transplant: analysis of postoperative periorbital function. J Surg Res. 2020;245:420–5.
11. Sosin M, Rodriguez ED. The face transplantation update: 2016. Plast Reconstr Surg. 2016;137:1841–50.
12. Shanmugarajah K, Hettiaratchy S, Butler PE. Facial transplantation. Curr Opin Otolaryngol Head Neck Surg. 2012;20:291–7.
13. Siemonov M, Gozel-Ulusal B, Engin Ulusal A, et al. Functional tolerance following face transplantation in the rat. Transplantation. 2003;75:1607–9.
14. Sosin M, Ceradini DJ, Hazen A, et al. Total face, eyelids, ears, scalp, and skeletal subunit transplant cadaver simulation: the culmination of aesthetic, craniofacial, and microsurgery principles. Plast Reconstr Surg. 2016;137:1569–81.
15. Mohan R, Fisher M, Dorafshar A, Sosin M, Bojovic B, Gandhi D, Iliff N, Rodriguez ED. Principles of

face transplant revision: beyond primary repair. Plast Reconstr Surg. 2014;134:1295–304.

16. Siemonow M, Bozkurt M, Zor F, Kulahci Y, Uygur S, Ozturk C, Djohan R, Papay F. A new composite eyeball-periorbital transplantation model in humans: an anatomical study in preparation for eyeball transplantation. Plast Reconstr Surg. 2018;141:1011–7.

17. Canavero S, Ren X. Advancing the technology for head transplants: from immunology to peripheral nerve fusion. Surg Neurol Int. 2019;10:240.

18. Ibid 10.

19. Ibid 9.

20. Cendales L, Kanitakis J, Schneeberger S, et al. The Banff 2007 working classification of skin-containing composite tissue allograft pathology. Am J Transplant. 2008;8:1396–400.

21. Morelon E, Petruzzo P, Kanitakis J, Dakpe S, Thaunat O, Dubois V, Choukroun G, Testelin S, Dubernard JM, Badet L, Devauchelle B. Face transplantation: partial graft loss of the first case 10 years later. Am J Transplant. 2017;17:1935–40.

22. Kanitakis J, Petruzzo P, Badet L, Gazarian A, Thaunat O, Testelin S, Devauchelle B, Dubernard J-M, Morelon E. Chronic rejection in human vascularized composite allotransplantation (hand and face recipients): an update. Transplantation. 2016;100(10):2053–61.

23. Lemogne C, Bellivier F, Fakra E, Yon L, Limosin F, Consoli SM, Lantieri L, Hivelin M. Psychological and psychiatric aspects of face transplantation: lessons learned from the long-term follow-up six patients. J Psychosom Res. 2019;119:42–9.

24. Ibid 3.

25. Moulin AM. Archaism and modenity: imagination and reality of the transplantation between orient and occident. p. 27–34. Transplanter: book edited by Hermann 2015, coordinated by B. Devauchelle and E. Fournier.